Presented to: Dr. Knapp
From: Mead Johnson

By: Bob Arend

D1708568

ADVANCES IN PEDIATRICS®

VOLUME 28

ADVANCES IN PEDIATRICS®

ADVANCES
in PEDIATRICS®

EDITOR

LEWIS A. BARNESS
University of South Florida College of Medicine
Tampa, Florida

ASSOCIATE EDITORS

ALFRED M. BONGIOVANNI
University of Pennsylvania
School of Medicine
Philadelphia, Pennsylvania

GRANT MORROW
Children's Hospital
Columbus, Ohio

FRANK OSKI
State University of New York
Upstate Medical Center
Syracuse, New York

ABRAHAM M. RUDOLPH
University of California School of Medicine
San Francisco, California

VOLUME 28 · 1981

YEAR BOOK MEDICAL PUBLISHERS, INC.
CHICAGO · LONDON

Library of Congress Catalog Card Number: 42-22236

International Standard Serial Number: 0065-3101

International Standard Book Number: 0-8151-0500-2

Editor's Preface

A REVIEWER commented that there was no theme to the choice of articles in last year's volume. The theme, ever since the inception of *Advances in Pediatrics,* has been to select those articles most likely to benefit the practitioner and to offer the investigator a source of topics that have reached a degree of concreteness outside the laboratory but that are still too controversial to be included in the newer textbooks. How concrete and controversial these topics may be is a matter about which the board of editors decides.

These goals have been at least partially realized, as many favorable comments from readers reflect. Last year's article by Stickler on how to use chemotherapeutic agents, for example, has been a real boon to students and practitioners. There have also been favorable comments concerning the chapters on abdominal pain, the several articles on immunity and infectious diseases, vitamin D, and tips on breast-feeding. We hope that this year's selections will be equally useful.

The chapter by MacDonald and Newton in this volume serves several purposes. MacDonald states that in 16 years of practice he made the diagnosis of alcohol abuse only once. Now he makes the diagnosis of drug abuse almost daily. How often have we academicians and practitioners missed or delayed making the diagnosis? How often do we make the proper observations or ask the leading questions outlined so well by MacDonald and Newton? Furthermore, this excellent paper has been written by physicians in full-time private practice, a habit to be emulated by others.

A revolution is occurring in the care of high-risk newborn infants. Excitement is generated by development of noninvasive techniques. One of the most far-reaching of these for this decade is transcutaneous oxygen monitoring. In an excellent review, Lucey describes its uses, accomplishments, and promise even, with bated breath.

When most of us went to medical school, vitamin K was thought to be something that had to do with blood clotting. The newer aspects of the importance of vitamin K are even more exciting, and may be more important in understanding human physiology. Corrigan brings these new vistas into focus for our understanding.

Block, Saltzman, and Block discuss problems and approaches to teenage pregnancy. Alternatives and care objectives are detailed, together with an excellent discussion of teen development. Hypotheses for prevention are explored.

Until recently, it was felt that everything about carbohydrate absorption was understood. Lebenthal, Hatch, and Lee review previous knowledge in this field and discuss in detail many data obtained since the availability of new techniques. Their discussion of ontogeny of enzyme development is especially important to all who care for newborns.

Brown has written a succinct summary of our present knowledge about infant botulism, a disease both old and new. He describes the possible pathophysiology of this apparently age-related phenomenon and suggests diagnostic and therapeutic modalities.

Gastroesophageal reflux, described many years ago, has hit pediatric literature like a tornado. Herbst and Meyers summarize our knowledge of this syndrome and tell us how to recognize, best diagnose, and treat it.

Sports participation, especially in organized sports, is becoming more and more common among children at an earlier age than ever. Smith provides an easy-to-read, easy-to-understand vade mecum with adequate anticipatory guidance and advice for all physicians who care for children and adolescents.

Thymosin is a factor with almost mysterious effects on the immune system. Present knowledge of thymosin and its effects is admirably summarized by Wara. The future of this material for therapy seems bright, and this furnishes an excellent basis for following its progress.

Left-handedness has fascinated genealogists, geneticists, paramedics, and social scientists for ages. Some light on the subject is beginning to appear. Galaburda and Geschwind are responsible for much of our understanding of left-handedness, and furnish a basis for study of some of the dyslexic problems in their lucid discussion of brain asymmetry.

Growth is a keystone of pediatrics. How growth occurs and what stimulates it are mysteries. The discovery of a group of chemicals, somatomedins, has taken us one step further toward the understanding of this process. Hintz, one of the active investigators in this area, has written an understandable article, not only on the basic chemistry of these substances but also on the clear indications of their clinical applicability.

Many special formulas have been created to treat gastrointestinal and some metabolic diseases. Lake, Kleinman, and Walker discuss some of the more common formulas available and suggest some of their uses.

One of the best, most complete discussions of lymphadenopathy in children has been written by Bedros and Mann. Our reviewers have been equally enthusiastic in recommending this chapter to students of physical diagnosis, practitioners frequently confronted with lymphadenopathy, and investigators in this area.

Singh has contributed a critical review of methods now used in the control of children with self-injurious behavior, including the autistic and retarded. His chapter will help pediatricians to understand some behavior-modification therapies. For others who care for children, and especially for physicians who work with these types of childhood problems, the needs and suggestions for better methodological studies are outlined.

Seizure disorders are problems for the child, the parents, and the physician. Recent changes in terminology further confuse the matter. Brill and Mitchell have selected pertinent data for a very readable, easy-to-follow guide to the proper diagnosis and treatment of all paroxysmal disorders and to the distinction of these from true seizure disorders.

As always, suggestions for topics to be included in future volumes will be much appreciated.

LEWIS A. BARNESS, M.D.
Professor and Chairman
Department of Pediatrics
University of South Florida
College of Medicine
Tampa, Florida

Contents

The Clinical Syndrome of Adolescent Drug Abuse

DONALD IAN MACDONALD, M.D.

Clinical Associate Professor of Pediatrics
University of So. Florida
College of Medicine
Tampa, Florida

AND

MILLER NEWTON, Ph.D.

Director, Straight, Inc.
St. Petersburg Program
St. Petersburg, Florida

THE CHILD WHO PRESENTS AT THE PEDIATRIC OFFICE with cough, fatigue, sore throat, stuffy nose, red eyes, chest pain, or other unexplained symptoms should be suspected of drug usage. No longer is it adequate to obtain a complete blood cell count, test for mononucleosis, ascertain the serum glutamic oxaloacetic transaminase level, and label the child as having fatigue just on the basis of insufficient sleep, an overly busy schedule, or mild adolescent withdrawal. No longer is it proper to order chest and sinus x-rays, nasal smears, allergy workups, antihistamines, and decongestants without suspecting smoking as a cause of the symptoms even in the elementary school child.

Asking a few key questions may lead to the correct diagnosis: How is your child doing in school? What is his attitude at home? Does he have dramatic swings of mood and behavior? Does he do his chores? Do you like his friends? Have his appearance and grooming changed?

Adolescent drug abuse, a disease of epidemic proportions, presents as a recognizable syndrome closely related to a wide

1

0065-3101/81/0028-0001-0025-$03.75

variety of other teenage problems, both serious and common. We will look at the characteristics of this clinical syndrome and the stages of chemical dependency and discuss probable causes of the problem, the solution to which must lie in prevention.

The use and abuse of chemicals in adolescence has changed markedly in recent years and continues to change. The chemicals presently in use are more varied, stronger, and more readily available than they were only five years ago. We use the words use and abuse interchangeably, for we feel that the use of any psychoactive chemical by children without strict medical supervision is an abuse. Not only are more children involved than ever, but involvement is heavier and occurs at younger and younger ages.

Trends in Adolescent Drug Use[17]

The surge in illicit drug use during the last decade has proved to be primarily a youth phenomenon. Onset of such use is most likely to occur during adolescence. From one year to the next, particular drugs rise or fall in popularity. Marihuana smoking has been increasing dramatically, as reflected by the figures in Table 1. The number of American high school seniors who smoked marihuana daily in 1978 (10.7%) almost doubled

TABLE 1.—HIGH SCHOOL SENIORS' DRUG ABUSE*

DRUG	1975 (%)	1978 (%)	1980 (%)
Marihuana			
Ever used	47	59	60
Used in past month	27	37	34
Use daily	6.0	10.7	9.1
Used by ninth grade	17	27	31
Alcohol—daily	5.7	5.7	6.0
In past month	68	72	72
Cigarettes—daily	27	28	21
Stimulants—past month	8.5	8.7	12.1
Methaqualone—past month	2.1	1.9	3.3
Cocaine—ever used	9.0	12.9	15.7
Perceive as great risk			
Marihuana	48	35	50
Tobacco	51	59	64

*Adapted from Johnston L.D., et al.: *Student Drug Use in America 1975–1980*. Rockville, Maryland: National Institutes on Drug Abuse, Division of Research, 1980.

the figure of three years earlier (6%) but did fall back some in 1980 (9.1%). This reduction may reflect an increasing concern among teenagers about the dangers of marihuana. The figure for boys was close to 13%, compared to about 6% for girls. The percentage of seniors who admitted to having smoked marihuana by the ninth grade had increased from 17% to 31% over the same five-year period and the age of first usage was decreasing. One child in six (16.7%), aged 12 to 17, was using marihuana on some regular basis. These figures may be low. They do not include alcohol, which has been tried by over 85% of all seniors. Consumption of alcohol has increased slowly; daily use among seniors has risen from 5.7% in 1975 to 6% in 1980.

Not only is the incidence of marihuana use increasing but so is its psychoactive strength. Also of concern is the fact that Δ-9-tetrahydrocannabinol (THC), the principal psychoactive ingredient of marihuana, is lipid soluble. This accounts for the fact that THC is stored in the body for long periods of time. Traces have been found after 30 days, and its half-life is seven to ten days.[41]

Marihuana is a plant (*Cannabis sativa*) from which over 421 chemicals have been isolated, many of which are cannabinoids or chemicals peculiar to cannabis. Of the drugs isolated, THC is the principal mind-altering component. Many varieties of cannabis are currently under cultivation at the legally run experimental farm of the National Institutes on Drug Abuse (NIDA) in Oxford, Mississippi. Experts there have been able to grow marihuana with higher and higher concentrations of THC, a feat also accomplished by illegal growers whose potent products make their way onto the streets.

In the early 1960s marihuana cigarettes ("joints") contained THC in concentrations of 0.1% to 0.2%. In 1975 the concentrations of street samples rarely exceeded 0.5%. Marihuana sold in school parking lots in 1980 commonly contained THC in concentrations ranging from 2% to 4%; concentrations of 5% to 6% were not unusual. This means that most joints nowadays are ten to 60 times stronger than they were. And worse is coming. At the Oxford farm, marihuana with a THC concentration of 11% has recently been assayed on material seized in northern California. Extracts of marihuana such as hashish (about 10% THC) and hash oil (on the average, 20% THC),[27] which were

not a part of the drug scene in the sixties, are common compan-
ions of the teenager of the eighties who experiments with
chemicals. Adulteration of joints with other psychoactive, often more deadly, drugs such as 1-(1-phenylcyclohexyl)piperidine
(PCP), LSD, "free-base" cocaine, and, more recently, heroin, is
an increasingly common practice. The heroin story is particularly frightening. Street heroin in this country is most often a
3.4% product (brown heroin) from Mexico. Newer heroin arriv-
ing from Iran and Afghanistan, where crops are flourishing,
has been assayed at over 20% strength (white heroin). This potent chemical may now be smoked for kicks (and addiction) and
sprinkled on joints by those who might refuse a needle. Such
joints have been recovered in Detroit and San Francisco, and
rates of addiction and waiting lines at treatment centers are
growing across the country.

The Clinical Syndrome

Drug-dependent teenagers are not all at the same level of
involvement and their symptoms and feelings vary. But as the
disease progresses the course is remarkably similar for each
child and a syndrome emerges in stages. Various forces push
the child into drug use, but once he is entrenched in it his drug-
induced feelings pull him further down. Miller Newton, who
works full time at Straight, Inc., a St. Petersburg, Florida, adolescent drug treatment program, has divided the syndrome
into stages by modifying the model proposed for alcoholics by
the Johnson Institute, a Minneapolis-based alcohol and drug
research and staff training center.[14] Looking at the teenage
chemical use syndrome in five stages allows us to follow the
young user on his downward path and gives us clinical clues
for evaluating the depth of his involvement. The stages are (0)
exposure to drugs, (1) learning the mood swing, (2) seeking the
mood swing, (3) preoccupation with the mood swing, and (4)
using drugs to feel normal.

STAGE 0: "THE CALL TO DO DRUGS"

Stronger and stronger forces are pushing our teenagers into
drug use and the defenses of the child and his family are crum-
bling (Table 2). For the 60% to 90% of adolescents who have

TABLE 2.—STAGE 0: THE CALL TO DO DRUGS*

PRESSURES	SUPPORTS
Hedonistic society	Laws and their enforcement
Sales pitches, high profits—legal and illegal	Education
Negative role models	Parents' attitudes and practices
	Awareness
	Caring communication and control
	Good personal example
Casual or ambivalent attitudes about drugs and alcohol	The strength to say no
	Strong coping mechanisms
	Appropriate attitudes
	Necessary life skills
"Normal" teenage attributes	
Respond to peer pressure	
Curiosity	
Like excitement	
Need to belong	
Quick to rebel	

*Fewer than 15% of high school seniors remain in Stage 0; more than 85% enter Stage 1.

tried drugs these pressures will not only continue but their resistance to them will be lowered as chemical escape is discovered. There is no one answer to the problem but prevention efforts must be aimed at decreasing both the supply of and demand for addictive drugs. Pediatricians and parents must be aware of these pressures and of ways to increase a child's resistance to them.

PRESSURES TO TAKE DRUGS

Hedonism.—Conspiring against the child of the eighties is an all too general societal message of "do it now" or "if it feels good, do it." This live-for-the-moment attitude leads to immediate gratification with little regard for long-term consequences.

Sales pitches, high profits (legal and illegal).—From an early age our children are exposed to media messages advertising relief in oral form for all sorts of "minor aches and pains." Television commericals promise relief from headache, tension, and sleep problems—relief, they say, no further away than the nearest pharmacy.

Alcohol is advertised not only as a social lubricant but as a reward. Weekends once made for Sabbath and family are now "made for Michelob." Climbing mountains is not primarily for exercise, views, or good times with friends, but to reach the cold beer at the top. Little wonder that the child who has some problem with his self image is tempted by the cigarette advertisement that implies a relationship between smoking and the macho on horseback.

The more active "do-drug" messages from the huge commercial industry dealing in illegal drugs are everywhere. Drugs are big business, second nationally only to Exxon and General Motors. Florida's largest industry is the importation of marihuana. California's largest crop is marihuana. The paraphernalia industry, unknown ten years ago, is booming with huge revenues. *High Life, High Times,* and other drug industry magazines are widely circulated and read by our children.

Negative role models.—The wealthy rock music industry is filled with musicians who look, dress, and act high and sing freely such songs as "I Get High with a Little Help from My Friends" and "Cocaine." A recent survey revealed that the average teenager in Atlanta spends from three to five hours daily listening to rock music. The "do-drug" and free sex messages seem more strongly to persuade the adolescent than the not infrequent reports of fatal overdose or suicide by the stars. Reports of widespread use of cocaine and amphetamines by professional ballplayers imply that drugs improve athletic performance. The widespread use of sports "heroes" in beer commercials presents a strong sales message.

Casual or ambivalent attitudes.—Parents, neighbors, teachers, police, and pediatricians do not help with attitudes that treat occasional use and experimentation as a part of growing up. The acceptance of drinking by adolescent boys is especially common.

"Normal" teenage attitudes.—Adolescents are a curious and experimenting group by nature. They want to belong. They are quick to share and their story of "super-highs" with "no side effects" is readily told. Marihuana is a sharing drug and the user wants to involve his friends in his great new experience. Former NIDA Director Robert DuPont has said: "The single main determinant of whether a particular young person uses drugs like marihuana is whether or not his best friend uses it [sic]."

Adolescents also feel other pressures. The temptation to deal with problems such as being too fat or too thin, being turned down for a date, or not making the team, by escape to chemical euphoria may be strong. Even stronger pressures may come from learning problems or family crises such as divorce. Other teenagers may be tempted to take drugs as a form of rebellion.

RESISTING THE PRESSURE AND REDUCING THE SUPPLY

Laws and their enforcement.—Stronger laws and stronger enforcement not only will decrease the drug supply but also give young people a message that adults do not feel ambivalent about drug use.

Education.—Children and their parents who know the dangers of drugs and alcohol are less likely to be involved in drug abuse. The 1980 NIDA figures (see Table 1), which show a decrease in daily marihuana and tobacco usage, are encouraging. This decrease was paralleled by an increased belief among teenagers that there are risks involved in smoking. Not encouraging is the fact that these improvements may be more than offset by increased use of cocaine, amphetamines, and methaqualone, about which adolescents are less well informed.

Parent's attitudes and practices.—These have a strong effect on children. Those who do not drink are less likely to have children who drink than those who routinely have two martinis before dinner. Parents who stay aware of the teen scene can provide their children with strong support and protection. They need to be actively involved in the lives of their children and exert the adequate but reasonable controls they feel are necessary. Achieving the necessary balance between being overprotective and not protective enough is a real parental challenge. At the same time they need to help their children learn to deal with their feelings and to develop drug-free alternative lifestyles.

The strength to say no.—The question, "What makes kids do drugs?" is frequently asked. In high school, where taking drugs and drinking have become so widely accepted, the question might better be phrased: "Why don't all kids do drugs?" The final answer has to lie within the child and his ability to resist saying yes.

Helpful inner defenses include feelings of self worth, identification with successful role models, and a positive relationship in which he feels himself a part of something greater than himself, such as family, country, and God. Belief in his ability to change the course of his life through his own actions helps.

Helpful coping skills are those of self-assessment, self-control, self-discipline, and the ability to listen and relate to others. Important also is the ability to analyze situations. He must be able to sort out the consequences of various courses of action and then make and carry out rational action in response to problems. The ability to analyze more abstractly and make moral decisions of wrong vs right provides strong support but is a skill often lacking.

The average teenage alcoholic and marihuana user scores poorly on tests for these perceptions and skills, as does his adult counterpart.[5, 13, 14] As "do drug" pressure builds, many children whose attitudes and skills might have been otherwise adequate now cannot defend themselves. Glenn[7] has studied the attitude and skill deficiencies and aimed his efforts in both prevention and treatment at building appropriate strengths in the child.

STAGE 1: LEARNING THE MOOD SWING

In this stage the child is introduced to a chemical that can make him feel good. His source may be a "friend," a sibling, or someone at a party under peer pressure. Most users say they have refused drugs three or four times before they first accepted any. Most teenagers do not like beer or marihuana any better at first exposure than they like cigarettes. But with practice one learns.

"Good feelings" and the excitement of a new and illicit experience are soon achieved. The user feels few if any aftereffects. As seen on the "feelings chart" (Table 3), his mood swings toward euphoria and returns to normal. Once the good feelings have been discovered, his urge to use drugs in times of stress will be increasingly tempting.

Tobacco is for many children the first illegal and potentially dangerous substance they try. In response to peer pressure, he has stepped over the line by smoking tobacco, and having few if any adverse reactions from it, will find it easier to proceed to other substances. In 1979, 27.5% of high school seniors in this country smoked tobacco daily. Although not strictly a psychoactive substance, a significant proportion of regular tobacco users are on their way into the drug culture.

Marihuana has been called the gateway drug that leads to others, but for many, alcohol or inhalants such as butyl nitrate ("Rush" or "Locker Room") may precede its use. At this stage, which is reached by approximately one third of all teenagers and over half of high school seniors in this country, there is little discernible behavior change except for some moderate "after the fact" lying. What makes the child go on the Stage 2 and beyond has not been fully established, but we do know that more and more children are escalating their habit to stages where return to nonuse or Stage 1 becomes increasingly difficult if not impossible.

STAGE 2: SEEKING THE MOOD SWING

No longer content to wait for someone at a party to offer him something to turn on with, the youngster begins to look for the drug and will beg or buy to meet his new desire. His usage progresses from occasional use, to regular weekend use, to occasional weekday use, to regular weekday use. He is developing pride in the way he handles drugs and his new "friendships" in the drug community. His new friends are often older and are frequently not brought home for parental inspection. Getting high is his object, and although he may have drug preferences he will use whatever drug is available. Polydrug use is the rule. (Of 104 clients questioned at Straight, 103 used both alcohol and marihuana on a regular basis.[23]) Escalation to harder drugs begins and he may now also use hashish, hash oil, and pills ("ups and downs"). What he uses will frequently depend on what is available or what he can afford. His ingenuity at trying out new things can be amazing. He leads a dual life, presenting one image to his parents and another to his peers. The pressures entailed in such duality increase his tension.

The physician who asks the key questions in the first paragraph of this chapter and notes the child's appearance and speech begins to get some clues as to what is going on. There is a move toward rock star appearance. In Stage 3 this appearance may include concert T-shirts, marihuana-leaf belt buckles, "coke" spoons on necklaces, longer hair often center-parted, and increasing use of slang expressions such as "cool" and

TABLE 3.—STAGES OF DRUG ABUSE

STAGE	MOOD ALTERATION	FEELINGS	DRUGS	SOURCES	BEHAVIOR	FREQUENCY
1: Learning the mood swing	Euphoria Normal Pain	Feel good Few consequences	Tobacco Marihuana Alcohol	"Friends"	Little detectable change Moderate "after the fact" lying	Progresses to weekend usage
2: Seeking the mood swing	Euphoria Normal Pain	Excitement Early guilt	All of the above plus: Inhalants Hash oil, hashish "Ups" "Downs" Prescriptions	Buying	Drop extracurricular activities and hobbies Mixed friends (straight and druggie) Dress changing Erratic school performance and "skipping" Unpredictable mood and attitude swings. "Conning" behavior	Weekend use progressing to 4–5 times per week Some solo use

3: Preoccupation with the mood swing	Euphoria Normal Pain	Euphoric highs Doubts including: Severe shame and guilt Depression Suicidal thoughts	All of the above plus: Mushrooms PCP LSD Cocaine	Selling	"Cool" appearance Straight friends dropped Family fights (verbal and physical) Stealing—police incidents Pathologic lying School failure, skipping, expulsion, jobs lost	Daily Frequent solo use
4: Using drugs to feel normal	Euphoria Normal Pain	Chronic Guilt Shame Remorse Depression	Whatever is available	Any way possible	Physical deterioration (weight loss, chronic cough) Severe mental deterioration (memory loss and flashbacks) Paranoia, volcanic anger, and aggression School drop-out Frequent overdosing	All day every day

"right on, man." In girls, well-worn skin-tight jeans, seductive halter tops or blouses, and overdone makeup and jewelry may be clues.

The amotivational syndrome[21] of marihuana may begin at this stage. There is a cutback in hobbies and extracurricular activities are given up. School performance may begin to dip, but stern parental action will often bring about a temporary improvement. Cheating may be a large part of this "improvement."

Personality changes occur. Questioning of a parent may reveal a child who is often moody and withdrawn. Tantrums and verbal abuse may be frequent and are often related to a parent's attempt to inquire about a child's whereabouts or activities or to suggest that he participate in family activities and chores. Appetite may decrease and meal skipping is common. The well-known "munchies" may occur at the same time. Although his periods of euphoria are more euphoric and more frequent, coming down involves some mild discomfort and guilt. He may be experiencing his first blackouts or periods of amnesia about part or all of his high.

STAGE 3: PREOCCUPATION WITH THE MOOD SWING

Now the child thinks of little else but getting high. Using the drug for social purposes or in response to peer pressure continues, but solitary use is increasing. He gets stoned daily and is openly identified as a "druggie," having dropped or been dropped by all his straight friends. Larger doses are required to get high and harder drugs may be used, such as cocaine, LSD, PCP, and mushrooms. Drug costs have gone up and the child is now dealing in drugs. He or she may turn to stealing or prostitution if necessary to support the habit. School may be a disaster, with low grades, suspension, skipping, or dropping out. If he does attend, sleeping or staring out the window takes the place of any real interest. Brushes with the law become frequent for such offenses as truancy, curfew violations, drunken driving, shoplifting, vandalism, possession of marihuana, sale of drugs, and breaking and entering. Sexual activity is high, with associated risks of venereal disease (VD) and pregnancy. In our study at Straight, 47% of those with a sexual history stated that they had their first sexual experience while they were high.[23]

The drug user is a confirmed liar and con artist. Volcanic anger and aggression have increased and paranoia is evident. This paranoia appears to be particularly related to the use of THC.[19] Blackouts and overdosing may occur. Certain drugs such as LSD may cause terror, not only during acute intoxication but later, in flashbacks. Experiences with overdosing disturb the child who thought he was in control of his "trips." His feelings of self worth progressively deteriorate as he loses control of his ability to quit taking drugs, begins to have encounters with the law, and feels shame for the things he is doing to support his drugs. When he comes down he feels dirty and ashamed. Physically and emotionally there is pain.

Family relations are terrible. They consist either of constant war or of the "pitstop" routine, where the child is home and in his room (frequently listening to high-volume rock music) until he goes out again with little family contact. Sneaking out the window is a common late-night activity. The family is often reduced to a position of avoiding conflict at all costs because of the violent outbursts of abuse, both verbal and physical, and fear that the child will run away, which he often does. Not knowing that drugs are the source of their child's problems or denying that possibility, they find some small comfort in the feeling that it is just a stage of adolescence that will pass with time.

Physical symptoms of red eyes, cough, sore throat, and fatigue are usual.

STAGE 4: USING DRUGS TO FEEL NORMAL

The euphoria is gone. Now the child wakes up in the morning and needs drugs to get him going. Coming down feels rotten so he takes drugs throughout the day to stay high. At home he becomes careless about any remaining efforts to hide the fact that he takes drugs. He has been expelled from school or dropped out. He is burned out.

THE BURNOUT.—Teens use the term burned out to describe the child who functions poorly, is almost always high, and has a characteristic blank zombie appearance. The exact causes of burnout are unknown but may involve a combination of factors: (1) Psychologic deterioration to Stage 4 when drugs are needed to feel okay and are used all day everyday; (2) saturation of lipid storage areas in the body (especially the brain). THC is a lipid-soluble substance with a half-life of seven days; traces may be found as long as 30 days after inhalation. The child who smokes frequently may reach a point of saturation and exhibit burnout; (3) of most concern are the findings of Heath in rhesus monkeys. Electrodes planted in the limbic area of the brain showed EEG changes with inhalation of marihuana smoke in amounts comparable to Stage 2 (less than two joints per week).[9] He also demonstrated intracellular changes after three months of such exposure that became permanent (cell destruction) after six months.[10] This may mean that Stage 2 and 3 smokers are doing themselves permanent damage physically as well as psychologically.

Characteristics of Chemical Dependency

Our experience with hundreds of adolescents treated for drug abuse has convinced us that chemical dependency has characteristics which must be understood to effectively diagnose and deal with the disease.

CHEMICAL DEPENDENCY IS A PRIMARY DISEASE.—Much time is spent on a variant of the old "Does the chicken precede the egg?" question. Do children with behavior problems resort to drugs or do drugs cause behavior problems? The answer to both questions is true but the answer is incomplete. Once the child begins to receive his orders from his feelings, as explained above, he is chemically dependent and drugs are the chicken *and* the egg. Efforts at control or treatment that do not comprehend this and the need for the child to be drug free will fail. Parents and counselors with inadequate understanding of the syndrome and its primary nature often waste time in behavior modification programs that ignore the basic etiology of the symptoms. Almost all of the clients at Straight have had previous unsuccessful experiences with psychiatrists, psychologists, or guidance counselors who were generally unaware of the depth of their drug involvement.

CHEMICAL DEPENDENCY IS A FAMILY DISEASE.[15, 16]—No one in the family of a chemically dependent person is not affected in some way. As the behavior of the affected teenager begins to change, each family member is drawn into responding, and until he knows the exact nature of the disease his response is likely to be inappropriate and harmful.

As these changes, which become increasingly apparent in Stage II, progress there is a natural tendency to want to believe they are just part of "normal" adolescent behavior. One parent, often the mother, has the feeling that the child needs more love and attention and may be tempted to chide the father for not spending enough time with his child. At the same time, the father may feel that things would be better all around if the mother would only be more consistent in discipline and setting of rules and regulations. As things worsen, and they will until it is understood that drugs are the cause of the negative attitudes and behaviors, the parents are apt to be in increasing conflict and in a lot of personal pain.

Parental denial and guilt often lead at least one parent to find excuses for the child's behavior and react with anger to suggestions that their child may be taking drugs. Others may reject the child as a "bad seed" and count the days until he leaves home. Rejection is especially easy if the child is adopted or is a stepchild.

The chemically dependent child, an expert at conning behavior, may use one parent against the other for his own purposes and by Stage III, divorce or separation are common. In many cases the child will actively promote divorce as an option that takes the heat off him.

Siblings are affected not only by the drug user's behavior and attitudes but by the changes they see in their parents. They are often taking drugs themselves or watching to see how their parents handle the more obvious offender. The most obviously involved child may become the scapegoat and shield for a child who is more deeply involved but whose behavior is less blatantly "druggie."

Success of treatment may depend to a large degree on family strength and involvement with their child's treatment program. Family members may also need extensive rehabilitation.

CHEMICAL DEPENDENCY IS A PROGRESSIVE DISEASE.—With increasing use the victim sinks lower into the syndrome (see Table 3) and finds it progressively more difficult to return to less serious usage. The drug use produces bad feelings and behavior that in turn lead to increased drug use. This leads to increasingly bad feeling and a "need" for more and stronger chemicals.

CHEMICAL DEPENDENCY IS A CHRONIC DISEASE.—Like the alcoholic, the "druggie" must learn to live with his disease. Giving up drugs isn't enough. He must alter his life-style. It is not unlike the chronic nature of diabetes, where in addition to taking insulin there are changes to be made in diet and life-style. When these changes are made a part of a daily pattern of living, the future can be long and rewarding.

An alcoholic is taught that he can never handle even one drink in a socially acceptable fashion without a strong drive to go on. Whether the drug-dependent adolescent will ever be able to have an occasional beer without returning to his previous stage of drug abuse is not known. In our experience even one joint is more than the "cured druggie" can handle without sliding back into his old pattern. Those who point out that the marihuana smoker will often turn to alcohol in his twenties are reminded that Alcoholics Anonymous estimates that there are already 16 million alcoholics in this country. Changing chemicals is not escaping dependency.

CHEMICAL DEPENDENCY IS A HARMFUL AND A POTENTIALLY FATAL DISEASE

Death.—The leading causes of death at age 15 to 24 today are accidents, suicide, and homicide. These are strongly drug-related, but frequent media reports of drug-related deaths rarely refer to chemical etiology. Marihuana alters reaction time in the young driver despite his claim that his driving skills improve while smoking. Massachusetts estimates that 16% of all highway fatalities in that state are related to marihuana. Nationally, 50,000 auto deaths occur annually, many of which are related to alcohol. Death from overdose accidentally and otherwise is especially obvious in reports from the rock music industry. Reported suicide rates in adolescence have tripled in 20 years. Suicide is the leading cause of death among college students.

Criminal activity.—The increasing cost of the drug habit, rebellion at authority, paranoia, and driving while intoxicated lead to brushes with the law. Drunken driving is obviously drug-related but newspaper reports of vandalism, shoplifting, and breaking and entering usually fail to relate these incidents to drugs.

Sexual problems.—Drug usage is closely related to looking for acceptance and to lowered moral resistance. Performing sex in exchange for drugs is common. Adolescent venereal disease and pregnancy, both national concerns, are increased in children who use drugs.

Child abuse.—More and more of the parents reported for child abuse are youngsters involved in the drug culture. These young people who are prematurely parents have not acquired the coping skills necessary for their new responsibility. Conversely, the exasperation of living with a child's "druggie" behavior may cause parents to react in a physical way.

School performance.—Scholastic Aptitude Test scores for students have fallen fairly consistently since 1964, when less that 2% of our population smoked marihuana. Discussion of this SAT problem rarely includes mention of adolescent drug use. Mental confusion, inability to concentrate, and diminished attention span have been reported as well as memory impairment.[33] All of these plus impulsive behavior lead to school failure, as does being stoned or absent.

Maturation.—Perhaps of greatest concern to pediatricians is arrest of the necessary adolescent experiences of learning to cope. Whether this essential period of development to full adult potential can ever be regained is not known. Psychiatrist Mitchell Rosenthal, president of Phoenix House, a New York rehabilitation program, has said: "If [adolescents] turn to marihuana they establish a pattern of escaping rather than dealing with reality. They do not learn to cope."[35] Mann deals with this problem at length in *Recovery of Reality.*[25]

Pharmacology and Physiology

Excellent clinical reviews of physiologic and pharmacologic studies on marihuana are available[1, 32, 37] and will not be presented in detail here. The detrimental effects on the fetus of alcohol, heroin, and tobacco are well known. Accidental poisoning of children with such things as PCP is being reported. Despite the fact that marihuana and other drug research is often anecdotal and uncontrolled, patterns of dysfunction are emerging. There are several reasons why marihuana research on humans is so hard to come by: (1) THC is an illegal drug that is dangerous for teenagers; (2) the great majority of drug users are involved in multiple drug usage, so effects may be synergistic and not related to a single substance; (3) trials with THC have yielded results different than trials with marihuana. It is believed that some effects of marihuana may be related to constituents of the smoke other than THC.

Even with research limitations, more and more adverse effects of marihuana are being reported. In addition to effects on brain and psyche, there are effects on the respiratory, reproductive, and probably the immune systems.

Effects on the respiratory system range from sinusitis and pharyngitis to chronic bronchitis and probably lung cancer.[22, 40] Low testosterone levels with associated delayed puberty,[4, 21] abnormal sperm mobility and number,[11, 12] gynecomastia,[8] and menstrual irregularity[2] are among the things most often reported about the use of marihuana. Disease has resulted from use of marihuana contaminated with Aspergillus[18] or Salmonella[3] organisms. Apologists for marihuana point to possible beneficial effects on glaucoma and chemotherapy-associated nausea. Neither of these afflications are common pediatric problems.

Diagnosis

Diagnosis is made primarily on the clinical picture of a child who has the appearance and behavior pattern of a "druggie." His overall manner, associated with poor school performance, nonstraight friends, loss of interest in family and extracurricular activities, hostile aggressive outbursts, brushes with the law, admission to tobacco smoking, and associated physical symptoms such as red eyes, cough, or lethargy make the diagnosis of the child in Stages 3 and 4 relatively easy. Identification of cannabinoids in the urine is helpful and may be done up to seven days after moderate exposure.[39]

Asking the parents of a child who is causing profound turmoil to all family members to search his room for drugs or paraphernalia is often met with great resistance. Their concern for the child's rights to privacy and trust must be weighed against his behavior change and an understanding of the importance of early diagnosis and treatment. Searches in such imaginative places as stereo speaker cabinets, the lining of drapes, the undersides of dresser drawers and behind electric switch plates and in toilet tanks is often diagnostic. It is not easy to lead parents to believe that a search may be as warranted in diagnosis as are the relatively common pediatric tools of venipuncture and lumbar puncture.

Of interest in our study at Straight[23] was the reticence of physicians to ask symptomatic teens about drug habits. Of 25 children taken to their physician because of concern about fatigue, only 11 were asked the threatening and well-remembered question about smoking or drugs. Six lied. The others minimized involvement and the diagnosis was not pursued. One practitioner who made the diagnosis of alcohol abuse just once in 16 years of practice, now makes the diagnosis of chemical abuse almost daily in the same practice. A diagnosis a day fits very well with what we now know about the incidence and depth of the problem. High index of suspicion and belief in the epidemic proportions of involvement are a must.

The physician who presents the diagnosis must realize that he is not only making a diagnosis but an accusation and is apt to be met with a full-blown grief reaction. Denial is usual and generally unresponsive to reason. Anger is real and often directed at the physician who does not understand the emotional impact of the diagnosis and the denial that asks him to prove his diagnosis. When dismissed from the office the child, who is an expert at conning his parents, may soon convince them that the doctor is overreacting. He has already conned himself. A study of high school students showed that although two thirds of them believed alcohol and other drugs could be harmful, there was a general feeling that marihuana was okay.

Temporary behavior changes will often satisfy the parent. But the disease will go on with incidents often kept from the parents by police, teachers, and friends who are either involved, see no deep problem, or fear their parents' wrath. Hopefully, with increased general awareness of the syndrome, more parents will accept the diagnosis in early stages. For those who won't, the physician who has presented his diagnosis in a nonblaming fashion will keep the lines of communication open. Perhaps many families will return for help before it is too late.

Treatment

Confidentiality is a key issue. How far must the physician go to treat the child and keep his confidentiality? Knowledge of the downward spiral of the disease, the user's emotional defense of marihuana as a good thing, and the accumulation of a drug that affects the user's thinking and willpower have shaped the authors' position. Success in treatment is unlikely unless the child can totally give up the drug long enough for his body to completely excrete it, a process that has been estimated to take from one to four months. Some feel that a month-long trial monitored by performance change and urine testing is worthwhile. We feel that the chances of the teenager accomplishing this are so slim as to be hardly worth trying. As with other diseases, delay in treatment can be associated with increased morbidity and a lowered success rate.

Occasional use of marihuana may produce no long-range effects other than its being a step on the road to more frequent use, but efforts aimed at having the frequent user smoke only moderately show a poor understanding of the process. Chemical dependency is a chronic and progressive disease from which there is no turning back to a stage of lesser involvement. For the emotionally labile and insecure adolescent, to return to occasional use is a more difficult feat than for the adult alcoholic to stop at one drink, or, for that matter, for the heavy tobacco smoker to cut back. Successful treatment requires total removal from psychoactive chemicals. For the physician this means more careful prescribing of analgesics, antihistamines, asthma medicines, and a variety of potentially psychoactive but frequently used medications.

Parents must be involved and the teenager informed of the reasons for the doctor's decision to involve them. Actually, little breach of confidence is involved because where the teen admits to regular usage the parents are already aware, and where he doesn't the diagnosis is made by the physician and does not involve disclosure of privileged information.

In his usual environment the chemically dependent teenager is constantly exposed to "do drug" messages and drug-using "friends" and has easy access to a wide variety of drugs. He has little willpower and no real interest in quitting. A few children with strong support may be able to quit, but for most, treatment demands complete removal from the environment to either a residential or strict foster care facility. Herculean efforts at supervision by dedicated parents have had some reported success, but for the advanced stages these efforts are unlikely to succeed. To be successful with this approach the parents must understand that drugs are found at school, in buses, at convenience stores, in stashes at home—nearly everywhere. The dependent child will find drugs if not monitored constantly. An excellent pamphlet by Menninger Clinic psychiatrist Harold Voth[40] describes the parental effort that is needed.

There are three phases of treatment. The first is to detoxify and help the patient to become drug free. The second is to expose and deal with the accumulated guilt and shame that blocks relationships with parents and others. This catharsis allows the child to experience feelings of guilt and shame that he has previously hidden with drugs and to deal with his feeling that he has no worth. The third is to rebuild those attitudes and skills that he either has lost or he has never had. Unless the program teaches coping skills, the recidivism rate will be high.

The treatment program at Straight Incorporated consists of removal of the child from his home with return dependent on the child. By the time he returns, the parents have had instruction in understanding chemical dependency and, where necessary, have altered the home environment. The emphasis on parent education is one of the program's strongest good points. Later in the program the child will return to work or school and afterward to leisure activity. The main part of his days will be spent in rap sessions led by peers who have completed the program. In these he will learn that he is not alone and that he was headed for destruction. As his self image improves he will learn techniques for dealing with problems and frustrations. He will learn the Serenity Prayer used by Alcholics Anonymous and seven steps for living that are modifications of the twelve used in AA. When he graduates he is expected to return for aftercare two evenings a week for at least six months. It is his understanding that for him drugs and alcohol will always be a trap.

Parents and Prevention

The answer to the drug epidemic has to lie in prevention. Treatment at best is far less than 100% successful and many who should reach treatment never will. Families with children have the most at stake and more and more of them realize that prevention is their responsibility. Across the country they are forming parent groups to fight for their children. A frequent beginning is for a concerned parent to call together the parents of their child's friends. These parents, who often have never met, are presented with information about drugs and their relationship to such things as behavior change, suicide, pregnancy, and accidental death. These parent groups then lay down guidelines, based on their own understanding and fears, for their children's behavior.

Hundreds of these parent groups banded together in April, 1980, to form the National Federation of Parents for Drug Free Youth.[30] This rapidly growing organization is mounting an attack on all of the forces discussed in "Stage 0: 'The Call to Do Drugs' " above. Their primary efforts however are still directed at helping their own children grow to maturation without drugs.

The National Federation was chartered at a Parent Resources in Drug Education (PRIDE)[34] meeting in Atlanta, where aroused parents from all over the country reported on what they were doing in their own communities. *Parents, Peers, and Pot*[38] served as a model for many of these families and is widely used by parents who want to organize groups for their own children.

The Role of the Pediatrician

Pediatricians have to reappraise their practice in light of what is happening to today's children. In 1940 the majority of deaths came from organic disease process. In 1980, 75% of deaths were related to life-style. It seems inappropriate to spend such great effort on such relatively minor problems as phenylketonuria testing and screening for urinary tract disease and so little on prevention of the major killers. Mothers who will bring a child for pediatric care at the first sign of a cold may not come in for help with temper tantrums and other behavior problems they see as normal phases of development.

PRIMUM NON NOCERE

The report of Roush et al.,[36] which shows a definite relationship between prescription of psychoactive medication to adolescents and subsequent illicit drug use, is disturbing. Not reported but worth consideration is the possible effect of using medication for symptomatic relief or placebo effect. Does this practice contribute to a general societal feeling that the way to feel good is to take drugs?

Ambivalence on the part of the pediatrician can also be harmful. Preaching moderation (rather than abstinence) and expecting teenagers to experiment as a part of growing up gives signals that may be harmfully permissive.

THE PEDIATRICIAN IN COMMUNITY AFFAIRS

The pediatrician will be increasingly called on by parent groups to offer support. He should keep current on the drug epidemic and be prepared to speak out. Little in his training or current pediatric literature prepares him for this task.

THE PEDIATRICIAN AS DIAGNOSTICIAN AND THERAPIST

The diagnosis of drug abuse will be made frequently by the alert pediatrician. His rapport with the child and his parents makes him particularly well suited for this task, as does his training in crisis management. He should familiarize himself with treatment resources available to his patients and be able to provide parents with an evaluation of such resources.

THE PEDIATRICIAN IN PREVENTION

Certainly the pediatrician should talk to adolescents and their parents about the dangers of drug abuse and provide them with literature freely. But is this enough? The prophylactic approach, so well outlined by Glenn and Warner[6] in their paper, "The Developmental Approach to Preventing Problem Dependencies," should speak directly to the pediatrician. Parents need specific help in teaching their children how to listen, communicate feelings, make rational decisions, defer gratification, and exert self-discipline. Children need to be made to feel they are responsible and useful members of their family and to be taught to identify with a higher power. The task is clear: we must build the child's coping mechanisms.

Summary

The current epidemic of teenage drug and alcohol abuse is wiping out parental and pediatric investment in early childhood care and protection. Pediatricians need to be aware of this epidemic, the clinical syndrome of such abuse, and the importance of its prevention, or, where necessary, its early diagnosis and treatment.

BIBLIOGRAPHY

1. American Academy of Pediatrics, Committee on Drugs: *Marijuana*. Evanston, Illinois: 1979.
2. Bauman J.: Effect of chronic marijuana use on endocrine function of the human female, in New York University Post Graduate Medical School and American Council on Marijuana, Second Annual Conference on Marijuana (1979): Marijuana: Biomedical Effect and Social Implications. Unpublished transcripts.
3. Center for Disease Control: Weekly report. *Morbid. Mortal. Weekly Rep.* 30:77, 1981.
4. Copeland K.C., Underwood L.E., VanWyk, J.J.: Marijuana smoking and pubertal arrest. *J. Pediatr.* 96:1079, 1980.
5. Donovan J.E., Jessor R.: Adolescent problem drinking: Psychological correlates in a national sample study. *J. Stud. Alcohol* 39:1506, 1978.
6. Glenn H.S., Warner J.W.: The developmental approach to preventing problem dependencies. Bethesda, Maryland: Family Development Institute, 1977.
7. Glenn H.S.: Toward an understanding of prevention. Proceedings, 28th annual meeting, Alcohol and Drug Problems Association of North America, September 25–29, 1977.
8. Harmon J., Aliapoulius M.A.: Gynecomastia in marijuana users. *N. Engl. J. Med* 287:936, 1972.
9. Heath R.G.: Testimony before the Senate Subcommittee on Internal Security, May 1974.
10. Heath R.G., Fitzjarrell A.T., Garey R.E., et al.: Chronic marijuana smoking: Its effects on function and structure on the primate brain. (See reference 27, p 713.)
11. Hembree W.C. III, Zeidenberg, P., Nahas G.G.: Marijuana's effect on human gonadal function, in Nahas G.G., et al. (eds): *Marihuana, Biological Effects—Analysis, Metabolism, Cellular Responses, Reproduction and Brain*. New York: Pergamon Press, 1979, p 521.
12. Hembree W.C. III, Nahas G.G., Zeidenberg P., et al.: Changes in human spermatozoa associated with high dose marijuana smoking. (See reference 27, p 429.)
13. Jessor R., Jessor S.L.: Adolescent development and the onset of drinking. *J. Stud. Alcohol* 36:27, 1975.
14. Jessor R., Chas J.A., Donovan J.E.: Psychosocial correlates of marijuana use and problem drinking in a national sample of adolescents. *Am. J. Pub. Health* 70:604, 1980.
15. Johnson V.E.: *I'll Quit Tomorrow*. San Francisco: Harper & Row, 1980.
16. Johnson Institute: *Chemical Dependency and Recovery Are a Family Affair*. Minneapolis: Johnson Institute (10700 Olson Memorial Highway, Minneapolis, MN), 1980.
17. Johnston L.D., Bachman J.G., O'Malley P.M.: *Student Drug Use in America 1975–1980*. Rockville, Maryland: National Institute on Drug Abuse, 1980.
18. Kagen S.L.: Aspergillus: An inhalable contaminant of marijuana. *N. Engl. J. Med.* 304(8):483, 1981.

19. Kolansky H., Moore W.T.: Effects of marijuana smoking on adolescents and young adults. *J.A.M.A.* 261:486, 1971.
20. Kolansky H., Moore W.T.: Toxic effects of chronic marijuana use. *J.A.M.A.* 222:35, 1972.
21. Kolodny R.C.: Testimony before the Senate Subcommittee on Internal Security (see reference 23). Washington, D.C.: U.S. Gov't. Printing Office, 1974.
22. Leuchtenberger C., Leuchtenberger R., Schneider, A.: Effect of marijuana and tobacco smoke on human lung physiology. *Nature* 241:137, 1973.
23. Macdonald D.I.: Survey of 104 adolescents in treatment for chemical dependency. Unpublished.
24. Malcolm A.: The amotivational syndrome—an appraisal. *Addictions* 23(3):28, 1976.
25. Mann G.: *Recovery of Reality.* New York: Harper & Row, 1980.
26. Marihuana-hashish epidemic and its impact on United States security: Hearings before the subcommittee to investigate the administration of the Internal Security Act and other internal security laws of the Committee on the Judiciary, United States Senate. Washington, D.C.: U.S. Gov't. Printing Office, 1974.
27. Marihuana-hashish epidemic and its impact on United States security: The continuing escalation. Hearings before the subcommittee to investigate the administration of the Internal Security Act and other internal security laws of the Committee on the Judiciary, United States Senate. Washington, D.C.: U.S. Gov't. Printing Office, 1975.
28. Marijuana: Biomedical effects and social implictions. Second Annual Conference on Marijuana, New York University Post Graduate Medical School and American Council on Marijuana, June 28–29, 1979. Unpublished transcripts.
29. Nahas G.G., Paton W.D.M., Idanpaan-Heikkila J.E. (eds): *Marihuana, Biological Effects—Analysis, Metabolism, Cellular Responses, Reproduction and Brain.* New York: Pergamon Press, 1979.
30. National Federation for Drug Free Youth, P.O. Box 57217, Pennsylvania Ave., Washington, D.C. 20037.
31. Newton M.: *Gone Way Down: Teenage Drug Use Is a Disease.* Tampa, Florida: American Studies Press, 1981.
32. Peterson R.C.: Marijuana, the continuing dilemma. Keynote address to American Academy of Pediatrics Annual Meeting, Oct. 1979.
33. Powelson D.H.: Testimony before the Senate Subcommittee on Internal Security, May 1974. (see reference 26.)
34. PRIDE (Parent Resources and Information on Drug Education), Georgia State University, Plaza, Atlanta, Georgia 30303.
35. Rosenthal M.S.: Statement before United States Senate Subcommittee on Criminal Justice, Jan. 16, 1980.
36. Roush G.C., Thompson W.D., Berberian R.M.: Psychoactive medicinal and nonmedicinal drug use among high school students. *Pediatrics* 66(5):709,1980.
37. Russell G.K.: *Marijuana Today,* rev ed. New York: The Myrin Institute Inc. for Adult Education, 1980.
38. Manatt M.: *Parents, Peers, and Pot.* Rockville, Maryland: Health and Human Services ADAMHA (5600 Fishers Lane, Rockville, MD), 1979.
39. SYVA Company: *New One-minute Emit-dau cannabinoid assay.* Palo Alto, California: SYVA Co. 3180 Porter Drive, Palo Alto, CA 94304), 1980.
40. Tashkin D.P., Shapiro B.J., Lee Y.E., et al.: Subacute effects of heavy marihuana smoking in pulmonary function in healthy man. *N. Engl. J. Med.* 294:125, 1976.
41. Turner C.S.: Personal communication, 1981 (R.I.P.S. School of Pharmacy, University, MS 38677).
42. Voth H.: *How to Get Your Child off Marijuana.* Stamford, Connecticut: Citizens for Informed Choices on Marijuana (300 Broad Street, Stamford, CT 06901), 1979.

Clinical Uses of Transcutaneous Oxygen Monitoring

JEROLD F. LUCEY, M.D., F.A.A.P.

Professor of Pediatrics
University of Vermont, College of Medicine
Burlington, Vermont

Introduction

THIS REVIEW is intended to bring the reader up to date on the wide variety of clinical uses of transcutaneous oxygen ($TcPo_2$) monitoring. This technique is relatively new. Physicians unfamiliar with it may consider it to be an interesting, expensive, and complicated research technique not yet suitable for routine clinical use. Those who have had experience with it realize that it can be quickly mastered, that it is cost effective, and that it is very useful in the care of sick infants. Indeed, some consider it indispensable.

One suggested analogy is that its use is comparable to the difference between watching a televised football game with instant replay ($TcPo_2$ monitoring) as compared to seeing one black and white photo every two hours during the game (intermittent arterial sampling)!

It is now realized that intermittent sampling of blood oxygen Po_2 is inadequate. It not only gives incomplete information but it does not reflect the true state of the infant's blood oxygen. Decisions based on this misinformation can be hazardous to the infant.

For those who are seriously interested in this technique, a complete history of its development is available in the proceed-

0065-3101/81/0028-0027-0056-$03.75

ings of the First International Symposium on Transcutaneous Blood Gas Monitoring, which was held in 1978 in Marburg,[1] and a textbook by Huch et al.[2] published in 1981.

History

In 1851, Gerlach,[3] a veterinarian, first reported that oxygen diffused through the skin of animals and man. Over a hundred years were to pass before this observation was used to benefit patients.

In 1956, the Clark Po_2 electrode[4] was developed. In the 1950s and early 1960s, Baumberger and Goodfriend,[5] Rooth et al.,[6] and Evans and Naylor[7] all reported that is was possible to measure Po_2 at the surface of the skin. Lubbers et al. began their work in 1967. This culminated in 1973 with the introduction of the prototype of the present clinical transcutaneous oxygen electrode. This device, and other similar models, were extensively clinically tested in Europe and Japan for six years prior to the introduction of the first commercial $TcPo_2$ monitors into the United States in January, 1978. The full significance and impact of this new technology is only now becoming apparent in the United States.

In the eight years since its introduction, this device has radically changed clinical practices, especially in intensive care nurseries, where they are now widely used. It marks the beginning of a new concept in patient monitoring: the use of the skin as a window through which to measure continuously and nontraumatically oxygen tension, which, under proper conditions, closely mirrors the arterial oxygen tension.

General Principles

The $TcPo_2$ electrode is a miniaturized, redesigned Clark electrode. The Clark electrode is the standard device used to measure blood oxygen tension in the laboratory.

The transcutaneous O_2 electrode consists of a ring-shaped silver anode heated by a coil to provide the required local hyperemia. It has three thin platinum cathodes, 15 mm in diameter, arranged in a triangle. All the elements are encased in plastic except for their working face, which is covered by a double membrane of Teflon and cellophane. A drop of electrolyte is

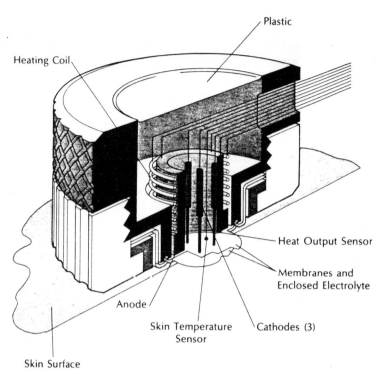

Plastic

Heating Coil

Heat Output Sensor

Membranes and
Enclosed Electrolyte

Anode

Skin Temperature
Sensor

Cathodes (3)

Skin Surface

Fig 1.—Cutaway view of TcPo$_2$ electrode shows ring-shaped silver anode, which is surrounded by heating coil, within anode are three thin platinum cathodes arranged in triangle. Current flow between anode and cathodes reflects amount of oxygen diffusing through skin into drop of electrolyte enclosed between the membranes. Heat output sensor regulates coil, maintaining preset temperature with high precision. Skin temperature sensor monitors cooling of skin by blood flow, i.e., relative local perfusion. (From *Hosp. Pract.* 6:43, 1976. Used by permission.)

placed between the double membrane and the face and another drop between the membrane layers. (The device is about 18 mm in diameter and about 9 mm high (Fig 1).

The device is connected to an electronic amplification unit that has three functions: (1) to measure oxygen tension in mm Hg directly by measuring the flow of current between the silver and platinum electrodes; (2) to vary the heat energy in the electrodes' core by feedback currents in order to maintain the temperature at any desired level; and (3) to measure the rate of skin cooling by capillary blood flow by monitoring the level of heat energy being expended. This is a sensitive indicator of the relative perfusion in the area.

The device is calibrated in vitro against either a humidified pure nitrogen atmosphere or a "null" solution and then against room air or a gas of known oxygen content corrected to barometric pressure, such as room air. It is then attached to the skin. To facilitate contact, a drop of water is placed at the point where the membrane will touch the skin. The heating coil is then activated with the thermostat set so that the silver electrode will reach a temperature of 44 C (Litton) for premature infants, 45 C for full-term infants and children.

The temperature settings are critical, as warming to these levels was determined by careful experiments to produce a degree of hyperperfusion sufficient to arterialize the skin blood.

TcPo$_2$ readings and arterial Po$_2$ readings are *not* identical but they correlate very closely. It should be remembered that: (1) O$_2$ consumption in the skin results in a TcPo$_2$ lower than Pa$_{O2}$; (2) the electrode heats *both* the skin and the capillaries, which causes a shift of the oxygen dissociation curve to the right. This means the Pa$_{O2}$ will be higher; therefore, TcPo$_2$ is higher than Pa$_{O2}$; (3) these two factors usually cancel each other out; (4) skin acts as a membrane through which oxygen must diffuse. The thickness of the skin determines the lag time, which is about ten seconds in a neonate.

The temperature settings are critical, as warming to these levels was determined by careful experiments to produce a degree of hyperperfusion sufficient to arterialize the skin blood.

The differences between these two values are not entirely due to inaccuracies of the TcPo$_2$ method. It is well known that considerable variation is possible among arterial values due to assay methods used and the skill of the assayer.

It should also be realized that to achieve these good correlations careful attention must be paid to the position of the electrode, the arterial sampling sites chosen for comparison, and the condition of the infant. (See "Causes of Poor Correlation between TcPo$_2$ and Pa$_{O2}$" below.)

Several modified commercial versions of the original Huch electrode have been produced. Considerable evidence exists to document that the Huch electrode (the Hellige-Litton version, Fig. 2) is accurate. Less evidence is available to document this same degree of accuracy of the other electrodes.[1]

AUTHOR	TYPE OF PATIENTS	TOTAL NO. OF PATIENTS	CORRELATION COEFF. - PAO2	COMPLICATIONS
PEABODY GREGORY TOOLEY LUCEY U.S.A.	PREMATURES - RDS SICK INFANTS	80	.98	2 BLISTERS
VERT FRANCE	NEWBORNS CONG. HEARTS	30	.94	NONE
REYNOLDS SOUTTER ENGLAND	PREMATURES - RDS	68	GOOD CORR. TO AORTIC DEVICE	2 BURNS
BUCHER DUC SWITZERLAND	PREMATURES - RDS CONG. HEARTS	68	.94	NONE
STRASSER GERMANY	ADULTS	50	.96	NONE
SCHANINGER GERMANY	PREMATURES - RDS	65	.92	NONE
YAMANOUCHI JAPAN	PREMATURES - RDS	276	.99	NONE
FENNER GERMANY	PREMATURES NORMAL, SICK	178	-	NONE
EMMRICH GERMANY	PREMATURES - RDS CHILDREN — CONG. HEARTS TRAUMA	48 11 34	.96	NONE
VESMOLD RIEGAL GERMANY	PREMATURES - RDS	73	.97	NONE
LONG LUCEY U.S.A.	PREMATURES RDS - NORMALS	86	.99	NONE
KOPPE HOLLAND	NEWBORNS	80	.98	NONE
HUCH HUCH GERMANY	NEWBORNS (SCREENING)	3200	NO LONGER DONE	NONE

Fig 2.—Summary of recent patient clinical experience with Huch (Litton-Hellige) TcPo$_2$ electrode, 1974–1978.

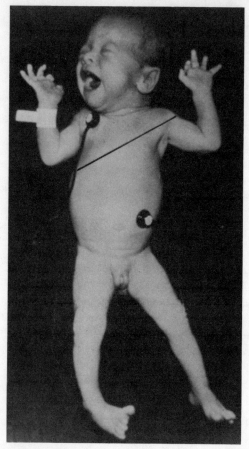

Fig 3.—An infant with a patent ductus arteriosus and a right-to-left shunt. In this situation the TcPo$_2$ electrode *above* the line will read 10–40 torr higher than the TcPo$_2$ electrode *below* the line on the abdomen. (From Lucey J.F.: *Hosp. Pract.,* February, 1981.)

Causes of Poor Correlation Between TcPo$_2$ and Pa$_{O2}$

Many careful studies have been reported confirming that under proper conditions with careful technique, the correlation coefficient for TcPo$_2$ vs Pa$_{O2}$ will be 0.9 or above. The following is a list of situations that may cause discrepancies.

1. *Presence of a patent ductus arteriosus with a right to left shunt.* In this situation the TcPo$_2$ electrode and the sampling site must be comparable, that is either both above or below the

ductus arteriosus. Figure 3 indicates the rough dividing line which is found in infants with a right-to-left ductal shunt. Preductal blood can have a Po_2 40 torr higher than postductal blood. The presence of an intermittent right-to-left ductal shunt in small low-birth-weight infants is quite common. In our experience 20% of infants of less than 1,500 gm can be demonstrated to have such intermittent shunts during the first week of life. These right-to-left shunts occur following large intravenous infusions, blood transfusions, respirator setting changes, apneic and hypoxemic spells (Fig 4). It appears that if the ductus is open, relatively small changes in pulmonary artery pressure can result in short intermittent periods of right-to-left ductal flow.

2. *Temporary local ischemia.* If the electrode is placed over a rib in a small infant and the skin is stretched taut, blood flow

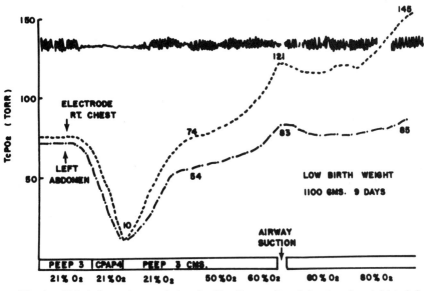

Fig 4.—This infant who was being double site-monitored developed a right-to-left shunt through a patent ductus arteriosus. Note very large difference between preductal $TcPo_2$ of 145 torr and postductal $TcPo_2$ of 85 torr. (Used with permission of I. Yamanouchi.)

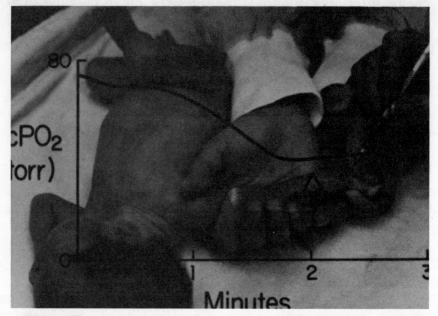

Fig 5.—When a resting sick infant cries during a peripheral arterial puncture, his arterial and $TcPO_2$ tension falls to 20 to 30 torr. This creates the false impression that the infant is hypoxemic.

under the electrode can be reduced and one will get a falsely low $TcPO_2$ reading. Any extra weight placed on the electrode can result in the same reading due to local ischemia.

3. *The use of peripheral arterial blood sampling after crying for comparision.* Crying in a sick infant lowers the true arterial O_2 tension. Therefore, such blood samples cannot be used to check the accuracy of the electrode. If they are used, a 20–30 second delay must be allowed for the $TcPO_2$ electrode to reflect the change in the resting arterial value created by the sampling trauma (Fig 5). It should be remembered that nearly all painful procedures in small sick infants result in injury, apnea, and some fall in arterial O_2 tension (Table 1).

4. *Temperature of the skin electrode is criticial.* This must be carefully watched. Most skin electrodes are designed to give their best correlations at 44 C in low-birth-weight infants and 45 C in full-term infants and children. If the electrode is run at lower temperatures, the correlations obtained will not be comparable to the original studies.

TABLE 1.—Causes of Hypoxemia in Sick, Low-Birth-Weight Infants

Feeding	Diagnostic procedures
Due to amount, quality, and	Head shaving
techniques	Lumbar puncture
Tube feeding—nasal or oral	Blood sampling—arterial or venous
Abdominal distension	Intravenous infusions
Hand under jaw feeding	Bladder catheterization
Neck flexion	Bladder puncture
Noise	Removal of urine bag
Crying—caused by any painful	Abdominal examination—palpation of
procedure or sudden noise	kidneys or liver
Diaper change	General
With neck flexion	Weighing an infant out of incubator
Bowel movements	Rough handling
Vulnerable airway	Removal from head box O_2 for "just a
Suctioning of airway	minute"
Pressure of face mask on lower	Abdominal distension
jaw	Poorly adjusted CPAP or leaks in
Poor positioning of nasal or	CPAP
endotracheal tube	Apnea
Nasal obstruction—partial,	Incubator temperature out of infant's
caused by mucous or eye	thermoneutral zone
blindfold	Convulsions
Neck flexion	Circumcision
Hyperextension of neck	

5. *Postcardiac surgery.* After extensive surgery the microcirculation of most infants is not normal and poor correlations between $TcPo_2$ and Pa_{O_2} are often found.[8] These infants are not in shock but neither are they "normal." It is probable that they represent minor disturbances in peripheral circulation previously undetectable by ordinary techniques. (See "Use of $TcPo_2$ in Shock" below.)

6. *Inaccuracies of the blood gas determinations.* Errors due to faulty technique or mechanical failure are not uncommon.

7. *Different electrodes.* Several $TcPo_2$ electrode systems are available. Some are not as accurate as the original Huch electrode (Hellige-Litton version). This electrode has been used in the majority of the clinical studies reported[1] (see Fig 2).

Clinical Uses of $TcPo_2$ Monitoring

Prior to the introduction of continuous $TcPo_2$ monitoring into the nursery, it was commonly assumed that an infant's arterial oxygen tension was relatively stable. This erroneous assumption occurred because intermittent arterial sampling supplied values that encouraged this thought. One of the first benefits to emerge with the advent of continuous $TcPo_2$ monitoring was the realization that the sick infant's arterial O_2 tension varied considerably. Indeed, it is quite unstable, varying 10–40 torr in a few seconds. It quickly became obvious that even simple routine procedures previously thought to be harmless could result in profound falls in arterial O_2 tension to hypoxemic levels, defined as a $TcPo_2$ of less than 40 torr. Table 1 is a list of the procedures and events that have been shown to result in hypoxemia in sick low-birth-weight infants. Several groups using $TcPo_2$ monitoring[9] and continuous intravascular monitoring[10] have confirmed these findings.

It has also been noted that if a sick infant is subjected to several therapeutic and diagnostic procedures, there may be a cumulative effect, as is demonstrated in Figure 6.

The final result of these well-intentioned maneuvers was to force the infant's arterial O_2 tension to hypoxemic levels that finally "required" that the infant be placed on assisted ventilation.

In many intensive care nurseries it has become accepted procedure to handle infants for "necessary care" one or two hundred times a day! It is now clear that this is not wise and should be avoided. Before handling a sick infant or subjecting him to a diagnostic procedure, the staff must ask themselves whether the procedure justifies the risk of a fall in the infant's $TcPo_2$ and if that risk can be minimized.

In one study, 75% of the hypoxemic episodes noted in sick

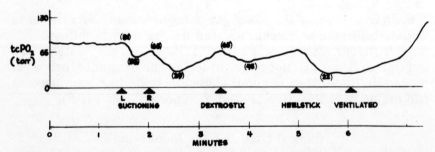

Fig 6.—The deleterious effect of repeated "routine" procedures upon an infant's $TcPo_2$ is demonstrated in this example. Note that the infant finally "required"(?) assisted ventilation! (Used by permission of James L.S., and L. Inckyk.)

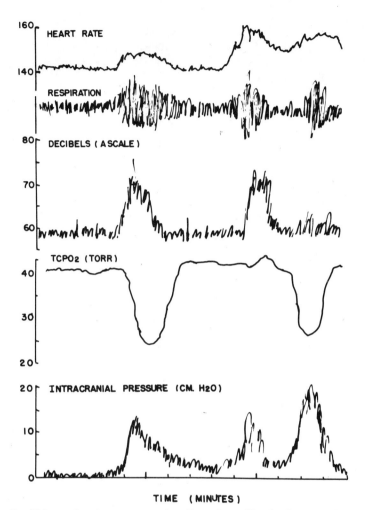

Fig 7.—This tracing demonstrates the effect of a sudden loud noise—the ring of a telephone—on infant's TcPo$_2$ intracranial pressure, respirations, and heart rate. Such events are not uncommon in noisy intensive care units.[12]

infants were related to procedures and considered to be iatrogenic.[11] One of the more unusual but not uncommon causes of hypoxemic episodes was sudden and loud noise. Long et al.[12] have demonstrated this very clearly in Figure 7.

Once TcPo$_2$ monitoring has been introduced into an intensive care nursery, one of the first things one notices is that the med-

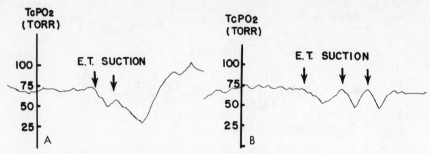

Fig 8.—Sample tracing of change in TcPo$_2$ vs time following endotracheal suctioning for control (A) and monitored (B) groups, respectively.[11]

ical and nursing personnel become more careful, gentle, and less aggressive in their handling of sick infants.

The presence at the cribside of a continuous, visible record that allows one to see immediately the effects of care on the infant's TcPo$_2$ is a very effective teaching tool. It literally allows the infant to immediately communicate his O$_2$ needs to the staff. As a result of this, any adverse effects of care are more rapidly detected, corrected, and hopefully avoided in the future.

Detection of Iatrogenic Hypoxemia

Thach and Stark[13] pointed out that small infants are especially vulnerable to upper airway obstruction. When their necks are flexed or pressure is placed on the lower jaw, air flow to the lungs can be completely blocked. Slight changes in the position of the neck can result in obstructions to breathing and the infants may then have repeated episodes of apnea.

Peabody et al.[14] have made similar observations and have documented the occurrence of previously undetected recurrent hypoxemia following the events and procedures listed in Table 1.

The treatment for such undesirable episodes is obvious. They should be avoided. Nurses who use the electrode quickly become aware of these problems and modify their care in numerous ways to avoid hypoxemia.

One technique is to pretreat the infant with small amounts of supplemental oxygen and raise the TcPo$_2$ to 80 torr before trying any therapy such as nasal or oral suction. Another is to modify the suctioning so that it is less stressful. This is shown in Figure 8. In the upper tracing labeled control, a routine endotracheal suctioning resulted in apnea and a TcPo$_2$ drop to 30 torr. The second tracing demonstrates the effect of three less traumatic suctionings.

The device is an invaluable aid for teaching purposes. The effects of a treatment or procedure can be immediately seen. Raval et al.[15] have carefully studied the effects of three techniques of tracheobranchial hygiene (chest physiotherapy, oral and nasal suction, and hand ventilation). They were unable to demonstrate any advantage in using these in different sequence. They found that initially each of these techniques resulted in a 20–30% decrease in the pretreatment TcPo$_2$ level.

The infant's eye bandages used during phototherapy may slip down over the nose and obstruct the nares. This is one of the commonest causes of hypoxemia and can cause profound hypoxemia.

Rough handling, physical examinations, and such stressful procedures as positioning and immobilizing a sick infant for a lumbar puncture can all result in severe hypoxemia (Fig 9).

Use During Assisted Ventilation

Arterial Po$_2$ varies greatly during assisted ventilation. If the infant is restless, struggling, or fighting the respirator, falls of 30 to 60 mm Hg in Pa$_{O_2}$ may be observed to occur within a few minutes (Fig 10).

Continuous TcPo$_2$ monitoring quickly reveals this and allows adjustments to be made. The infant may be sedated or given Curare to improve his ventilation. One can quickly judge whether suctioning or repositioning of an endotracheal tube is effective. The effects of respirator setting changes in rate or pressure can be observed within minutes. No longer is it necessary to wait 30 minutes to an hour for a blood gas reading. The ability to "fine-tune" assisted ventilation this way is a great advantage.

Weaning an infant from respiratory support can be very difficult. With continuous monitoring this transition can be carried out safely and smoothly: time is saved and risks are minimized. The potential benefits from this use alone are of major importance. These should include a decrease in the total time

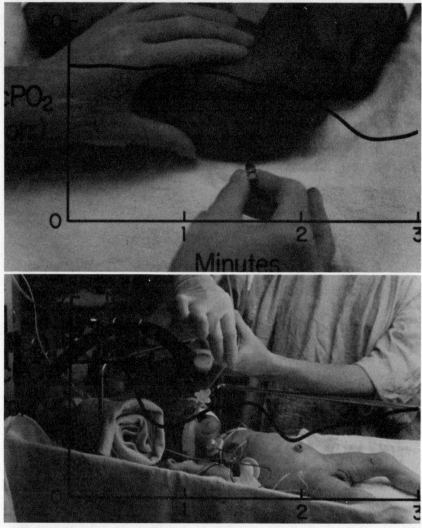

Fig 9 (top).—Note effect on TcPo$_2$, which fell from approximately 60 torr to 40 torr during a two-minute immobilization for a lumbar puncture. Longer periods of "holding" for such a procedure can result in much greater falls of TcPo$_2$.

Fig 10 (bottom).—Note that repeated suctioning can cause hypoxemia. This technique allows nurses to judge the effectiveness of their suctioning. If it is too stressful or ineffective this can be detected.

infants spend on assisted ventilation and a decrease in the incidence of complications directly related to the use of respirators, such as bronchopulmonary dysplasia and pheumothoraces. Significant savings in patient care costs can be expected to occur from shorter hospital stays and fewer complications of oxygen therapy.[16]

Superiority Over Conventional Apnea Alarms

During their studies, Peabody et al.[14] noted long (60-second) and repeated episodes of hypoxemia ($TcPo_2 = 20$ to 40 mm Hg) that occurred during active and transitional sleep or following excessive handling. These infants were also being monitored by conventional impedance-type apnea alarms and cardiac rate monitors. The alarms were set to go off at 15 or 20 seconds but missed these episodes of hypoxemia completely.

Conventional apnea alarms are designed to report *only* chest *movement* and when it stops. They are not designed to report air flow or to detect obstructed breathing. The alarms are also

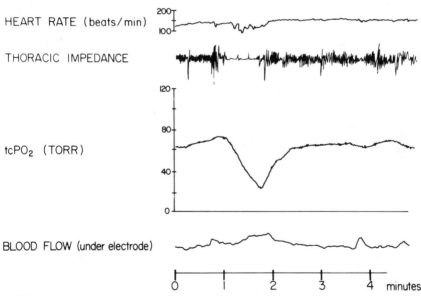

Fig 11.—During broken apnea notice that the thoracic impedance indicates a respiration that has "fooled" the alarm into not going off. The infant, however, has experienced a bout of hypoxemia. This type of spell is not detected by the conventional apnea alarms.

usually disconnected during many of the activities listed in Table 1 and so are not capable of detecting hypoxemia—the single most important effect of apnea. In observations of more than 500 apnea spells in sick newborns, Peabody et al. found two types of apneic attacks missed by conventional apnea alarms. In one—"broken apnea" (Fig 11)—an infant's chest moves slightly during the apneic spell, enough to deceive the alarm but not enough to move very much air. As a result, the infant becomes hypoxemic, although the alarm has not gone off. This is common. This type of apnea comprised more than 50% of the observed attacks.

The second type of apnea can be called disorganized breathing (Fig 12). During this spell the infant is usually sleeping. Often, but not always, there is rapid eye movement (REM) or transitional sleep. The infant appears to be breathing deeply but no air moves into his lungs, as is shown by the lack of air flow past a special detector thermistor at the nose. In this situation the pharyngeal muscles have apparently become hypotonic and collapsed and have obstructed the upper airway. During these episodes, an infant's $TcPo_2$ drops abruptly and may remain low for two or three minutes. These spells are very similar to the sleep-apnea, upper airway obstruction pattern seen in adults. Should these episodes occur repeatedly, they may have serious sequelae. Some preliminary studies indicate that, during these episodes of hypoxemia, blood pressure increases and intracranial pressure may also rise. Studies are in progress to determine if these episodes might be a factor contributing to intracranial bleeding.[17]

It should be emphasized that neither of these types of apnea, and the hypoxemia they cause, have been previously detectable. The results are not due to an artifact of transcutaneous monitoring. They have also been observed with continuous intravascular O_2 monitoring.[10]

Some episodes of "disorganized breathing" are iatrogenic and can be avoided by allowing the infant to remain undisturbed in quiet sleep as long as possible. Unnecessary procedures and diagnostic tests should be avoided. Necessary procedures should be carried out when the infant is awake and has been pretreated with oxygen to slightly raise the arterial O_2 tension prior to the procedures.

A study by Long et al.[11] indicated that if all personnel are

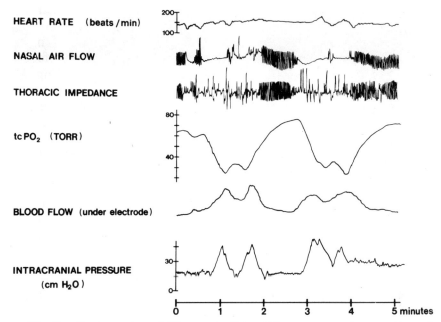

Fig 12.—During prolonged "disorganized" breathing an upper airway pattern of obstruction occurs. The infant appears to be breathing normally but no air flow occurs past the nose. These spells result in significant hypoxemia. They are not detected by apnea alarms.

made aware of the problems of iatrogenic hypoxemia and hyperoxia, they can be virtually eliminated. In their studies of a small group of 15 infants when personnel used TcPo$_2$ monitoring, "undesirable time," defined as a TcPo$_2$ of over 100 torr or under 40 torr, could be reduced to six minutes in a day, as compared to their control group of 15 infants without TcPo$_2$ monitoring-modified care, who spent 40 minutes a day in an "undesirable" range.

As continuous monitoring techniques are more widely used, one can anticipate that the care of sick infants will become less hectic and intensive and probably more gentle, quiet, and effective.

Prevention of Hyperoxia

Many nurses and physicians are unaware as to how rapidly an infant with normal lungs or one who is recovering from the

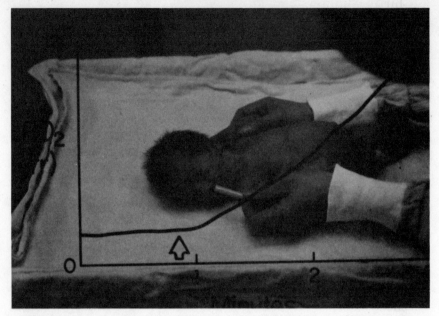

Fig 13.—Note the effects of a short period of 100% nasal oxygen. Hyperoxemia can rapidly occur and may last several minutes.

respiratory distress syndrome can raise his arterial Po_2 when given a few "whiffs" of oxygen via a nasal catheter or funnel (Fig 13). This form of mild resuscitation is commonly used in nurseries and should be watched carefully.

Abrupt changes in blood flow to the lungs can occur during improvement in the respiratory distress syndrome. When these occur the supplemental oxygen requirements of the infant change rapidly. This rapidly changing situation is easily detected during continuous O_2 monitoring.

It has been claimed, on the basis of little evidence, that retrolental fibroplasia (RLF) can occur as a result of very brief periods of hyperoxemia. The use of continuous $TcPo_2$ monitoring might enable researchers to answer this question. Preliminary evidence suggests that $TcPo_2$ monitoring will be effective in lowering the incidence of RLF in low-birth-weight infants but not in completely avoiding this dreaded complication. Yamanouchi[18] has transcutaneously monitored O_2 tension in 55 low-birth-weight (< 1,500 gm) infants and observed four infants with Grade I RLF. His control group of 46 conventionally monitored infants included 12 infants with Grade I RLF.

Use to Improve Feeding Techniques in Sick Infants

Sick infants often have feeding problems. Nurses frequently report apneic spells and cyanotic episodes after and during feedings. Feeding may have important effects upon an infant's arterial O_2 tension, usually resulting in drops of 10 to 30 torr shortly after the feeding.[19] The infant may become quite hypoxemic if its feeding is too long or if it is fed too much too fast. Nurses quickly realize that disinterest in feeding may not be due to the infant's being "full" but rather to the effect of the feeding efforts on his blood O_2 tension. Improvements in feeding can occur when proper attention is paid to avoiding hypoxemia *during* feeding.

Nonnutritive sucking has the interesting effect of usually improving an infant's blood O_2 tension.[20] This behavior should be encouraged in infants by offering them something to suck on, such as a pacifier, which will decrease crying and restlessness.

Complications

Erythema occurs at the electrode site in all infants. Minor thermal injury commonly occurs in infants of less than 1,500 gm birth weight. These red spots may last for several days. Blisters rarely occur, probably in less than 0.1% of the infants monitored[1, 2] (see Fig 2). We have observed that septic infants who are either hyperthermic or hypothermic seem to be the most prone to thermal injury. It is probable that the presence of endotoxemia plus hyperthermia or hypothermia constitute a vascular injury. In such situations we recommend that the electrode be moved every one or two hours in order to decrease the risk of burns. To date we have not observed serious burns in over four years of experience of monitoring over 1,200 infants.

Recently, Golden[21] has reported that minor skin craters or pits can be observed in very small infants who have been monitored. This is a rare complication.

In judging the risk of these complications one should remember the serious risks of peripheral arterial sampling, such as nerve damage, arterial thrombosis, and gangrene. Umbilical artery sampling carried a risk of some serious complication occurring in at least 3% of the catherizations. It has been estimated that death from a catheter complication occurs in approximately one in every 250 catherizations.[22]

Use During Pediatric Surgery

It is surprising to realize that during surgery on infants and children arterial oxygen tensions are usually not monitored. The majority of anesthesia machines deliver only 100% oxygen. When no inhalant anesthetic agent is mixed with this the infant may become markedly hyperoxemic. A case of retrolental fibroplasia in a premature infant whose *only* exposure to an elevated F_{IO_2} occurred during surgery has been reported.[23] Welle et al.[24] have reported that significant periods of hypoxemia and hyperoxemia occur during routine pediatric surgery and that these undesirable periods can be detected by using $TcPO_2$ monitoring during surgery.

Because marked fluctuations occur in the infant's $TcPO_2$ during surgical manipulations, it is probable that $TcPO_2$ monitoring will become routine during pediatric surgery. Its use will make surgeons aware of the profound effects of some of their manipulations upon an infant's $TcPO_2$. It should be possible to modify these manipulations and avoid the deleterious effects probably associated with them.

Necrotizing Enterocolitis

A major problem known to be associated with necrotizing enterocolitis is impaired peripheral perfusion. Traditional methods for the early detection of impaired peripheral perfusion, such as a falling blood pressure or X-ray demonstration of free peritoneal air, are not entirely satisfactory. Burtain et al.[25] have proposed that this poor perfusion can be detected by using the $TcPO_2/Pa_{O2}$ ratio. Under normal circumstances this ratio is .97 ± 0.4 in their hands. In a group of infants with necrotizing enterocolitis and poor perfusion, this ratio was 0.5 or less. They suggest that the response of this ratio could be used to judge fluid therapy in patients. They found no survivors if the ratio could not be corrected to above 0.6 before surgery.

This ingenious use of the new technique to improve patient care should be quite helpful. It requires confidence in your $TcPO_2$ technique, in addition to an understanding of the physiology involved.

Double Site TcPo₂ Monitoring

Japanese researchers have explored the use of two electrodes on different skin areas of the same patient.[26, 27] "Double-site" monitoring appears to be an important new use of transcutaneous monitoring.

In a tour de force of logical thinking, Professor Yamanouchi has applied one electrode above the ductus arteriosus on the right chest and another electrode on the left side of the abdomen, below the ductus arteriosus. Electrodes applied in these positions will give the same $TcPO_2$ readings, within 2 to 5 torr, unless the ductus arteriosus is open and shunting R > L is occurring. If this is the case and blood is shunting right to left through the ductus, the $TcPO_2$ on the abdomen will give a read-

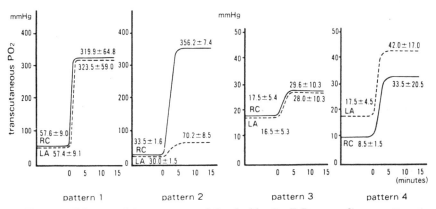

Fig 14.—Schemes of four patterns of the double-site $TcPO_2$ recordings: *pattern 1,* case of healthy newborn infant or with simple left to right shunt such as ventricular septal defect (VSD) or patent ductus arteriosus (PDA); *pattern 2,* patient with coarctation of aorta complex (Co/Ao) or interruption of aorta complex (Int/Ao) with normal aortic root; *pattern 3,* patient with markedly cyanotic heart disease; *pattern 4,* patient with cyanotic heart disease with reversed ductal shunt, i.e., Co/Ao or Int/Ao complex with conotruncal malformation. (From Tateishi K., Yamanouchi I.: *Pediatrics* 66:22, 1980. Used by permission.)

ing of 10 to 50 torr lower (see Fig 3). This simple technique allows physicians to noninvasively follow the opening and closing of the ductus areteriosus. Yamanouchi et al.[26, 27] have shown that such common events as excessive crying and struggling or positive airway pressure can reopen a previously closed ductus arteriosus. It is now possible to follow the effects of routine procedures in the intensive care nursery upon the status of the ductus arteriosus.

The incidence of patent ductus arteriosus in low-birth-weight infants—those under 1,500 gm at birth—is 30% to 40% in some intensive care nurseries. In others the problem is very rare. At the University of Vermont and Dartmouth Medical School nurseries only six patients with patent ductus arteriosus have been diagnosed and treated surgically or with indomethacin among 360 infants under 1,500 gm. It seems highly likely that these very different incidence rates are due not to diagnostic problems but rather to iatrogenic factors that affect the ductus arteriosus. Tateishi and Yamanouchi[27] have also pointed out that double-site $TcPo_2$ monitoring can be used very effectively to diagnose some types of congenital heart disease. These patterns are demonstrated in Figure 14.

This technique can also be used to document the closure by medical or surgical therapy of a patent ductus arteriosus with a right-to-left shunt. In other types of congenital heart disease, such as pulmonary artery atresia, transposition of the great vessels, and tricuspid atresia, it is an advantage for the infant to maintain a patent ductus arteriosus. Tateishi and Yamanouchi[27] have demonstrated that prostaglandin E can be used to accomplish this.

It can also be used to follow the effects of balloon septostomy.

Use of $TcPo_2$ Electrode in Shock

It is well known that when an infant is seriously ill he will usually have some degree of peripheral vasoconstriction. It was, therefore, anticipated that $TcPo_2$ monitoring might give an inaccurate reflection of central arterial oxygen tension in very sick infants. This has proven to be at least partially true, but only if the infant is *severely* ill.[28] The clinical conditions in which $TcPo_2$ monitoring may generally, but not always, produce "falsely" low O_2 values are as follows: (1) Shock—blood pressure (2 to 3 SD below normal); (2) severe acidosis (pH < 7.15); (3) hypothermia—temperature (< 35 C); (4) postcardiac surgery—(open heart) possibly due to conditions one, two, or three or to anesthetic effects; (5) infant's receiving high-dosage tolazoline, usually for persistent fetal circulation syndrome; (6) severe edema or anemia, usually in combination in hemolytic disease; (7) hyperthermia of bacteremic shock; and (8) cyanotic congenital heart disease (Pa_{O_2}, 30 mm Hg).

The basic mechanism by which these conditions interfere with $TcPo_2$ monitoring appears to be by producing a severe disturbance in the microcirculation of the skin. The failure to obtain good agreement between the $TcPo_2/Pa_{O_2}$ value in these situations should *not* be considered a lack of reliability of $TcPo_2$ monitoring. Indeed, $TcPo_2$ is providing a *true* reflection of the situation in the peripheral skin, where the microcirculation is disturbed.

These conditions are all usually clinically easily recognizable. It can be argued that once the limitations of the method are recognized it is easy to avoid errors by simply realizing that under these conditions the method should not be relied upon to reflect central arterial Po_2. When one suspects that the clinical status of the patient may interfere with the accuracy of the $TcPo_2$ measurement, a central PA_{O_2} should always be checked. If a poor correlation is found and no technical problem is apparent, then a diagnosis of early shock or a disturbed peripheral microcirculation should be considered and appropriate measures to treat this should be instituted.

Failure to obtain good agreement between $TcPo_2$ and PA_{O_2} values in shock situations should not be considered to reflect a lack of reliability of $TcPo_2$ monitoring. Indeed, under these conditions $TcPo_2$ accurately reflects the real situation in the peripheral circulation.

This has important physiologic significance. One can use this information to establish a diagnosis of shock and follow the effects of treatment. If an infant has one $TcPo_2$ electrode on a limb and one on the right chest plus a central arterial line being used for intermittent sampling and blood pressure monitoring, initially all values recorded from these sites will be in close agreement. If the infant has a severe grade 4 intracranial hemorrhage, hypotension will occur with an abrupt fall in the limb $TcPo_2$ from the 75-torr range to 45 torr. The other moni-

toring sites will show only a small decrease. In this situation
the peripheral limb $TcPO_2$ will give an indication of the disturbed peripheral circulation seen early in shock. As the infant's blood pressure improves, the discrepancy between the
monitoring sites regresses. It is possible that this double-site
peripheral vs central $TcPO_2$ might prove to be a valuable
method for the early detection of shock, one that could be carried out noninvasively. Further research on this point is
needed. Tremper et al.[29-31] have made similar observations in
animals and human adults. They point out that the difference
between $TcPO_2$ and Pa_{O2} is *not* a shortcoming of the device. In
shock, Pa_{O2} has been shown to be a poor measure of the patient's status and an unreliable variable to follow during resuscitation.[32] A more clinically relevant variable may be the tissue
oxygen tensions, because their restoration may be considered
the ultimate goal of the peripheral circulation. The $TcPO_2$ is a
sensitive indicator of peripheral perfusion. These researchers
found that in adults $TcPO_2$ no longer correlates with the Pa_{O2}
when the cardiac output falls to about 65% of the normal level.
They believe that $TcPO_2$ monitoring is "a significant break-
through in continuous monitoring of critically ill patients" and
"an effective way of guiding therapy with almost real time responses."

Our own experience agrees with this. We have observed
abrupt falls of $TcPO_2$ readings to zero in two patients several
minutes before they had cardiac arrests during exchange transfusions. It may be possible to use this window on the complex
microcirculation to improve care of such seriously ill patients.

Prenatal Use of $TcPO_2$ Monitoring

One of the most promising developments has been the introduction of transcutaneous monitoring into the field of obstetrics. A specially modified electrode has been developed that
permits its attachment to the fetal scalp.[34] The first extensive
clinical trial has been reported.[1, 34, 37] This experience, which
amounts to over 200 maternal-fetal studies, has produced some
interesting results. The technique is not difficult to master. Fetal $TcPO_2$ monitoring will be introduced into the United States
in the next few years for research puposes. Using this technique it has been possible to directly observe the effects of ma-

ternal pain, irregular breathing with transient apnea, hypoventilation, analgesic drugs, and tranquilizers on the fetal scalp oxygen tension. All of these events and treatments lower fetal O_2 tension. The most important feature of fetal $TcPo_2$ monitoring is not so much that it provides precise data, which it does, but that it allows changes in Po_2 resulting from procedures or medications to be seen *immediately*. The obstetrician is thus able to correct deteriorations very rapidly and to prevent or avoid treatments or maneuvers that produce hypoxemia.

The deleterious effects of the maternal supine position during labor on fetal oxygenation are obvious. The beneficial effects of a change to the lateral position can be easily and rapidly seen. When the fetus is hypoxemic (fetal $TcPo_2 < 15$ torr) and oxygen is administered to the mother, the nearly instantaneous fetal response is visible as one observes the fetal $TcPo_2$ to rise 10 torr or more.[34, 37, 38] No longer will an obstetrician have to guess whether a procedure or treatment has improved the status of fetal oxygenation. The early studies indicate that some of the pathologic fetal heart rate patterns observed by fetal EKG monitoring are not actually related to fetal hypoxemia. One can anticipate a great deal of new information emerging about the fetal oxygen environment.

Blood Pressure Measurements by Use of the Heating Power "Relative Perfusion Flow Channel"

One of the great advantages of the Huch electrode is its heating element, which is used to produce local vasodilatation. This feature enables you to detect when the electrode has become detached from the skin (the heating power increases) or when pressure on the electrode produces local ischemia (the heating power decreases). This information is essential in the use of any transcutaneous monitoring device. The electrical power required to maintain and produce a skin temperature of 44 to 45 C is recorded and displayed. Under conditions of maximal vasodilatation blood flow is largely dependent on blood pressure. It has often been suggested that it might be possible to correlate the heating power required to produce and maintain vasodilatation with the blood pressure. Peabody et al.[33] have recently demonstrated that if the electrode is *properly insulated* from environmental temperature changes, the flow channel power requirements can be used to accurately reflect changes in blood pressure. We can expect to see further developments and improvements in the use of the Huch electrode to monitor blood pressure. The clinical advantages of having a continuous noninvasive electrode that monitors oxygen tension and blood pressure are many. This development potentially represents a major advance in simplifying neonatal intensive care.

TcPO$_2$ to Study Drug Effects

Relatively few studies have been reported in which TcPO$_2$ monitoring has been used to judge the effects of drugs.

The depressing effects of diazepam and pethidine on maternal and fetal oxygenation have been reported.[34] It has also been possible to demonstrate the beneficial effects of a change in the mother's position from supine to lateral and to show the benefits of maternal O$_2$ breathing of fetal TcPO$_2$. The response of neonatal patients with patent ductus arteriosus to indomethacin has been followed with TcPO$_2$ monitoring,[26] as has the response of patients with severe congenital heart disease (pulmonary atresia, transposition of the great vessels, and tricuspid atresia) to prostaglandin infusions.[27] It would appear to be an effective way to judge therapy in these situations.

A study of low-birth-weight infants receiving theophylline for recurrent apneic attacks revealed that TcPO$_2$ values during therapy were stabilized by the regular breathing pattern produced by this substance.[35]

Some studies of the effects of preanesthetic agents and N$_2$O have been carried out.[36]

Evans and Naylor,[7] in one of the earliest studies of TcPO$_2$, performed some interesting experiments in which they applied solutions of barbiturates to stripped adult skin. They observed marked changes in the O$_2$ utilization of the treated skin areas, which they attributed to the O$_2$ sparing effect of barbiturates. These observations suggest that TcPO$_2$ monitoring may provide a convenient method for studying O$_2$ consumption of whole limbs and skin area in vivo. It certainly deserves further study.

One fairly obvious future application of TcPO$_2$ monitoring in older children and adults will be in judging the response of patients with obstructive airway problems such as asthma, croup, or chronic pulmonary disease such as cystic fibrosis to various bronchodilators, oxygen, or chest physiotherapy. In asthma patients the effect of an allergy challenge on $TcPo_2$ can be seen. This may prove to be a more meaningful way to measure a patient's response to a suspected pulmonary allergen than other types of testing. One report indicates that the technique can be useful in long-term home management of a patient with bronchopulmonary dysplasia. By using the technique it should also be possible to answer questions about the effects of therapies such as Intralipid on O_2 and about the use of diuretics to decrease lung fluid.

Use of Huch "Trough" Electrode For Bedside Blood O_2 Tensions

The Huch electrode can be modified to run on batteries and used at 37 C to determine blood Po_2 directly on arterial blood. The whole unit is slightly larger than a package of cigarettes and is very portable. This allows one to rapidly check, at the bedside, values reported by the central laboratory, which often take 30 to 60 minutes to arrive. Long et al.[39] demonstrated that under field trial conditions the electrode has an excellent correlation coefficient with the commonly used blood O_2 tension machines.

The simplicity and accuracy of doing O_2 tensions with this device is impressive. It can be easily operated by resident physicians and nurses. When this device is commercially available it should prove very useful.

Combined Microprocessor and Continuous $TcPo_2$ Monitoring

Continuous $TcPo_2$ monitoring generates a huge amount of data that create record storage problems. To solve these problems, a microprocessor-based device (Oxygram) that can be attached to the $TcPo_2$ monitor (Litton) has recently been introduced.[40] This device keeps track of the time spent by an infant in each of ten preset $TcPo_2$ ranges. This enables research workers to accurately assess the total amount of time an infant spends in either a hyperoxic or hypoxic state. It will enable meaningful comparisons to be made between one hospital and another as to the quality of their oxygen care. Figure 15 is an example of the type of data comparison which can be made.

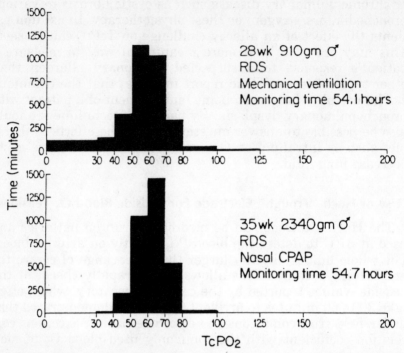

Fig 15.—The Oxygram of the infant in the upper figure indicates he has spent a considerable amount of time in an undesirable TcPo$_2$ zone. The infant in the lower figure was much better controlled.[40]

The 28-week-old infant spent considerably more time in an "undesirable" O$_2$ range than did the 35-week-old infant.

The safe limits for arterial Po$_2$ in the newborn and the effects of varying degrees of hypoxemia and hyperoxemia are not known. In the future, the Oxygram and similar devices should permit much better studies of this question.

REFERENCES

1. Huch A., Huch R., Lucey J.: Continuous transcutaneous blood gas monitoring. *Birth Defects* 15:1, 1979.
2. Huch A., Huch R., Lubbers D.: *Transcutaneous Blood Gas Monitoring.* In press.
3. Gerlach P.: Uber das Hautathmen. *Arch. Anat. Physiol. Wissenschoftl. Med.* (1851), pp. 431–555.
4. Clark L.C. Jr.: Monitor and control of blood and tissue oxygen tension. *Trans. Am. Soc. Artif. Intern. Organs* 2:41, 1956.
5. Baumberger J.P., Goodfriend R.B.: Determination of arterial oxygen tension in man by equilibration through intact skin. *Fed. Soc.* 10:10, 1951.

6. Rooth G., Sjostedt S., Caligara F.: Bloodless determination of arterial oxygen tension by polarography *Science Tools, The LKW Inst.* 4:37, 1957.
7. Evans N.T.S., Naylor P.F.D.: Steady states of oxygen tension in human dermis. *Respir. Physiol.* 2:46, 1966.
8. Indyk L., Raker R., Kull C., et al.: Transcutaneous PO_2 monitoring in pediatric patients following cardiac surgery. *Birth Defects* 15:365, 1979.
9. Lucey J.F., Peabody J.L., Philip A.G.S.: Recurrent undetected hypoxia and hyperoxia: A newly recognized iatrogenic problem of intensive care. *Pediatr. Res.* 11:537, 1977.
10. Pollitzer M.J., Reynolds E.O.R., Morgan A.K., et al.: Continuous comparison of in vitro and in vivo calibrated transcutaneous oxygen tension with arterial oxygen tension in infants. *Birth Defects* 15:295, 1979.
11. Long J.G., Philip A.G.S., Lucey J.F.: Excessive Handling as a cause of hypoxemia. *Pediatrics* 65:203, 1980.
12. Long J.G., Lucey J.F., Philip A.G.S.: Noise and hypoxemia in the intensive care nursery. *Pediatrics* 65:143, 1980.
13. Thach B.T., Stark A.R.: Spontaneous neck flexion and airway obstruction during apneic spells in preterm infants. *J. Pediatr.* 94:275, 1979.
14. Peabody J.L., Gregory G.A., Willis M.M., et al.: Failure of conventional monitoring to detect apnea resulting in hypoxemia. *Birth Defects* 15:275, 1979.
15. Raval D., Yeh T.F., Mora A., et al.: Changes in transcutaneous PO_2 during tracheobronchial hygiene in neonates. *Perinatol. Neonate* 4:41, 1980.
16. Lucey J.F., Dehner L.: $TcPO_2$ monitoring reduces costs of blood gas monitoring. *Pediatr. Res.* 14:604, 1980.
17. Horbar J., Lucey J.F.: Hypoxia and intracranial bleeding. In press.
18. Yamanouchi I.: Effect of continuous oxygen pressure monitoring on the incidence of retrolental fibroplasia. *Proc. 16th Int. Congress of Pediatrics*, Barcelona, Spain, September, 1980.
19. Bodefeld E., Schachinger H., Huch A., et al.: Continuous $TcPO_2$ monitoring in healthy and sick newborn infants during and after feeding. *Birth Defects* 15:503, 1979.
20. Burrows A.K., et al.: The effect of nonnutritive sucking on transcutaneous oxygen tension in noncrying preterm infants. *Res. Nursing Health* 1:69, 1978.
21. Golden S.: Skin craters, a complication of transcutaneous monitoring. *Pediatrics* 67:514, 1981.
22. Rao M.H.K., Elhassani S.B.: Iatrogenic complications of procedures performed on the newborn. *Perinatol. Neonate* 4:25, 1980.
23. Bettes E.K., Downes J.J., Schaffer P.B., et al.: Retrolental fibroplasia and oxygen administration during general anesthesia. *Anaesthesia* 47:518, 1977.
24. Welle P., Hayden W., Miller T.: Continuous measurement of transcutaneous oxygen tension of neonates under general anesthesia. *J. Pediatr. Surg.* 15:257, 1980.
25. Burtain W.L., Conner E., Emrico J., et al.: Transcutaneous oxygen measurements as an aid to fluid therapy in necrotizing enterocolitis. *J. Pediatr. Surg.* 14:728, 1979.
26. Yamanouchi I., Igarashi I.: Ductal shunt in premature infants observed by $TcPO_2$ measurements. *Birth Defects* 15:323, 1979.
27. Tateishi K., Yamanouchi I.: Noninvasive transcutaneous oxygen pressure diagnosis of reversed ductal shunts in cyanotic heart disease. *Pediatrics* 66:22, 1980.
28. Versmold H.T., Linderkamp O., Holtzmann M., et al.: Transcutaneous monitoring of PO_2 in newborn infants: What are the limits? *Birth Defects* 15:285, 1979.
29. Tremper K.K., Waxman K., Shoemaker W.C.: Effects of hypoxia and shock on transcutaneous PO_2 values in dogs. *Crit. Care Med.* 7:526, 1979.
30. Tremper K.K., Waxman K., Shoemaker W.C.: Transcutaneous oxygen sensors for continuous monitoring in shock and resuscitation. *Crit. Care Med.* 7:136, 1979.

31. Tremper K.K., Waxman K., Bowman R.: Continuous transcutaneous oxygen monitoring during respiratory failure, cardiac decompensation, cardiac arrest, and CPR. *Crit. Care Med.* 8:377, 1980.
32. Maxwell T.M., Lim R.C., Fuchs R.: Continuous monitoring of tissue gas tension and pH in hemorrhagic shock. *Am. J. Surg.* 126:249, 1973.
33. Peabody J., Willis M., Gregory G.A., et al.: Reliability of $TcPo_2$ electrode heating power as a continuous noninvasive monitor of mean arterial pressure in sick infants, *Birth Defects* 15:127, 1979.
34. Huch A., Huch R., Schneider H.: Continuous transcutaneous monitoring of fetal Po_2 during labor. *Br. J. Obstet. Gynaecol.* 84(suppl 1):1, 1977.
35. Peabody J., Neese A., Philip A., et al.: Transcutaneous oxygen monitoring in aminophyline-treated apneic infants. *Pediatrics* 62:698, 1978.
36. Gothgen I., Jacobsen E.: Transcutaneous oxygen during halothane and neurolept anesthesia, *Birth Defects* 15:549, 1979.
37. Huch A., Huch R.: Transcutaneous noninvasive monitoring of Po_2. *Hosp. Pract.* 6:43, 1976.
38. Huch A., Huch R., Schneider H., et al.: Monitoring fetal arterial oxygen continuously during labor. *Contemp. Obstet. Gynecol.* 12:73, 1978.
39. Long J.G., Lucey J.F., Huch A., et al.: Blood Po_2 analysis at the bedside, *Birth Defects* 15:585, 1979.
40. Horbar J.D., Clark J.T., Lucey J.F.: The newborn oxygram: Automated processing of transcutaneous oxygen data. *Pediatrics* 66:848, 1980.

The Vitamin K-Dependent Proteins

JAMES J. CORRIGAN, JR., M.D.

Professor of Pediatrics
Chief, Section of Pediatric Hematology-Oncology
University of Arizona Health Sciences Center
Tucson, Arizona

Introduction

ADVANCES IN BIOCHEMICAL AND IMMUNOLOGIC TECHNIQUES have given rise to rapid progress in our understanding of vitamin K metabolism and function. These advances have also allowed the discovery of a specific vitamin K-dependent biochemical reaction, a new amino acid, the presence of precursor coagulation proteins, and many new vitamin K-dependent proteins. Terms such as osteocalcin, protein C, protein S, a-carboxy proteins, and γ-carboxyglutamic acid (Gla) may even seem foreign to the reader. The purpose of this chapter is to review current data and concepts on the vitamin K-dependent proteins, show that not all of them are coagulation proteins, and indicate their clinical relevance where it is known.

Historical Review

There are a number of excellent reviews on vitamin K metabolism and function.[1-6] Vitamin K and its use in the treatment of hemorrhagic disease of the newborn has been reviewed twice in *Advances in Pediatrics*—by Poncher in 1942[7] and Dam and his colleagues in 1952.[8] The history of the discovery of vitamin K and its involvement in health and disease is fascinating, but only some of the historical highlights are empha-

0065-3101/81/0028-0057-0074-$03.75

sized here. Although the disease we now call hemorrhagic disease of the newborn (HDNB) had been known for many years, perhaps centuries, it was not until the 1930s that two significant advances were made that allowed us to understand this entity in more detail. The first was the discovery of a new vitamin, vitamin K, and the second, the development of specific coagulation tests designed to measure prothrombin (factor II). In 1929 Dam, studying cholesterol metabolism in chicks, noted that when the animals were placed on a diet free of sterols they bled to death. However, it was not until 1934 and 1935 when he published his classic work on the bleeding problem, which he reported was due to a deficiency of a newly unidentified chemical that he called vitamin K.[9] Dam and associates subsequently identified prothrombin deficiency in the plasma of hemorrhagic chicks and were able to correct the deficiency in vitro with a very crude factor II preparation but not with vitamin K. Other investigators noted that mammals could develop a similar bleeding disorder in obstructive jaundice and when the bile was excluded from the intestinal tract.[10, 11] During this period, Quick was developing the one-stage prothrombin time, which was thought to measure prothrombin. It is now known that prothrombin time actually measures five coagulation factors (fibrinogen, II, V, VII, and X). In addition, investigators at the University of Iowa devised a two-stage clotting test that subsequently has been shown to be a specific coagulation test for factor II coagulant activity. During the 1930s the application of these two coagulation tests demonstrated that certain infants had prolonged prothrombin times. Furthermore, factor II coagulant activity was low in normal newborns, and in hemorrhagic disease of the newborn these levels were reduced even further. Another significant advance made in the early 1940s was the isolation of a material that caused hemorrhagic disease in cattle that had eaten spoiled sweet clover. This material, called dicumarol, was subsequently found to antagonize vitamin K's action and thus the era of anticoagulation by means of vitamin K antagonists emerged.[3, 5] During the next couple of decades, clinical and animal studies confirmed that to prevent avitaminosis K one had to have a diet containing vitamin K or intestinal bacteria capable of synthesizing vitamin K, bile in the intestine (since vitamin K is fat soluble), a normal absorptive surface in the intestine, and a normal liver function.

As early as the 1950s and 1960s, precursor proteins were thought to exist for the vitamin K-dependent proteins. Quick suggested that for prothrombin such a precursor existed and he called it prothrombinogen.[12] Hemker and his associates studied patients who lacked vitamin K or were receiving vitamin K antagonists and suggested the confusing term preprothrombin in 1963 and then, in 1968, PIVKA to describe these proteins.[5, 13] (The letters stand for *Protein in Vitamin K Absence* or due to *Vitamin K Antagonists*.) This was based on the finding that prothrombin times were longer than expected in comparison to the measured levels of factors II, VII, and X in patients with a vitamin K deficiency or with coumarin-induced hypocoagulability. The explanation for the discrepancy was hypothesized to be the interaction of precursor molecules of the prothrombin complex factors in the coagulation process. In 1968, Ganrot and Niléhen demonstrated by immunochemical methods the presence of an abnormal prothrombin in plasma from coumarin-treated patients.[14] Josso and associates, also using a precipitating antibody against factor II, showed excess cross-reacting material in such patients relative to the amount of factor II coagulant activity.[15] Other investigators have subsequently shown similar abnormalities for the other vitamin K-dependent coagulation factors. In 1969 Suttie and his colleagues approached the possibility of a precursor protein in a different way.[16] The precursor protein to prothrombin was suggested to them by the nature of the response observed when vitamin K was administered to severely hypoprothrombinemic rats. In their studies they noted a short lag during which there was no increase in prothrombin, followed by a very rapid increase in plasma prothrombin occurring 30 to 60 minutes after administration of the vitamin. The same response was noted whether the hypoprothrombinemia was produced by a nutritional deficiency of the vitamin or by administration of one of the coumarin anticoagulants. In addition, they showed that the appearance of prothrombin in plasma was preceded by a transient increase of prothrombin in liver microsomal preparations. This increase peaked about ten minutes after vitamin K had been administered to hypoprothrombinemic rats, and the microsomal content decreased as prothrombin appeared in the plasma. The nature of these responses strongly suggested to these investigators that the hypoprothrombinemic rat had a pool of precursor that could be converted to prothrombin in a vitamin K-dependent step. When the pool was depleted the rate of synthesis would slow. The precursor hypothesis was strengthened by a number of investigators whose data have recently been reviewed by Suttie et al.[17, 18] Table 1 summarizes the characteristics of the precursor and functional protein for factor II.

In 1974 a new era was ushered in when three groups independently reported that functional prothrombin contained several residues of a new amino acid, γ-carboxyglutamic acid (Gla), which was not present in the precursor protein.[19, 20, 21] It was subsequently determined that carboxylation of the γ-methylene carbon atom of certain glutamic acid residues was a vitamin K-dependent reaction that allowed the formation of a functional coagulation protein. The resulting γ-carboxyglutamate residues chelate calcium ions and aid in the activation of prothrombin to thrombin by factor Xa, factor V, and phospholipid.[22] This vitamin K-dependent carboxylation is now known to modify the other vitamin K-dependent coagulation factors (VII, IX, and X). Other Gla-containing proteins have been subsequently identified from bone (osteocalcin), kidney, spleen, placenta, pancreas, lung, and other tissues.[23] Current investigation suggests that they too are dependent on vitamin K for their formation and probable physiologic effects. It seems fairly certain that the 1980s will show what role this reaction plays in the normal physiology of coagulation and noncoagulation proteins and its involvement in certain diseases.

TABLE 1.—SIMILARITIES AND DIFFERENCES BETWEEN PRECURSOR AND FUNCTIONAL FACTOR II

ITEM	PRECURSOR	FUNCTIONAL
Immunoreactive protein	Similar	Similar
γ-Carboxylated residues	0	+
Bind calcium ions	0	+
Bind to phospholipid membrane surfaces	0	+
Requires vitamin K	0	+
Thrombin formed by:		
Nonphysiologic activators	+	+
Physiologic activators	0	+
Requires:		
Normal hepatic function	+	+
Bile salts	0	+
Normal intestinal absorption	0	+

Vitamin K Function

Vitamin K is a fat-soluble vitamin found in many plants and vegetable oils.[24] Bacteria, including those that colonize the human gut, also synthesize vitamin K. The vitamin found in vegetables is chemically different from the one formed by bacteria. The vitamin found in vegetables is called vitamin K1 (phylloquinone) and the one synthesized by bacteria is called vitamin K2 (menaquinone). The major site of absorption appears to be the small intestine; absorption will not take place in the absence of bile. Vitamin K depletion as a result of dietary deficiency alone is exceptionally rare. Depletion caused by dietary lack associated with a change in the gut flora (such as diarrhea or treatment with broad-spectrum antibiotics) can result in a deficiency of vitamin K. After its absorption, vitamin K1 is initially concentrated in the liver, but within 24 hours the concentration there declines significantly. The body's capacity to store vitamin K is extremely limited, and deficiency, as evidenced by hypoprothrombinemia, may be produced within 24 hours in animals by diversion of intestinal lymph or by biliary fistulas. The exact human requirement for vitmin K is difficult to assess because of the two sources of supply. It apparently is extremely small and ranges between 8 and 10 µg/kg daily in man.[25, 26] Current biochemical data suggests that there is a vitamin K cycle important in the carboxylation reaction of vitamin K-dependent proteins, as shown in Figure 1.[17, 27] After absorption, vitamin K must be reduced to the naphthoquinone form (KH_2) and then there is a stepwise oxidation to vitamin K epoxide (KO); it is this reaction that is coupled with the protein carboxylation. Following this there must be enzymatic reduction of the epoxide to regenerate the native vitamin K and the reduced vitamin K form. These reactions appear to take place in the microsomal fraction of liver parenchymal cells. The significance of the vitamin K reaction can be illustrated best with one of the vitamin K-dependent coagulation proteins, prothrombin. Patients treated with vitamin K-antagonistic drugs (coumarins) demonstrate an abnormal protein in their plasma (PIVKA) that does not have coagulant activity. Unlike normal prothrombin, the abnormal protein cannot bind calcium ions but it does have the same main antigenic determinants as normal or functional prothrombin. The purified abnormal pro-

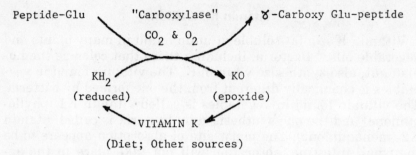

Fig 1.—The vitamin K cycle and its association with the carboxylation reaction. γ-
Carboxy Glu-peptide: coagulation factors II, VII, IX, and X, bone protein (osteocalcin),
and other Gla-containing proteins.

thrombin has no prothrombin activity in coagulation tests using physiological activators, but like normal prothrombin it
can be activated to form thrombin by nonphysiological activators such as venom from the snake *Echis carinatus* (Fig 2).[18, 28]
Biochemical comparisons between normal and abnormal prothrombin resulted in the discovery of the new amino acid, γ-
carboxyglutamic acid (Gla), in normal prothrombin. In normal
prothrombin the first 10 glutamic acid residues in the amino
terminal end of the molecule are carboxylated, whereas warfarin-induced prothrombin lacks carboxylated residues and has
ordinary glutamic acids in the corresponding positions. In people rendered vitamin K-deficient, this precursor does spill over
into the plasma and can be measured by immunologic methods
or by using *Echis* venom. The formation of γ-carboxyglutamate

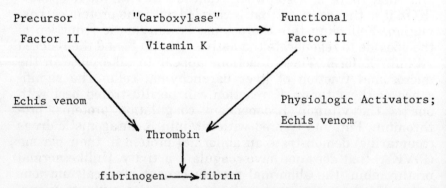

Fig 2.—Activation of precursor and functional factor II with physiologic and nonphysiologic (*Echis* venom) activators to form prothrombin.

in the vitamin K-dependent blood coagulation factors allows these proteins to specifically bind calcium ions, which then permit the calcium-mediated absorption of these proteins to phospholipid membrane surfaces. Thus, proteolytic (coagulation) activation can occur in vivo.

Suttie and his colleagues noted that the initial peak of prothrombin production following the administration of vitamin K in the hypoprothrombinemic intact rat was decreased only slightly by prior administration of the protein-synthesis inhibitor cycloheximide.[16] They also showed that the additional increase of plasma prothrombin seen between the first and second hours after vitamin K administration, which presumably would require continued synthesis of the precursor, was blocked by administration of cycloheximide. These findings strongly supported their idea that protein synthesis was not required for the vitamin K reaction. Thus, the vitamin K-dependent step follows synthesis of the protein component of clotting factors, and the vitamin has no activity in the formation of the precursor protein.

This particular reaction, although noted here for prothrombin, has also been found for the other vitamin K-dependent coagulation proteins (VII, IX, and X) and the more recently discovered plasma proteins (protein C, protein S), and the vitamin K-dependent proteins in other organs such as the bone, kidney, spleen, and placenta. Evidence suggests that the vitamin does not affect the precursor synthetic phase but only the conversion of the precursor to functional protein.

Vitamin K-Dependent Proteins

Vitamin K-dependent proteins include plasma proteins—coagulation factors II, VII, IX, and X, and Proteins C and S—and other Gla-containing proteins in bone (osteocalcin), the kidney, spleen, placenta, pancreas, lung, and other tissues. Of all such proteins, those that are most familiar are the coagulation factors. From the above discussion it is clear that these proteins are synthesized by the liver in precursor form and require the presence of reduced vitamin K, a carboxylase enzyme, a source of oxygen, and carbon dioxide to produce the Gla residues, which is characteristic of the functional protein. Factors II, VII, and X are important in the extrinsic or tissue coagulation mechanism, and factors II, IX, and X are essential in the intrinsic or plasma coagulation mechanism. A newly discovered vitamin K-dependent plasma protein, protein C, has been recently described.[29, 30, 31] Protein C appears to be a potent anticoagulant; it inhibits prothrombin activation by reactions mediated by both plasma and platelets. Its role in normal physiology, however, is not clear at this time. Protein S has recently been discovered and its function is still unknown.[32] Similarly, proteins that depend on vitamin K and the carboxylase reaction have been found in kidney and other tissues, but their roles have yet to be defined. One exciting area of research has been the demonstration of vitamin K-dependent protein in bone. Gallop and his associates have demonstrated proteins rich in Gla residues in mineralized tissues, bone, tooth, dentin, ectopic calcifications, kidney, and other tissues.[33, 34] The Gla-containing protein in bone has been termed osteocalcin by these investigators. Its function is not completely understood at this time; however, it is known that it abounds in bone and has specific calcium-binding properties. This suggests that it may have an active role in mineralization. The Gla protein in the kidney may be involved with reabsorption of calcium in the renal tubule. What role this may play in normal human physiology or disease is unknown.

Clinical Application

From the above discussion it is apparent that new coagulation and immunologic techniques can now be applied to study the normal development of vitamin K-dependent proteins and their role in the pathophysiology of various diseases. The most obvious area is that involved with the human neonate.

NORMAL HUMAN NEONATE

Normal human neonates have a reduction in the vitamin K-dependent coagulation proteins.[35-39] This reduction is gestational-age-dependent in that the more preterm the baby the more severe the reduction in these coagulation proteins. Because findings in hemorrhagic disease of newborn and other vitamin K-deficient states showed similar data, it was presumed that all human newborns began extrauterine life with a vitamin K deficiency. Recent data, however, suggest that normal newborns are not vitamin K deficient but do not synthesize the same amount of coagulant protein that normal older children or adults do. Analysis of cord blood has not confirmed a deficiency of vitamin K.[40-44] It has been found that the normal human newborn's coagulant activity is directly proportional to the amount of immunoreactive protein present (Table 2). In vitamin K deficiency one would find a reduction in coagulant activity in comparison to the amount of immunoreactive protein, as is shown for patients treated with warfarin (see Table 2). This should not be interpreted to mean that vitamin K deficiency cannot occur at the time of birth. In 1952, Dam[8] noted that infants who suffered intrauterine asphyxia (to the extent that amniotic fluid was stained by meconium) had prothrombin levels lower than those of infants without complications. Corrigan and Kryc[43] reported that newborns with low one-minute Apgar scores (mean, 6.0) and meconium staining had lower factor II coagulant activity and higher antigen levels than in infants with high Apgar scores (mean, 8.2) (groups A and B, respectively, in Table 3). Their study showed, further, that the ratio of coagulant activity to antigen was very low in group A and normal in group B newborns. These results suggested an impairment in the vitamin K mechanism in group A newborns. Nevertheless, the uncomplicated normal human neonate (term and preterm) appears to have no vitamin K deficiency at birth.

TABLE 2.—FACTOR II (PROTHROMBIN) COAGULANT ACTIVITY (CA) AND ANTIGEN (AG) IN CORD BLOOD FROM NORMAL NEWBORNS*

STUDY GROUP	FACTOR II CA†	Ag†	RATIO CA:Ag
Term (40)‡	39±2	44±2	0.89
Preterm (17)	30±1	31±4	0.97
Warfarin (30)	25±2	87±8	0.29
Controls (50)§	83±3	91±4	0.91

*Compared with warfarin-induced vitamin K deficiency.[28, 43]
†CA and Ag expressed as percent of normal plasma pool.
‡Numbers in parentheses indicate number of patients.
§Controls = hematologically normal adults.

TABLE 3.—FACTOR II COAGULANT
ACTIVITY (CA) AND ANTIGEN (AG) IN
CORD BLOOD*

NEWBORNS	FACTOR II CA†	FACTOR II Ag†	RATIO CA:Ag
Normal			
Term (40)‡	39 ± 2	44 ± 2	089
Stressed			
Group A (7)	32 ± 2	58 ± 3	0.55
Group B (12)	39 ± 2	44 ± 3	0.89

*Comparison of normal and stressed-term
newborns.[43]
†CA and Ag expressed as percent of normal.
‡Numbers in parentheses indicate number of
patients.

HEMORRHAGIC DISEASE OF THE NEWBORN

It has been clearly shown by numerous investigators that vitamin K-dependent coagulation factors decline after birth and
do not begin to rise until the third to fifth day postpar-
tum.[8, 35, 45-48] This decline is especially marked in breast-fed infants, breast-fed infants who have had intrauterine anoxia, and
infants born of mothers who have taken anticonvulsants or
coumarin anticoagulants before parturition.[8, 43, 46, 49, 50] In some
cases the levels drop below hemostatic levels and the patient
demonstrates a hemorrhagic disease that has been termed
hemorrhagic disease of the newborn (HDNB). Hemorrhagic disease of the newborn is probably the first hemorrhagic state to
come to the attention of man.[12] It is possible that in antiquity
HDNB had something to do with Mosaic law, which required
circumcision of males on the 8th day of life. In 1694 Mauriceau
reported the first clinical description of bleeding in the neonate.
Bowditch in 1850 and Minot in 1852 suggested that such bleeding was due to an abnormal blood condition and noted that coagulation was delayed or absent. It was not until 1894 that
Townsend described HDNB as a self-limiting coagulopathy distinct from hemophilia. In 1910 Schwartz and Ottenburg
showed an increased clotting time in newborns with HDNB
and suggested that it was caused by a deficiency of thromboki-
nase. In 1911 Schloss and Commiskey attempted to classify
hemorrhage on the basis of its clinical picture and separated
HDNB from hemophilia, sepsis, and syphilis.[51] They assumed

that HDNB was due to an unknown cause and showed in one case that adding defibrinated blood to the infant's blood corrected the clotting time. They therefore suggested that bleeding was not due to a lack of fibrinogen. Whipple, in 1912, and Gelston, in 1921, felt that the entity was caused by decreased "prothrombin" in blood. Brinkhouse and his associates noted in 1934 that the newer two-stage assay technique showed newborns to have reduced prothrombin. In 1939 Waddell et al. related hypoprothrombinemia to a deficiency of vitamin K. After this era, a number of papers confirmed that vitamin K deficiency was involved in the clinical picture of HDNB. Quick suggested in 1958 that the newborn was prone to develop a deficiency of vitamin K because of a lack of fetal storage reserves, a low intake during the first few days of life, and a high metabolic demand for the vitamin. In 1962 Aballi and de Lamerens separated HDNB from the other coagulopathies acquired during the newborn period. They also reviewed the world literature on the efficacy of the prophylactic use of vitamin K and the use of vitamin K with those infants with HDNB.[52] Recent studies using immunologic and coagulation techniques in vitamin K-deficient newborns have shown the same laboratory pattern as that described in older children and adults. That is, these infants have a low level of functional prothrombin, as shown by physiologic activators, and higher levels of precursor protein, as measured by immunoprecipitation techniques or by *Echis* clotting assays.[42-43, 48]

Hemorrhagic disease of the newborn is rarely seen in infants given cow's milk formula or artificial milk supplemented with vitamin K or in those given vitamin K prophylactically at birth. The development of a vitamin K deficiency after birth appears to be related to a decrease in dietary intake of vitamin K and the fact that the infant's gastrointestinal (GI) tract is free of bacteria. The amount of vitamin K in breast milk is considerably less than that found in cow's milk and there is some evidence to suggest that organisms that colonize the GI tract of breast-fed babies may not produce vitamin K. It should be noted that when vitamin K is given to infants with HDNB, their coagulation defect is promptly corrected and their bleeding ceases, but their coagulation factors return only to the level of what one would expect of the normal newborn.[53] The level for these factors does not usually increase into the adult range until after the first year of life.[36, 40, 44, 55] Although numerous reports suggest that the prophylactic use of vitamin K prevents HDNB, other studies doubt its efficacy.[45, 54] The available evidence, however, would suggest that vitamin K should continue to be used prophylactically, particularly in those infants who are at high risk.

VITAMIN K DEFICIENCY BEYOND THE NEWBORN PERIOD

Children may lack vitamin K after the newborn period because of disease in the hepatobiliary tract, malabsorption syndromes, drugs that may interfere with vitamin K absorption or metabolism, or a reduced dietary intake in association with diarrhea and/or the use of an antibiotic.

Vitamin K deficiency as a cause of bleeding should be suspected in children who have cholestasis secondary to biliary atresia or cholelithiasis involving the common bile duct. This deficiency has also been noted in patients with hepatocellular disease associated with cystic fibrosis, fructose intolerance, Reye's syndrome, hepatitis, Wilson's disease, and other forms of hepatic disease.[28, 56-58, 61] Malabsorption of fat-soluble vitamins can lead to avitaminosis K in patients with cystic fibrosis, a-β-lipoproteinemia, and other steatorrheas, regional enteritis, ulcerative colitis, and poor dietary intake associated with gastroenteritis or the use of antibiotics.[59-70] Dietary deficiency alone is unheard of unless it is associated with some other abnormality, such as a change in the gut flora or malabsorption of vitamin K due to entities noted above. Coumarin drugs used therapeutically as anticoagulants act by inhibiting the function of vitamin K. A number of drugs can either enhance or suppress the anticoagulant effect of coumarin. For example, barbiturates can suppress, and chloral hydrate, chloramphenicol, and salicylates can enhance, the hypoprothrombinemic effect of oral anticoagulants.[71] A deficiency in the vitamin K-dependent coagulation factors has also been noted in children with gram-negative septicemia.[72] The clinical picture of vitamin K deficiency beyond the newborn period consists of easy bruisability, delayed onset bleeding after deep cuts and surgical procedures, and, on occasion, mucous membrane bleeding. Perhaps one of the most frightening and significant complications in children under the age of two is a high frequency of spontaneous bleeding of the central nervous system.[66, 68, 69, 73] Bleeding of the central nervous system can result in significant morbidity and mortality.

Hemorrhagic disease that occurs in patients with an inadequate absorption or supply of vitamin K can easily be corrected by the administration of vitamin K, which will result in prompt correction of the coagulopathy. Patients with liver disease, however, may or may not respond to vitamin K administration. In those patients with an obstructive disease of the biliary tract or without significant hepatic cell damage, correction of the defect will occur. However, in those with significant hepatic cell damage, the precursor may not be synthesized and thus vitamin K will be of no benefit. In those patients who have a fat malabsorption, such as those with cystic fibrosis, steatorrhea or a-β-lipoproteinemia, a water analogue may be beneficial and can be given orally. In view of the fact that vitamin K is not stored to any significant degree, it is recommended that the vitamin be given once a day or once every other day for adequate prophylaxis. In the child who becomes over anticoagulated, or if there is accidental ingestion of coumarin derivatives, then the use of vitamin K will counteract the warfarin effect. Vitamin E has been noted to benefit animals and a few human beings with a deficiency of vitamin K.[74-77] Evidence suggests that large doses of vitamin E are nontoxic and have no effect on the coagulation mechanism of normal humans. However, those who are deficient in vitamin K may undergo a significant change in their vitamin K-dependent coagulation factors, a change that does not appear to depend on the effect of vitamin E on warfarin metabolism. It is recommended that if patients have a vitamin K deficiency and are to receive vitamin E (such as patients with cystic fibrosis), they be supplemented with vitamin K.

CLINICAL RELEVANCE OF THE NONCOAGULATION VITAMIN K-DEPENDENT PROTEINS

As mentioned above, there is no known role for the other vitamin K-dependent proteins at the present time. The most interesting studies, however, have to do with osteocalcin, the vitamin K-dependent protein in bone. More and more evidence appears to implicate vitamin K in the biological mineralization process. This vitamin K-dependent Gla-containing protein has an affinity for insoluble calcium salts and may participate in the regulation of calcium salt deposition in mineralized tissue. A number of investigators have shown that osteocalcin is formed de novo in bone tissue and that bone microsomes can carry out the posttranslational vitamin K-dependent carboxylation reaction. In developing chick bone and in the rat bone-matrix implant system, osteocalcin formation coincides with histologically detectable mineralization. Although animals given anticoagulants for long periods of time demonstrate undercarboxylated forms of osteocalcin, their bones appear to be histologically normal and the content and composition of the mineral appears grossly unaffected. In warfarin-treated embryonic chicken bone, however, there is a substantial increase in low-density low-mineral material and a decrease in high-density high-mineral material.[34] In the human fetus, serious bone defects are seen in the so-called fetal warfarin syndrome.[78-80] Here, women who take warfarin during the first trimester of pregnancy expose their fetuses to the risk of defective bone development with stippled epiphysis, punctate calcifications (chondrodysplasia congenita punctata), saddle nose, frontal bossing, and other bone anomalies. Although the development of the fetal warfarin syndrome may involve defective osteocalcin biosynthesis, the placenta has a Gla-containing protein mechanism that may also be impaired. If the placental system is likewise affected, the transport of calcium from maternal to fetal circulation may be inhibited, which would likewise delay mineralization of fetal bone. A vitamin K-dependent protein carboxylase system has also been demonstrated in kidney microsomes. The properties of the kidney Gla protein apparently include calcium binding and membrane localization in the renal tubular cell. Its function regarding calcium hemostasis and its role in disease is unknown. Likewise, synthesis of Gla proteins has been demonstrated in a variety of other organs. The role of these proteins has yet to be determined.

Summary

A new class of proteins has emerged, the so-called vitamin K-dependent calcium binding proteins, which are uniquely characterized by the presence of α-carboxyglutamic acid residues. These proteins have been identified in a variety of tissues and body fluids. The specialized nature of calcium binding by Gla residues promotes protein phospholipid interaction, which is important not only in blood coagulation but in many tissue processes involving calcium metabolism. What role other than the blood coagulation mechanism the vitamin K reaction may play in diseases in children is still unclear.

REFERENCES

1. Brinkhouse K.M. Plasma prothrombin; Vitamin K. *Medicine* 19:329, 1940.
2. Almquist H.J.: Vitamin K. *Physiol. Rev.* 21:194, 1941.
3. O'Reilly R.A., Aggeler P.M.: Determinants of the response to oral anticoagulant drugs in man. *Pharmacol. Rev.* 22:35, 1970.
4. Suttie J.W.: Vitamin K and prothrombin synthesis. *Nutr. Rev.* 31:105, 1973.
5. Mann K.G., Owen C.A. Jr.: Symposium on Vitamin K. *Mayo Clin. Proc.* 49:911, 1974.
6. Olson R.E.: Discovery of Vitamin K. *Trends Biochem. Sci.* 4:118, 1979.
7. Poncher H.G.: The role of vitamin K in hemorrhage in the newborn period. *Adv. Pediatr.* 1:151, 1942.
8. Dam H., Dyggve H., Larsen H., et al.: The relation of vitamin K deficiency to hemorrhagic disease of the newborn. *Adv. Pediatr.* 5:129, 1952.
9. Dam H.: The antihemorrhagic vitamin of the chick. *Biochem. J.* 29:1273, 1935.
10. Greaves J.D., Schmidt C.L.A.: Nature of the factor concerned in loss of blood coagulability of bile fistula rats. *Proc. Soc. Exp. Biol. Med.* 37:43, 1937.
11. Warner E.D., Brinkhous K.M., Smith H.P.: Bleeding tendency of obstructive jaundice: Prothrombin deficiency and dietary factors. *Proc. Soc. Exp. Biol. Med.* 37:628, 1938.
12. Quick A.J.: Hemorrhage in the newborn. *Lancet* 85:222, 1965.
13. Hemker H.C., Veltkamp J.J., Hensen A., et al.: Nature of prothrombin biosynthesis: Preprothrombinaemia in vitamin K deficiency. *Nature* 200:589, 1963.
14. Ganrot P.O., Niléhn J.-E.: Plasma prothrombin during treatment with dicumarol: II. Demonstration of an abnormal prothrombin fraction. *Scand. J. Clin. Lab. Invest.* 22:23, 1968.
15. Josso F., Lavergne J.M., Gouault M., et al.: Différents états moléculaires du facteur II (prothrombine): Leur étude à l'aide de la staphylocoagulase et d'anticorps anti-facteur II. I. Le facteur II chez les sujets traités par les antagonistes de la vitamine K. *Thromb. Diath. Haemorrh.* 20:88, 1968.
16. Suttie J.W.: Control of clotting factor biosynthesis by vitamin K. *Fed. Proc.* 28:1696, 1969.
17. Jackson C.M., Suttie J.W.: Recent developments in understanding the mechanism of vitamin K and vitamin K antagonist drug action and the consequences of vitamin K action in blood coagulation. *Prog. Hematol.* 10:333, 1977.
18. Suttie J.W., Jackson C.M.: Prothrombin structure, activation, and biosynthesis. *Physiol. Rev.* 57:1, 1977.
19. Magnusson S., Sottrup-Jensen L., Peterson T.E., et al.: Primary structure of the vitamin K-dependent part of prothrombin. *FEBS Lett.* 44:189, 1974.
20. Nelsesteun G.L., Zytkovicz T.H., Howard J.B.: The mode of action of vitamin K: Identification of α-carboxyglutamic acid as a component of prothrombin. *J. Biol. Chem.* 249:6347, 1974.
21. Stenflo J., Fernlund P., Egan W., et al.: Vitamin K-dependent modifications of glutamic acid residues in prothrombin. *Proc. Natl. Acad. Sci. U.S.A.* 71:2730, 1974.

22. Nelsestuen G.L.: Interactions of vitamin K-dependent proteins with calcium ions and phospholipid membranes. *Fed. Proc.* 37:2621, 1978.
23. Suttie J.W. (ed): *Vitamin K Metabolism and Vitamin K-Dependent Proteins.* Baltimore: University Park Press, 1980.
24. Woolf I.L., Babior B.M.: Vitamin K and warfarin: Metabolism, function and interaction. *Am. J. Med.* 53:261, 1972.
25. Frick P.G., Riedler G., Brogli H.: Dose response and minimal daily requirement for vitamin K in man. *J. Appl. Physiol.* 23:387, 1967.
26. Anonymous: Vitamin K deficiency in adults. *Nutr. Rev.* 26:165, 1968.
27. Bell R.G.: Metabolism of vitamin K and prothrombin synthesis: Anticoagulants and the vitamin K-epoxide cycle. *Fed. Proc.* 37:2599, 1978.
28. Corrigan J.J. Jr., Earnest D.L.: Factor II antigen in liver disease and warfarin-induced vitamin K deficiency: Correlation with coagulant activity using *Echis* venom. *Am. J. Hemat.* 8:249, 1980.
29. Stenflo J.: A new vitamin K-dependent protein: Purification from bovine plasma and preliminary characterization. *J. Biol. Chem.* 251:355, 1976.
30. Comp P.C., Esmon C.T.: Activated protein C inhibits platelet prothrombin-converting activity. *Blood* 54:1272, 1979.
31. Kisiel W.: Human plasma protein C.: Isolation, characterization and mechanism of activation by α-thrombin. *J. Clin. Invest,* 64:761, 1979.
32. DiScipio R.G., Davie E.W.: Characterization of protein S, an γ-carboxyglutamic acid containing protein from bovine and human plasma. *Biochemistry* 18:899, 1979.
33. Hauschka P.V., Lian J.B., Gallop P.M.: Vitamin K and mineralization. *Trends Biochem. Sci.* 3:75, 1978.
34. Gallop P.M., Lian J.B., Hauschka P.V.: Carboxylated calcium-binding proteins and vitamin K. *New Engl. J. Med.* 302:1460, 1980.
35. Bleyer W.A., Hakami N., Shepard T.H.: The development of hemostasis in the human fetus and newborn infant. *J. Pediatr.* 79:838, 1971.
36. Norén I., Carlsson E., Kretzschmar G., et al.: Prothrombin in newborns and during the first year of life. *Acta Paediatr. Scand.* 60:269, 1971.
37. Jensen A.H-B., Josso F., Zamet P., et al.: Evolution of blood clotting factor levels in premature infants during the first 10 days of life: A study of 96 cases with comparison between clinical status and blood clotting factor levels. *Pediatr. Res.* 7:638, 1973.
38. Sell E.J., Corrigan J.J. Jr.: Platelet counts, fibrinogen concentrations, and factor V and factor VIII levels in healthy infants according to gestational age. *J. Pediatr.* 82:1028, 1973.
39. Barnard D.R., Simmons M.A., Hathaway W.E.: Coagulation studies in extremely premature infants. *Pediatr. Res.* 13:1330, 1979.
40. Schettini F., de Mattia D., Mautone A., et al.: Post-natal development of factor II (pre-prothrombin and prothrombin) in man. *Biol. Neonate* 29:82, 1976.
41. Van Doorm J.M., Muller A.D., Hemker H.C.: Heparin-like inhibitor, not vitamin K deficiency, in the newborn. *Lancet* 1:852, 1977.
42. Dreyfus M., Lelong-Tissier M.C., Lombard C., et al.: Vitamin-K deficiency in the newborn. *Lancet* 1:1351, 1979.
43. Corrigan J.J. Jr., Kryc J.J.: Factor II (prothrombin) levels in cord blood: Correlation of coagulant activity with immunoreactive protein. *J. Pediatr.* 97:979, 1980.
44. Schettini F., de Mattia D., Altomare M., et al.: Post-natal development of factor IX. *Acta Paediatr. Scand.* 69:53, 1980.
45. Fresh J.W., Ferguson J.H., Stamey C., et al.: Blood prothrombin, proconversion and proaccelerin in normal infancy: Questionable relationships to vitamin K. *Pediatrics* 19:241, 1957.
46. Sutherland J.M., Glueck H.I., Gleser G.: Hemorrhagic disease of the newborn:

Breast feeding as a necessary factor in pathogenesis. *Am. J. Dis. Child.* 113:524, 1967.
47. Keenan W.J., Jewett T., Glueck H.I.: Role of feeding and vitamin K in hypopro-thrombinemia of the newborn. *Am. J. Dis. Child.* 121:271, 1971.
48. Muntean W., Petek W., Rosanelli K., et al.: Immunologic studies of prothrombin in newborns. *Pediatr. Res.* 13:1262, 1979.
49. Bleyer W.A., Skinner A.L.: Fatal neonatal hemorrhage after maternal anticonvul-sant therapy. *J.A.M.A.* 235:626, 1976.
50. Stevenson R.E., Burton O.M., Ferlauto G.J., et al.: Hazards of oral anticoagulants during pregnancy. *J.A.M.A.* 243:1549, 1980.
51. Schloss O.M., Commiskey L.J.J.: Spontaneous hemorrhage in the newborn. *Am. J. Dis. Child.* 1:276, 1911.
52. Aballi A.J., de Lamerens S.: Coagulation changes in the newborn period and in early infancy. *Pediatr. Clin. N. Am.* 9:785, 1962.
53. Wefring K.W.: Hemorrhage in the newborn and vitamin K prophylaxis. *J. Pediatr.* 61:686, 1962.
54. Denton R.L.: Vitamin K for the newborn: *Pediatr. Clin. N. Am.* 8:455, 1961.
55. Glueck H.I., Sutherland J., Gleser G.: Prothrombin levels during the first year of life. *Am. J. Dis. Child.* 107:612, 1964.
56. Roberts H.R., Cederbaum A.I.: The liver and blood coagulation: Physiology and pathology. *Gastroenterology* 63:297, 1972.
57. Pegelow C., Goldberg R., Turkel S., et al.: Severe coagulation abnormalities in Reye's syndrome. *J. Pediatr.* 91:413, 1977.
58. Doering E.J. III, Savage R.A., Dittmer T.E.: Hemolysis, coagulation defects, ful-minant hepatic failure as a presentation of Wilson's disease. *Am. J. Dis. Child.* 133:440, 1979.
59. Torstenson O.L., Humphrey G.B., Edson J.R., et al.: Cystic fibrosis presenting with severe hemorrhage due to vitamin K malabsorption: A report of three cases. *Pediatrics* 45:857, 1970.
60. Walters T.R., Koch H.F.: Hemorrhagic diathesis and cystic fibrosis in infancy. *Am. J. Dis. Child.* 124:641, 1972.
61. Odievre M., Gentil C., Gautier M., et al.: Hereditary fructose intolerance in child-hood. *Am. J. Dis. Child.* 132:605, 1978.
62. Caballero F.M., Buchanan G.R.: Abetalipoproteinemia presenting as severe vita-min K deficiency. *Pediatrics* 65:161, 1980.
63. Corrigan J.J. Jr., Taussig L.M., Beckerman R., et al.: Factor II (prothrombin) co-agulant activity and immunoreactive protein: Detection of vitamin K deficiency and liver disease in patients with cystic fibrosis. *J. Pediatr.* In press.
64. Rapoport S., Dodd K.: Hypoprothrombinemia in infants with diarrhea. *Am. J. Dis. Child.* 71:611, 1946.
65. Goldman H.I., Deposito F.: Hypoprothrombinemic bleeding in young infants: As-sociation with diarrhea, antibiotics, and milk substitutes. *Am. J. Dis. Child.* 111:430, 1966.
66. Goldman H.I., Amadio P.: Vitamin K deficiency after the newborn period. *Pediat-rics* 44:745, 1969.
67. Moss M.H.: Hypoprothrombinemic bleeding in a young infant: Association with a soy protein formula. *Am. J. Dis. Child.* 117:540, 1969.
68. Nammacher M.A., Willemin M.T., Hartmann J.R., et al.: Vitamin K deficiency in infants beyond the neonatal period. *J. Pediatr.* 76:549, 1970.
69. Bhanchet P., Tuchinda S., Hathirat P., et al.: A bleeding syndrome in infants due to acquired prothrombin complex deficiency. *Clin Pediatr. (Phila.)* 16:992, 1977.
70. Minford A.M.B., Eden O.B.: Haemorrhage responsive to vitamin K in a 6-week-old infant. *Arch. Dis. Child.* 54:310, 1979.
71. Anonymous: Adverse interactions of drugs. *Med. Lett. Drugs Ther.* 21:5, 1979.

72. Corrigan J.J. Jr., Ray W.L., May N.: Changes in the blood coagulation system associated with septicemia. *N. Engl. J. Med.* 279:851, 1968.
73. Visudhiphan P., Bhanchet M.D., Lakanapichanchat C., et al.: Intracranial hemorrhage in infants due to acquired prothrombin complex deficiency. *J. Neurosurg.* 41:14, 1974.
74. Mellette S.J., Leone L.A.: Influence of age, sex, strain of rat and fat soluble vitamins on hemorrhagic syndromes in rats fed irradiated beef. *Fed. Proc.* 19:1045, 1960.
75. Doisy E.A. Jr.: Nutritional hypoprothrombinemia and metabolism of vitamin K. *Fed. Proc.* 20:989, 1961.
76. March B.E., Wong E., Seier L., et al.: Hypervitaminosis E in the chick. *J. Nutr.* 103:371, 1973.
77. Corrigan J.J. Jr.: Coagulation problems relating to vitamin E. *Am. J. Pediatr. Hem. Oncol.* 1:169, 1979.
78. Pettifor J.M., Benson R., Congenital malformations associated with the administration of oral anticoagulants during pregnancy. *J. Pediatr.* 86:459, 1975.
79. Becker M.H., Genieser N.B., Finegold M., et al.: Chondrodysplasia punctata: Is maternal warfarin therapy a factor? *Am. J. Dis. Child.* 129:356, 1975.
80. Shaul W.L., Emery H., Hall J.G.: Chondrodysplasia punctata and maternal warfarin use during pregnancy. *Am. J. Dis. Child.* 129:360, 1975.

Teenage Pregnancy

ROBERT W. BLOCK, M.D.
STEVEN SALTZMAN, M.D.
AND
SHARON A. BLOCK, R.N.

The Departments of Pediatrics and Ob-Gyn
University of Oklahoma Tulsa Medical College
Tulsa, Oklahoma

Introduction

ASSESSING GROWTH TASKS[1] or developmental levels of adolescence is helpful in understanding a young person's behavior, attitude, or medical problem. As discussed by Katchadourian,[2] three developmental issues must be resolved during adolescence: establishing a personal identity, developing interpersonal relationships, and enhancing self-esteem. Piaget[3] adds a fourth area: representative intelligence by means of formal operations. Understanding the sexual behavior of an adolescent becomes somewhat easier if that behavior is analyzed in the context of resolution of developmental tasks.

Part of one's identity is sexual, so that following hormonal effects toward sexual exploration and experimentation is developmentally correct. As identity becomes less diffuse, more true intimacy and responsibility appear, and sexual behavior becomes more responsible.

Interpersonal relationships are partly sexual, especially during mid-adolescence. Reacting to someone sexually may well be necessary for completion of a growth task. Obviously, sexual reaction need not include intercourse and pregnancy, but the unprepared adolescent often finds that consequence to what is otherwise a normal behavior.

75

0065-3101/81/0028-0075-0098-$03.75

Self-esteem is another critical issue. Peer pressure responses of adolescents are more readily understood in the context of preservation of ego. Parents often anguish over their adolescent's lost "respect" for their moral teachings and role modeling, but fail to accept the incredible pressure of adolescent society on an individual's sense of esteem. Sexual acting out may be a requirement for some adolescents' generation of ego-strength.

Eventually a child develops enough to come to grips with formal operational thinking, including subjective or abstract reasoning. At this time he or she is able to make appropriate decisions about behavior and can balance emotion with fact. Now sexuality becomes easier to deal with and behavior becomes more planned, assuming that the person has appropriate facts and answers to questions. Unfortunately, for many, pregnancy has already taken place. The occurrence of this otherwise healthy and natural happening out of developmental sequence becomes a distinct problem that disrupts development, interferes with life-style, and can totally change the future for many people. Consequently, pregnancies that occur prior to completion of adolescent development are a formidable challenge for physicians and others who work with young people.

This article will not deal with the morality of teenaged sexual behavior. To argue about morality, as one response to the American Academy of Pediatrics' statement on "pregnancy and abortion counseling"[4] attempted to do,[5] is to ignore individual conscience and deny variation of opinion on morality. Regardless of one's personal response to a pregnant twelve-year-old and abortion, contraception, rights of parents, rights of minors, or other issues, acceptance of teen pregnancy as an immediate problem of great magnitude is one area in which we can all agree.

The Scope of the Problem

The statistics verifying adolescent pregnancy as a major problem in the United States have been well documented.[6,7] The oft-quoted figure of one million teenage pregnancies remains valid. Of great concern is the 61% increase in the total number of births to girls aged 15 and younger between 1960 and 1977.[8] Even more dramatic are some figures generated from a local study in Oklahoma, the state now listed ninth in the nation for "excess" unwanted births to teenagers.[9] Tulsa County, Oklahoma, has a population of adolescents aged 12–19 of about 50,000. Data from the Guttmacher report and other sources[10] indicate that from 10% to 55% of the teen population's female subpopulation are sexually active, depending on age. Assuming that about one half of the 50,000 teenagers in Tulsa County are girls, it was determined that about 8,000 may be sexually active. In 1979 there were 1,562 live births to girls less than 20 years of age in Tulsa County. Given an estimated abortion rate of 33% for teen pregnancies, there would probably have been about 2,400 pregnancies in 1979 in that age group. Therefore, 30% of all at-risk (sexually active) girls in the county probably became pregnant, 20% of the at-risk population gave birth, and one in every ten girls, disregarding sexual activity, became pregnant.

Admittedly, many teen pregnancies are planned. Many 18- and 19-year-old girls are married and intend to begin families early. Of concern, however, is the fact that in Oklahoma 39% of teen births are to girls under 18, and 31% of all teen births are out of wedlock. National figures are comparable.[11, 12]

Teenage pregnancy is not a new problem. However, in the last 20 years several factors have influenced our awareness of the problem and its consequence. Furstenberg lists several reasons for increased attention recently focused on teen pregnancy.[13] They are: (1) An increase in the teenage population; (2) more awareness of population control; (3) more liberal teenage sexual behavior, coupled wih a disdain for early marriage, resulting in increased illegitimate birth; and (4) governmental concern about socioeconomic conditions vis-à-vis teenage parenthood and poor educational, vocational, and social stability.

As early as 1930, the dollar cost of unregulated parenthood was recognized.[14] A recent estimate for the state of Oklahoma alone indicated that the cost to taxpayers for teen pregnancies and the consequences of welfare, medicaid, food stamps, subsidized day care, etc., was greater than $19,000,000 every year.[15]

Who is the Pregnant Teenager?

Our experience shows she is unlikely to have completed growth tasks, especially the acquisition of independent thinking and a mature understanding of self. She often has failed to remain in school, especially if alternative school programs are inaccessible. Most often she is black and comes from a lower socioeconomic background. However, this represents a danger- ous misrepresentation of the facts about who *becomes* pregnant versus who *remains* pregnant. White girls from higher socio- economic backgrounds also become pregnant, but usually have greater access to first trimester abortion. Backed by a Supreme Court ruling denying federal dollars for abortion, American so- ciety has purposefully skewed the teenage parent population toward a poor black majority. The consequence of this action will undoubtedly be greater costs, both in dollars and in human needs, to us all. Already we see that the teenage parent has a greater than two to one chance of being on welfare. As illegiti- macy rates continue to rise, the teenage parent is destined to face the burdens of single parenthood. Despite that burden, she has at least a 70% chance of becoming pregnant a second time during adolescence if no services are available to her.

Causes of Teenage Pregnancy

A discussion of etiologies of teenage pregnancy is, by defini- tion, diffuse and not always logical. Adolescents themselves are often illogical, and their behavior, especially sexual behavior, is not and cannot be expected to be rationally controlled. Mul- tiple causative factors can be grouped into four areas: biological factors, the role of peers, societal influences, and contraception.

BIOLOGIC FACTORS

During the last century the age of menarche has decreased by 3 to 4 months each decade.[16] Some investigators feel this trend has slowed or stopped, signalling an arrival at physical care, nutrition, and environment that may be collectively as close to optimal as we might expect for a while.[17] In any case, recent studies show a mean age of menarche at 12.9 years, with a two-standard deviation range from 10.5 to 14.1 years.[18] The much heralded secondary sex characteristic of breast develop- ment usually begins about two years prior to menarche. There- fore, the early sexual developers may begin to show physical changes as early as eight and a half years of age. By 13 years of age these girls have menstruated and have waists, hips, thighs, calves, and buttocks that appear very feminine. They are two years past the age of peak height velocity and have breast maturation (not size) that may be 80% to 100% of final stages.[18] Within one or two years after menarche, most girls have ovulatory periods and are fertile.

Consequently, there is a significant population of girls aged 12.5–15 years who biologically and physically are close to being mature women and are capable of becoming pregnant. That population grows larger monthly throughout the school-age years.

THE ROLE OF PEERS

Over the last three years, the authors have encountered large numbers of adolescents, both male and female, in practice, clinics, and an outreach educational project. Time and again teenagers relate that peer pressure is their single greatest motivator. Children from "good families" as well as those from broken homes, foster care, poor socioeconomic situations, etc., all agree that parent-taught morality, lessons from school (rare in our state), facts from books, church group discussions, and the like, all take a back seat to real or perceived pressure to conform to peer standards. Sometimes the standards are difficult. As several seventh-grade girls told us, "You're either gay, a prude, or a slut."

It is interesting that standards are not set by the majority. Only about 24% of 15-year-old girls are sexually active. Upon graduation from high school, only one half of the girls are sexually active. However, sexual activity is defined as having sexual intercourse. The number of girls who have almost reached that point is much higher.

Other factors in adolescent peer relationships foster the chance of a premature pregnancy. Physical appearance has always been important to teenagers. In the '70s, physical appearance was closely aligned to sexual appearance; there is no sign that this will change in the '80s. Sex appeal and foxiness are key factors in the determination of physical appearance for teenagers.

Teenage drug abuse, especially abuse of marihuana and alcohol, probably creates atmospheres where sexual acting out is less inhibited and more generally tolerated. Gatherings and parties for junior-high-aged youth where beer, wine, marihuana, and other drugs are common signal an atmosphere of poor judgment and diminished responsibility where sexual acting out can occur.

SOCIETAL INFLUENCES

Having looked briefly at the impact of peer pressure on an adolescent's behavior, one might ask how the prevailing attitude among our young is determined. What impact does society have on an individual adolescent? Large advertising investments made by companies corroborate the notion that attitudes can be fostered through the sale of concepts to a gullible public. In the last 20 years, concurrent with the rearing of a generation, the concept has been sex and the attitude has been acceptance of sexuality. Typical examples are bikini-clad volleyballers of the "Pepsi generation," sexy models who sell cigarettes and toothpaste presumably with sex appeal, and naked-to-the-waist women wearing brand-name blue jeans, all of whom promote products that appeal to adolescents.

In addition, the sex appeal of TV, movie, and singing stars has been widely promoted. Posters are "in" and many teens' rooms are decorated with large photos of their favorites in bikinis or macho poses. The movies and TV shows in which these heroes and heroines play have overt sexual themes. Younger and younger children are appearing in sexual roles, like Brooke Shields in "Pretty Baby."

If society acquiesces to the constant exposure of its young to sex, it must carefully provide a support system to enable the adolescent to deal effectively with sexuality. A support system must provide factual information, a chance for counseling and discussion, appropriate presentation of alternatives, and medical guidance and treatment. Such a system is discussed later in this chapter.

Family structure is a societal phenomenon that also has an impact on teenagers. More and more adolescents are being raised by something less than the traditional two-biologic-parent family. Single parenthood is no longer unusual. Exposure to separation and divorce is commonplace and the adolescent is often without family support. Just as pediatricians emphasize "parenting" to parents of young children, so we should perhaps emphasize the importance of "familying" to families of older children. Although the term family may need to be redefined for the 1980s, support systems within whatever family structure remains are essential.

CONTRACEPTION

Two recent reviews thoroughly discuss contraception in the adolescent.[19, 20] In addition, we have found useful a book entitled, *Contraceptive Technology*.[21] For the physician familiar with contraceptive techniques, it is frustrating to deal with the large percentage of teenagers who fail to use adequate protection. Adolescents often deny that they can become pregnant[22] and consequently some of them do not even consider contraception. Other reasons for nonuse that are commonly reported include a desire not to plan ahead, boyfriends who do not want to use condoms, and the contention that contraception often interrupts sex.[23, 24]

Opponents of contraception for teenagers often cite the Pill as a cause of increased sexual activity. To our knowledge, no data to substantiate this claim has been produced. It is well known that the overwhelming majority of adolescents who request contraceptive information has already been involved in unprotected sex; the provision of contraceptive devices does not increase their sexual activity.[25]

Obviously, there is no easy answer as to why the problem of teenage pregnancy looms so large. As pointed out by McAnarney,[6] we need a broader understanding of the adolescent as a person and adolescents of the '80s as a group and effective methods of reaching them. The physician can at least attempt to bring some insight into emotional discussions about teenage sex, sex education, and teen pregnancy.

We must accept the fact that many girls are now fertile at 12 years of age, some even before that. Their peers usually condone sexual intercourse and almost always approve and encourage sexual activity that stops short of intercourse. Now we have a 12–15-year-old girl, often matched with a male partner about two years older than she, who is sexually developed and fertile and whose friends encourage her to "hang loose." Society then tells her to have sex appeal and to be sexy. The fashions, cosmetics, popular dance, music, TV, movies, and magazines to which she is exposed all tend to advance sexual themes. She may come from a supportive family, but many teenagers do not come from a two-parent, secure home. Sex education is usually *not* available to her. Consequently, she is fertile and determined to be sexually attractive and popular among peers, but she is emotionally immature, lacks facts and a sense of self-worth, and is terribly confused. We should wonder, not why so many teens become pregnant, but why so many do not.

The Teenage Father

Professionals who work with adolescent boys are well aware of the influence of sexuality on the teenager's conscious thought, his fantasies, body image, and social interactions. In our own adolescent clinic we often hear how sexual intercourse is better than drugs and is the ultimate good time. Often overlooked, however, is the stress placed on a teenaged boy who is not yet comfortable with his own sexuality and sexual relations. These boys are afraid of tarnishing their developing male identity if on Monday reports circulate that on their weekend date they didn't even try to make strong sexual advances. Teenage girls need to be told how to inform their dates that it would be better for both if intimate sexual action did not occur. Teenage boys need to be told that sexual acting out, even if condoned by their partner, is not the only road to masculinity and self-respect. Restraint might also be a measure of manhood and self-control a respected trait.

Adolescent boys should be informed about the consequences of sexual activity in their own lives. These consequences are often overlooked because the boy's activity is not the "rate-limiting" factor. If conception follows intercourse, the boy is usually not a party to decisions about abortion or adoption, so his sexual act has no bearing on his subsequent role as a father. He is usually not consulted about options, but is sometimes held accountable for financial and sociologic support of a new mother and child. It is the girl who determines her own motherhood and her male partner's fatherhood. Frank discussions about the implications of this fact, as dramatically shown in the film "Teenage Father,"[26] is essential in counseling the adolescent.

The consequences of pregnancy are not limited only to mothers. Identification of teenaged fathers is certainly more difficult than finding the teen mother, but the potential father can be easily found and must be prepared by education and counseling for either appropriate delay of his role as a father or coping with its premature occurrence.

Complications of Teenage Pregnancy

During the early part of this century, obstetric complications were referred to solely as a function of parity and/or illegitimacy.[27] Teenage pregnancy was rarely alluded to, and only infrequent cases of pregnancy in the very young, such as Lina Medina, who gave birth at age five, were reported.[28]

As the number of teenagers increased in the 1950s and 1960s, the subject of adolescent pregnancy began to appear in the literature; studies described increased frequencies of both maternal and perinatal complications. The problems most frequently found were prematurity, nutritional deficiencies, toxemia, abruptio placentae, cephalopelvic disproportion, and increased neonatal death rates.[29, 30, 32] The United States Obstetrical Statistical Cooperation Study of 1960–1969 confirmed the findings of these complications in the pregnant adolescent.[7]

It has become increasingly apparent that it may be too simplistic to group complications of pregnancy as a function of the teenage years. The very young adolescent may behave very differently than the 17- to 19-year-old. As Beric[32] in Yugoslavia found, premature deliveries in girls ages 10 to 14 were 32.9% of total deliveries, compared with 9% in women 17 to 18 years old. In an effort to further separate these differences, other studies have limited their patient populations to adolescents aged 15 and younger.[29, 33, 34]

Two areas of concern have developed since the earliest reports of teenage pregnancy: problems of pregnancy strictly related to maternal age and not due to other, confounding criteria; and conflicting reports on adolescent pregnancy complications.[29] These concerns are being resolved by means of control groups, the exclusion of the older teenager from patient populations, and alterations in study design.

Young women would be expected to have increased complications of delivery because of a lack of full development of the bony pelvis. In fact, Duenhoelter did find a statistically significant difference in the presence of contracted pelvis in pregnant patients under age 15, as compared to patients aged 19 to 25.[29] This would lead one to expect a cesarean section rate in adolescents higher than that of the general population. However, this does not seem to be the case. In a retrospective review of 4,224 deliveries to patients aged 19 or younger, Hutchins et al. reported a cesarean section rate of 5.5% for girls less than 17 years of age and 7.9% for the entire patient population.[35] Duenhoelter compared 412 patients under the age of 15 with matched controls aged 19 to 25, and although the cesarean section rates were 10.4% and 7%, respectively, the differences were not statistically significant.[29] Spellacy et al.[33] reviewed 1,021 pregnancies in girls aged 10 to 15 and women 20 to 24 and reported similar cesarean section rates for the adolescents (10.4%) and the older group (12.2.%). These findings were supported by Ryan and Schneider,[36] who found cesarean section rates for adolescents to be consistent with the total patient population.

Perhaps any increased frequency of cephalopelvic disproportion in teenagers leading to cesarean section is counterbalanced by a decreased frequency of other complications that also lead to that procedure. For example, the frequency of twinning increases with maternal age,[37] as does placenta previa, breech presentation, and oblique or transverse lie of the fetus.[28, 32, 33]

The occurrence of preeclampsia and eclampsia is a function of parity. Primiparas have up to three times the frequency of this disease over multiparas.[38] Some authors have even stated that the finding of preeclampsia in any multipara should be suspect.[28] It has been theorized that preeclampsia may be caused by an "immature immunologic system" and a lack of blocking antibodies of chorionic villi.[28] Consequently, it could be speculated that the propensity to develop this disease might, in addition to parity, be a function of low maternal age. But one study comparing the frequency of preeclampsia in black girls aged ten to 15 versus black women aged 20 to 24 showed no change in the frequency of the disease.[33] Dott[34] stated in 1976 that the risk of preeclampsia may be greater if pregnancy occurs within the first 24 months of menarche. This problem remains somewhat controversial and is compounded by the lack of prenatal care received by many adolescents.

Other problems such as the development of prolonged premature rupture of the membranes does not seem to be increased in the adolescent.[33] The presence of anemia in teenagers compared to the general population is debatable. Hutchins[35] found an 11% frequency of anemia in pregnant adolescents less than 17 years of age, compared with 6.6% in pregnant women aged 20 to 34. At variance with this, Spellacy[33] found the problem not to be significantly affected by maternal age.

Maternal mortality in the United States in 1978 was 9.9 per 100,000 live births, representing a total of of 320 maternal deaths.[28] For the adolescent who becomes pregnant before age 15, the frequency of death is reportedly 60% higher, and for teenagers who become pregnant between ages 15 and 19, 13% higher. In the Maternal Mortality Study in New York State, the leading causes of death were anesthesia, eclampsia, ectopic pregnancy, trauma, cerebrovascular disease, and cardiovascular disease.[39]

The pregnant teenager is prone to deliver premature infants.[35] Spellacy[33] compared adolescents with women aged 20 to 24 and found a prematurity rate of 20.2% versus 8.7%. Hutchins[35] showed slightly higher prematurity rates in pregnant women less than 17 years of age as compared with women 20 to 34 years of age. Ryan reported the incidence of premature deliveries in adolescents to be almost twice that of the general population.[36] However, not all studies support these findings. In a controlled study of pregnant girls under age 15 versus women aged 19 to 25, Duenhoelter[29] did not show a significant difference in mean birth weights for the two groups. The adolescent study group had mean birth weights of 2,914 ± 30.3 gm versus 2,948 ± 29.2 gm for the older control group. Perhaps this difference could be explained by comparing mean values with absolute frequencies. Aside from this difference, in 1975 mothers age 15 and under had 14.9% of their infants with birth weights less than 2,500 gm versus 7.1% for women aged 20 to 24.[6]

Stillbirths comprise nearly one half of perinatal deaths. Although the etiologies are protean and often remain unknown, deaths in utero tend to decline as prenatal care improves. Hutchins et al.[35] reported that the tendency for infant mortality rate to rise as maternal age decreases. In a study of 414 births to girls under age 15, Dott and Fort[34] reported the stillbirth rate for mothers aged 10 to 14 to be 31.9 compared to 10.3 for women aged 20 to 24. However, other studies have not demonstrated this increased incidence of stillbirths in adolescents.[29, 33, 35]

Neonatal deaths and total perinatal mortality have been reported to be higher in the teenager. Ryan and Schneider[36] reported a perinatal mortality rate of 54 per 1,000 births, which was approximately twice that of the general population. Dott's study was comparable: it found perinatal death rates for girls aged 10 to 14 to be 56.5 versus 23.4 for women aged 20 to 24.[34]

Congenital anomalies have generally not been found to be increased in infants of teenage mothers. It is interesting to note, however, that of the 26 patients with septo-optic dysplasia, the five mothers whose maternal ages were reported were all teenagers.[40]

Of all countries that report legal abortions, the United States had the highest percentage of teenagers who obtained abortions in 1976.[41] Although maternal mortality from elective abortion during the first eight weeks of pregnancy is only about 0.6 per 100,000 procedures,[28] the question of long-term effects may be important. As the teenager uses this means of dealing with an unwanted pregnancy, problems may develop that should be discussed as a part of overall complications of teenage pregnancy. Bulfin[41] reported the development of postabortion infection and/or uterine trauma in 23 of 54 teenage patients who had legal abortions. Although Daling and Emanuel[42] and Cates[43] did not find increases in fertility problems or perinatal morbidity and mortality following elective abortion, the area remains somewhat controversial. If complications of abortion do exist, they may become less frequent, because it appears that a substantial number of women who would have obtained publicly funded abortion before the 1977 restrictions of Medicaid and Title XX monies are now more likely to continue their pregnancies.[44] The effect of this phenomenon on pregnancy complications for young girls who otherwise would have aborted will be worthy of observation.

An infrequent but important complication of teenage pregnancy is maternal suicide attempts. In 1970 Gabrielson[45] reported 14 cases of suicide attempts in pregnant teenagers. All of these pregnancies involved some degree of obstetrical complications, and it was stated that problems in general could be decreased by a more accepting attitude toward these pregnancies.

The literature continues to demonstrate that maternal and perinatal complications of teenage pregnancy are protean. While the etiologies of some of these problems are well elucidated, others remain enigmatic. The mitigation of many maternal and perinatal complications is no doubt a function of prenatal care. Since it is apparent that antenatal care of pregnant teenagers is grossly deficient, an analysis of their problems is compounded. However, it appears as if, with the exception of preeclampsia and a small bony pelvis in the adolescent, the majority of complications of teenage pregnancy are more a function of lack of prenatal care than they are of maternal age, at least if the mother has a gynecologic age of more than two years.[46]

Nutrition in Teenage Pregnancy

The eating habits of teenagers vary considerably, so that generalizations are prone to discrepancies, but it is safe to say that deviations from optimum nutrition are so numerous that poor dietary self-regulation places many pregnant girls at risk. A recent study of a population of pregnant teenagers identified several problems with nutrition, including: limited food availability, diets that provided less than two thirds of the RDA for major nutrients, suboptimal protein intake in 75% of the study group, poor diet habits such as skipping breakfast or eating mainly junk food, and the prevalence of anemia.[47]

Another study of adolescents in Kentucky showed that 41% of white girls and 43% of black girls received less than two thirds of the recommended daily allowances (RDA) for total energy (calories).[48] For specific nutrients, the percentages of those who received less than two thirds the RDA were 12% and 19% (white and black) for protein, 76% for calcium, 78% and 76% for iron, 73% and 67% for vitamin A and 57% and 48% for vitamin C.

Although the data is not clear on the effect of nutrition on an infant's birth weight, length, length of gestation, and overall condition at birth,[49] and although we have been recently reminded of the "noble gift of moderation"[50] during supplementation, it is probable that sound prepregnancy nutrition and

ROBERT W. BLOCK, STEVEN SALTZMAN, AND SHARON A. BLOCK

attention to an adequate diet during pregnancy with supplementation when necessary can only benefit the often still developing teenage mother and her fetus.

The prepregnancy nutritional status of a teenager is a result of dietary behaviors that are often in concordance with other adolescent rebellious behaviors. Teens often view meals and food habits as family-centered[51] and therefore purposefully create poor eating habits for themselves as an assertion of independence or an identification with peer groups.[52] If any education about nutrition is offered to teens, it is offered in school and is often associated negatively with other unliked academic subjects and/or with authority figures (teachers) from whom the teen feels compelled to remain distant. Consequently, the pediatrician must find a way to relate nutritional information to parents and children and later to adolescent patients to assure a better nutritional status, especially for girls who may become pregnant. Relating nutrition to weight control, energy levels (stamina), clear skin, optimum height, or other body-image areas with which the adolescent is always concerned may be one way to gain the attention and cooperation of teens. Once a girl is pregnant, gently challenging her to produce a baby of appropriate gestational age and weight, maintain a normal hemoglobin, and keep her weight at optimal levels with positive reinforcement of interval successes by a physician, nurse, or nutritionist who is not viewed as a disciplinarian or authority figure may be helpful.

Factors related to nutrition that place the adolescent at risk during pregnancy include low prepregnancy weight (10% or more under the standard weight for height), insufficient weight gain (24–28 pounds),[53, 54] obesity (20% or more over the standard weight for height), existing medical complications, dietary faddism, pica, and low income or ethnic variances.

Recent reviews have documented the need for protein,[49] vitamins, minerals,[55] and calories[56] during pregnancy. We will summarize current recommendations as a guide for management. Girls aged 11 to 14 need 2,200 calories a day. Girls aged 15 to 19 need 2,100 calories a day. The range for calories is between 1,500 and 3,000 calories per day; 300 calories per day should be added for pregnancy.[57] Normally active pregnant females need 45 calories per kg of body weight per day (compared to 50 calories per kg per day for normally active nonpregnant girls) plus 300 calories per day for pregnancy. A gain of 2 to 4 lb during the first trimester of pregnancy is appropriate. During the second and third trimesters a gain of 0.9 lb per week is appropriate. Weight gain ought to total 24 to 28 lb. Appropriate weight gain is probably the best indicator of optimal caloric intake.

PROTEIN REQUIREMENTS

Most recent reviews agree that the pregnant adolescent who has not yet completed her own linear growth needs extra protein.[57, 58] Linear growth is not usually complete until four years after menarche. The mean age for linear growth completion is now 16.9 years. Consequently, most girls 17 and younger (the high-school-age female population) are at risk and must receive adequate protein (and calories). For the girl 11 to 18 years old, 46 gm of protein per day are recommended, with an additional 30 gm per day added for pregnancy. The 76-gm total supplies 304 calories, or approximately 12% of the total daily calorie intake. The 76 gm per day of protein equals 1.6 to 1.4 gm of protein/kg/day based on ideal prepregnancy mean weights of 46 kg (101 lb) at 11–14 years and 55 kg (120 lb) at 15–18 years.

Protein requirements are based on the variability of the population and the efficiency of converting food to tissue protein (utilization).[49] There is an average utilization rate of 75% in the American diet, but at the end of pregnancy the rate falls to 26%, which creates a need for extra protein. If the above recommendations are followed, protein intake during pregnancy should be adequate.

VITAMINS

FAT SOLUBLE VITAMINS

Vitamin A.—The current recommended dietary allowance (RDA) is 1,000 retinol equivalents, or 5,000 international units (IU), during pregnancy, which is 25% more than the RDA for nonpregnant females.[59] This amount can be supplied by a good diet, and supplementation is unnecessary.

Vitamin D.—The current RDA is 10 μg as cholecalciferol (400 IU)[57]; some sources call for an additional 5 μg (200 IU) for pregnancy. This amount is supplied in 6 cups of milk daily (see

"Calcium" below) and no supplement is needed if milk intake is adequate.

Vitamin E.—A slight increase in this vitamin is recommended during pregnancy to supply fetal storage needs. The RDA is 15 IU or 10 α-tocopherol equivalents. Again, complete diets supply vitamin E and no supplement is necessary.

Vitamin K.—This vitamin is produced by intestinal bacteria and does not have an RDA.

WATER SOLUBLE VITAMINS

Vitamin B_6.—The RDA for vitamin B_6 for the pregnant teenager is 2.6 mg per day and for the nonpregnant teenager is increased from 1.8 to 2 mg per day. Although pregnancy creates biochemical findings consistent with vitamin B_6 deficiency, those findings probably represent an altered metabolism.[55] Consequently, the 6–10 mg of vitamin B_6 needed to normalize the biochemistry do not have to be supplemented. Vitamin B_6 requirements do increase with high protein diets.[59] The RDA for vitamin B_6 is adequate in complete diets.

Other B complex vitamins.—The RDA for thiamine is 1.5 mg per day and for riboflavin, 1.6 mg per day; 16 mg of niacin and 4 μg of vitamin B_{12} are recommended. These amounts are adequate in complete diets. Folacin (folic acid) requirements double in pregnancy because of increased maternal erythropoiesis and fetal placental growth.[59] The RDA becomes 800 μg with pregnancy; supplementation may be necessary.[56, 59] Pantothenic acid has an RDA of 5–10 mg; supplementation may be necessary.[60]

Vitamin C.—Recommendations vary from 60–80 mg/day. In 1980 the RDA for pregnant teens aged 11–14 was 70 mg and for those aged 15–18 it was 80 mg. All sources agree that a complete diet supplies adequate vitamin C.

MINERALS

CALCIUM.—The fetus accumulates about 300 mg per day during the last trimester (a total of about 30 gm).[55] Although that only accounts for approximately 2%–3% of the maternal body content, and although the fetus could be supplied by maternal stores, depletion of stores in a teenager is inappropriate. Fortunately, cow's milk contains about 1,150 mg of calcium per quart. The 1980 RDA for calcium is 1,600 mg, an increase of

400 mg over nonpregnant states. Therefore, a quart of milk daily plus some cheese (800 mg calcium per 100 gm) adequately supplies this nutrient. As mentioned above, this intake also supplies adequate vitamin D.

PHOSPHORUS.—The RDA for this mineral follows calcium, as does the dietary supply, so usually no problems are encountered. Interestingly, a common problem of teenagers is leg cramps, a problem also more common in pregnant women. Consequently, teenagers who happen to be pregnant often complain of this problem. Although some investigators have postulated an association between decreased serum calcium with increased serum phosphate and cramps, the data does not support the theory. However, if leg cramps are a serious problem, a judicious trial of no milk (milk is high in phosphorus) with calcium lactate or gluconate supplementation and an aluminum hydroxide antacid to bind phosphates may be useful.

IRON.—All current sources recommend a daily supplementation of 30–60 mg of iron as ferrous salts to provide the 750–800 mg gestational iron requirement. About 500 mg of elemental iron is needed for maternal erythropoiesis, and 250–300 mg for placental and term fetal needs.[59]

TRACE MINERALS

The RDA for zinc is 20 mg during pregnancy, an amount readily supplied by animal protein in an adequate diet. Other elements such as copper, chromium, and manganese have no RDA, as no data are available with which to formulate one. However, all important trace minerals can be provided in a complete diet. Health food storekeepers might disagree, but the best assurance of adequate attention to the essential traces is a sound diet, not expensive supplementation, especially during an adolescent's pregnancy.

Nutrient Summary

An excellent food guide and nutrition handbook is available from the California Department of Health.[58] The physician will be a better nutrition counselor if he or she knows some tips to make proper eating more acceptable to adolescents. For example, it helps to know that peanuts, milk shakes, hamburgers, hotdogs, and pizza are good sources of protein. A meal at a fast-food restaurant may not be so bad after all if it includes a milk shake, French fries, and a quarter-lb beef hamburger with lettuce, cheese, and tomato. Salads and casseroles combine nutrients and are usually acceptable. Lastly, the physician must be interested in nutrition so that the great importance of this area will be obvious to his or her teenage patients.

From the previous discussion we learn that only iron and maybe folacin and pantothenic acid need to be added to the diet of the pregnant teen. Recent literature supports this concept.[56] Of much greater importance than routine vitamin and mineral supplementation is attention to the overall improvement of adolescent nutrition and prepregnant nutritional status. During pregnancy, adequate total caloric intake and good weight gain, optimum protein intake, and a balance of fruits, vegetables, and other food groups will maintain optimum nutritional status. A supplemental pill may give a teenager the false impression that she need not pay attention to the rest of her diet. Encouraging her to create proper nutrition naturally is more acceptable and healthy.

Obviously, we have been referring to an ideal state of acceptance of nutrition by teenagers. The physician must recognize the lack of reality in phrases such as complete diet. If the teenager has not maintained optimum nutrition prior to her pregnancy, she is unlikely to change during a time of added stress. If she managed to arrive at pregnancy with an adequate nutritional status, she may well not comply with advice about added needs any more than she did with advice about abstinence or contraception. Consequently, vitamin and mineral supplements may well be required and total calories must be closely monitored. But, to restate a point, if supplements are used, they must not be allowed to become substitutes for sound, basic nutrition.

What Are the Options for a Pregnant Girl?

The physician who may deal with pregnant teenagers should be knowledgeable about their choices and the consequences of each. The first option is abortion. Although abortion is legal during the first trimester, accessibility varies from state to state depending on expense and laws about parental consent.

We recognize that some physicians are opposed to abortion and feel compelled to extend their personal morality to the general public. We agree with them that they have a right and an obligation to tell their patients what their personal belief is. They also have an obligation to refer their patients who need information about abortion to a resource that can offer information on abortion, so that the patient (and her parents and male partner, if appropriate) can make an informed decision.

The second option is adoption. Only about 7% of the teenagers who carry a pregnancy to delivery follow through with adoption. Recognition of this fact is important to physicians who might assume adoption to be an easy solution for the girl who becomes pregnant. Counseling about adoption is difficult and must be done by someone who is cognizant of peer, family, and cultural pressures on a girl to keep her baby. Postadoption counseling is also important to help the relinquishing mother cope with her loss. Counselors must also keep current with changing adoption laws, especially as they relate to the adoptee's right at the age of majority to know his or her parentage and to gain access to adoption procedure records. We feel that most girls who keep their babies do so without a full understanding of the meaning of parenthood. They always ask about adoption, "How can I be sure my baby will go to really good parents?" but fail to ask the same question of themselves before keeping their baby. Consequently, the more information about parenthood we can give teenagers before they must choose options, the better their choices might be. They need to know the constraints on time, self, money, and other life-style areas that a child places on a parent. They need to consider 3 A.M. feedings, diarrhea, and persistent crying. The realities of parenthood include difficult times as well as joy, and we should convey this fact to teenagers to help them choose.

The next two options follow the choice to carry the pregnancy to term and to keep the baby. They are marriage versus single parenthood. Both can be done with or without family support. The options available to one girl may vary considerably to those available to another, depending on parental attitude, the male partner's attitude, family economics, and future life goals for all involved. The decision should not be made in a void. A physician is often the first, sometimes the only, professional to become involved. We should be aware of community resources to which we can refer adolescents for counseling about options, or we can develop knowledge and skills in adolescent counseling and offer services ourselves in conjunction with comprehensive programs.

Prevention

Education and services are the two major components in the prevention of teenage pregnancy.[6] We must also deal with the fact that teens now comprise about 20% of mothers who deliver. Prevention of the undesirable consequences of teen parenthood must be part of services to infants and adolescents. Preventative education can be effective in two areas. A recent study demonstrated an increase in knowledge obtained by a group of teenage girls exposed to a comprehensive curriculum designed to teach decision-making skills, facts about gynecological health, venereal disease, birth control, and parenthood.[61] The same study documented retention of information and positive behavior one year after the course was given. Goals of the curriculum included development of a trusting relationship between adolescents and responsible adults, comfortable attitudes toward oneself and others, self-awareness, decision-making skills, an awareness of values and value systems, communication skills, and information about human sexuality. The second area of effectiveness for preventative education can be increased communication between parents and adolescents. We feel a real need for parents to become more informed about sex education so that they can assume more of their responsibility as primary sex educators. If parents abdicate that responsibility, it should be assumed by churches, youth organizations, and schools using competent and thoroughly trained sex educators. We have found that effective education of youth relies on an interchange among peers, so even families who attempt to educate their children about sex can have their effort augmented by organized curricula requiring teen group participation.

Services to pregnant teens must be comprehensive. Several points regarding the structure of services were recently made by Hollingsworth and Kreutner.[62] They emphasize the need for reasonable, accessible prenatal care, access to first trimester abortion, continuation of schooling, access to social support systems, vocational training, and counseling about reproduction and contraception. Brann et al.[63] have recently demonstrated the success of several programs that achieved as high a reduction in fertility rates as 56% among teen participants. A model program in Tulsa, Oklahoma, has been growing in scope for the last ten years. The Margaret Hudson Program for Teenage Parents emphasizes services in the areas of continuing academic education, vocational training, social services, health, contraception counseling, adoption counseling, nutrition, and avocation. A vital component of the program is a parent education laboratory where pregnant teenage students act as a day-care staff under direct supervision. Hand-on contact with neonates and toddlers allows a more realistic and practical parenting education.

What about the consequences of teen parenthood? Merritt et al.[64] state that, from a medical point of view, the optimal age to give birth is between the ages of 16 and 19. Yet, as they caution, we must also consider the psychosocial outcomes of premature parenthood. Sahler[65] has pointed out that conflicting reports on the quality of teen parenthood cannot be analyzed until more data is available. While we await additional information, support services must be provided to the teenager, male as well as female, who becomes a parent. The Margaret Hudson Program has adequately demonstrated the ability of many teenage parents to become good parents and attain personal growth toward success. However, this success cannot occur without accessible services similar to those mentioned above. Punishing the adolescent for his or her action does not prevent a repeat pregnancy and jeopordizes both teenage parents and their baby. Purposefully withholding services so as not to appear to condone teen parenthood is a grave error.

Summary

The pediatrician's role in teenage pregnancy is multifaceted. The problem is a sociologic phenomenon with medical consequences. The pregnant teenager actually represents three patients: the mother, the baby, and the adolescent herself. Prepregnancy nutrition can be improved through pediatric education and advice. Sex education can be improved through the advocacy of pediatricians, who can discuss postponing parenthood until the end of adolescence with many of their patients.

Services to prevent pregnancy can be offered by pediatricians. Unfortunately, in Oklahoma it is illegal to dispense contraceptives to minors without parental consent. Pediatricians should work to gain acceptance of laws modeled after the American Academy of Pediatrics' health care for minors policy. Lastly, support services to promote proper parenthood and establishment of families can be developed with pediatric input. The entire problem must be viewed in the context of current social patterns, an understanding of adolescent development, the significance of peer pressures, and the biological changes that make it possible for children to bear children.

REFERENCES

1. Felice M., Friedman S.: The adolescent as a patient. *J. Continuing Education Pediatr.* 15, October, 1978.
2. Katchadourian H.: Adolescent sexuality. *Pediatr. Clin. North Am.* 27(1):17, 1980.
3. Piaget J.: Intellectual evolution from adolescence to adulthood. *Hum. Dev.* 15:1, 1972.
4. American Academy of Pediatrics: Pregnancy and abortion counseling, Committee on Adolescence. Pediatrics 63:920, 1979.
5. Miller J.: Letter. *Pediatrics* 65(6):1193, 1980.
6. McAnarney E.: Adolescent pregnancy—A national priority. *Am. J. Dis. Child.* 132:125, 1978.
7. Alan Guttmacher Institute: *11 Million Teenagers.* New York: Planned Parenthood Federation of America, Inc., 1976.
8. American College of Obstetricians and Gynecologists: *Adolescent Perinatal Health.* Chicago, American College of Obstetricians and Gynecologists, 1980.
9. Brann E.: Teenage pregnancy project preliminary report. Program Evaluation Branch, Family Planning Evaluation Division, Bureau of Epidemiology, C.D.C., 1976.
10. Zelnik M., et al.: Sexual and contraceptive experience of young unmarried women in the U.S., 1976 and 1971. *Fam. Plan. Perspect.* 9(2):55, 1977.
11. Fielding J.: Adolescent pregnancy revisited. *New Engl. J. Med.* 299(6):893, 1978.
12. American Academy of Pediatrics: Statement on teenage pregnancy, Committee on Adolescence. *Pediatrics* 63(5):795, 1979.
13. Furstenberg F.: *Unplanned Parenthood.* New York: Free Press, 1976.
14. Malinowski B.: The principal of legitimacy, in Coser R. (ed): *The Family: Its Structure and Functions.* New York: St. Martin's Press, 1930.
15. Jodar N.: Teenage pregnancy in Oklahoma: An overview. The Youth Task Force of the Governor's Committe on Children and Youth, 1979.
16. Anyan W.: *Adolescent Medicine in Primary Care.* New York: John Wiley & Sons, 1978.
17. Zacharias L., et al.: A prospective study of sexual development and growth in American girls: The statistics of menarche. *Obstet. Gynecol. Surv.* 31(suppl):325, 1976.
18. Petersen A.: Female pubertal development, in Sugar M. (ed): *Female Adolescent Development.* New York: Brunner/Mazzel, 1979.
19. Greydanus D., McAnarney E.: Contraception in the adolescent: Current concepts for the pediatrician. *Pediatrics* 65(1):1, 1980.
20. Greydanus D.: Contraception in adolescence: An overview for the pediatrician. *Ped. Ann.* 9(3):111, 1980.

21. Hatcher R., et al: *Contraceptive Technology 1978–1979*, ed 9. New York: Irvington Publishers, 1978.
22. Litt I., Cohen M.: Adolescent sexuality. *Adv. Pediatr.* 26:119, 1979.
23. Nadelson C., et al.: Sexual knowledge and attitudes of adolescents: Relationships to contraceptive use. *Obstet. Gynecol.* 55(3):340, 1980.
24. Miller W.: The use and non-use of contraception by teenagers. *Transitions* 2(2):10, 1979.
25. Reichelt P.: Contraception: A cause of teen sex activity? *Transitions* 3(4):3, 1980.
26. DeArmond C., Hackford T. (producers): *Teenage Father,* a film distributed by Children's Home Society of California, 1978.
27. Hirst B.C.: *A Textbook of Obstetrics.* Philadelphia: W.B. Saunders Co., 1918, pp 592–593.
28. Pritchard J.A., MacDonald P.C.: *Williams Obstetrics,* ed 16. New York: Appleton-Century-Crofts, 1979.
29. Duenhoelter J.H., Jimenez J.M., Baumann G.: Pregnancy performance of patients under fifteen years of age, *J. Obstet. Gynecol.* 46:49, 1975.
30. Evrard J.R., Gold E.M.: Adolescent pregnancy. *Perinatal Care,* June, 1977.
31. Hassan H.M., Falls F.H.: The young primipara: A clinical study, *Am. J. Obstet. Gynecol.* 88:256, 1964.
32. Beric B., Bregun N., Bujas M.: Obstetrics aspects of adolescent pregnancy and delivery. *Int. J. Obstet. Gynaecol. Obstet. (Stockholm)* 15:491, 1978.
33. Spellacy W.N., Mahan C.S., Cruz A.C.: The adolescent's first pregnancy: A controlled study. *South. Med. J.* 71(1):768, 1978.
34. Dott A.B., Fort A.T.: Medical and social factors affecting early teenage pregnancy. *Am. J. Obstet. Gynecol.* 125(4):532, 1976.
35. Hutchins F.L., Kendall N., Rubino J.: Experience with teenage pregnancy. *Obstet. Gynecol.* 54(1):1, 1979.
36. Ryan G.M., Schneider J.M.: Teenage obstetric complications. *Clin. Obstet. Gynecol.* 21(4):1191, 1978.
37. Hendricks C.H.: Twinning in relation to birth weight, mortality and congenital anomalies. *Obstet. Gynecol.* 27:47, 1966.
38. Long P.A., Abell D.A., Beischer N.A.: Parity and pre-eclampsia. *Obstet. Gynecol. Surv.* 35:435, 1980.
39. McLean R.A., et al.: Maternal Mortality Study. *N.Y. State J. Med.* 79(2):226, 1979.
40. Elster A.B., McAnarney E.R.: Maternal age re: Septo-optic dysplasia (letter). *J. Pediatr.* 94(1):162, 1979.
41. Bulfin M.J.: A new problem in adolescent gynecology. *South. Med. J.* 72(8):9628, 1979.
42. Daling J.R., Emanuel I.: Induced abortion and subsequent outcome of pregnancy in a series of American women. *New Engl. J. Med.* 297:1241, 1977.
43. Cates W.: Late effects of induced abortion: Hypothesis or knowledge? *J. Reprod. Med.* 22:207, 1979.
44. Center for Disease Control: *Morbidity & Morality Weekly Report.* 29(22):2, 1980.
45. Gabrielson I.M.: Suicide attempts in a population pregnant as teenagers. *Am. J. Public Health* 60:2289, 1970.
46. Zlatnik F., Burmeister L.: Low "gynecologic age": An obstetric risk factor. *Am. J. Obstet. Gynecol.* 128(2):183, 1977.
47. Alton I.: Nutrition services for pregnant adolescents within a public high school. *J. Am. Diet. Assoc.* 74:667, 1979.
48. Lee C.: Nutritional status of selected teenagers in Kentucky. *Am. J. Clin. Nutr.* 31:1453, 1978.
49. King J.: Protein metabolism during pregnancy. *Clin. Perinatol.* 2(2):243, 1975.
50. Barness L.: Moderation, the noblest gift of Heaven. *Pediatrics* 65(4):834, 1980.
51. King J., Jacobson H.: Nutrition and pregnancy in adolescence, in Zackler J., et al.

98   ROBERT W. BLOCK, STEVEN SALTZMAN, AND SHARON A. BLOCK

(eds): *The Teenage Pregnant Girl*. Springfield, Ill.: Charles C Thomas, Publisher, 1975.
52. American Academy of Pediatrics: Health assessment and health maintenance for the adolescent, Committee on Adolescence. Unpublished, 1980.
53. Jacobson H.: Weight and weight gain in pregnancy. *Clin. Perinatol.* 2(2):233, 1975.
54. Worthington B.: Nutrition during pregnancy, lactation and oral contraception. *Nurs. Clin. North Am.* 14(2):269, 1979.
55. Pitkin R.: Vitamins and minerals in pregnancy. *Clin. Perinatol.* 2(2):221, 1975.
56. Heald F., Jacobson M.: Nutritional needs of the pregnant adolescent. *Pediatr. Ann.* 9(3):95, 1980.
57. Food and Nutrition Board, National Academy of Sciences—National Research Council: *Recommended Dietary Allowances*. Washington, D.C., 1980.
58. California Department of Health: *Nutrition During Pregnancy and Lactation.* 1975.
59. Pitkin R.: Nutritional influences during pregnancy. *Med. Clin. North Am.* 61(1):3, 1977.
60. Cohenour S., Calloway D.: Blood, urine and dietary pantothenic acid levels of pregnant teenagers. *Am. J. Clin. Nutr.* 25:512, 1972.
61. Block R., Block S.: Outreach education: A possible preventer of teenage pregnancy. *Adolescence* 14(59):657, 1980.
62. Hollingsworth D., Kreutner A.: Teenage pregnancy—solutions are evolving. *N. Engl. J. Med.* 303(9):516, 1980.
63. Brann E., et al.: Strategies for the prevention of pregnancy in adolescents. *Adv. Plan. Parent.* 14:68, 1979.
64. Merritt T., et al.: The infants of adolescent mothers. *Pediatr. Ann.* 9(3):100, 1980.
65. Sahler O.: Adolescent parenting: Potential for child abuse and neglect? *Pediatr. Ann.* 9(3):120, 1980.

Carbohydrates in Pediatric Nutrition—Consumption, Digestibility, and Disease

EMANUEL LEBENTHAL, M.D.

Professor of Pediatrics
State University of New York at Buffalo
Chief, Division of Gastroenterology and Nutrition
Children's Hospital of Buffalo
Buffalo, New York

TERRY F. HATCH, M.D.

Assistant Professor of Clinical Sciences (Pediatrics)
University of Illinois School of Clinical Medicine
Director of Medical Education
Carle Foundation Hospital
Urbana, Illinois

AND

P.C. LEE, PH.D.

Associate Professor of Pediatrics and Biochemistry
State University of New York at Buffalo
Director, Gastroenterology Laboratories
Children's Hospital of Buffalo
Buffalo, New York

Introduction

THE TERM CARBOHYDRATES refers to a group of compounds primarily composed of carbon, hydrogen, and oxygen with the last two elements in the proportion of two to one. Carbohydrates exist in many forms, from simple sugars (monosaccharides) with a molecular weight of 100 to complex polymers (polysaccharides like starch and cellulose) with a molecular weight well over 1,000,000. Carbohydrates occur in both plant and an-

99

0065-3101/81/0028-099-139-$03.75

imal tissues. In animals carbohydrate is stored in the form of glycogen. In plants there exists a wide variety of simple to complex carbohydrates; the major storage product is starch.

Carbohydrates serve as an important source of calories in the diets of infants and young children. Though not established as an obligatory nutrient, carbohydrate in its many forms is an inexpensive, useful, and readily available source of calories. Interest in carbohydrate digestion arises from three principal concerns. The first relates to the bioavailability of the constituent sugar itself. The second is the potential that undigested carbohydrates may have for producing diarrheal symptoms, malabsorption, and changes in gastrointestinal flora. The third is the recent implication of dietary sucrose in the genesis of several medical problems including dental caries, obesity, and atherosclerotic heart disease.

This chapter treats recent practices in nutritional counseling and the consumption of carbohydrates, particularly in infants and children. These are correlated with the ontogeny and development of the hydrolytic capacities for starches, other polymers of glucose, and disaccharides and the ability to transport monosaccharides into the mature epithelial cell in the small intestine. Carbohydrate malabsorption and its pathophysiology, clinical presentation, and related diagnostic tests are briefly reviewed. The metabolism and use of carbohydrates are discussed only with reference to several clinical states of current concern that are potentially related to excess carbohydrate consumption. Finally, a critical assessment of the current consumption of carbohydrate is presented and appropriate recommendations are given.

A Historical Perspective—Carbohydrates as Nutrients

Carbohydrate serves as a principal nutrient in the diet of the Western world and provides the largest percentage of calories in the adult diet. Of the 360 gm of carbohydrate ingested daily, approximately 60% is starch, 30% sucrose, and 10% lactose.[1] The diet of infants fed mainly by breast or with commercial formulas based on cow's milk provides 35 to 55% of calories as carbohydrates in the form of lactose. The amount and composition of carbohydrate calories is dramatically altered by the introduction of infant solids, or "Beikost." (This German term, for which no equivalent word may be found in the English, was introduced and popularized by Dr. Samuel Fomon. It refers to infant food other than milk or formula.) These calories may be in the form of sucrose, amylose, amylopectin, modified food starches, or other complex carbohydrates. In order to examine the current role of carbohydrates in the diet of the young and gain a perspective from which to understand the direction of current and potential change in their use, a short review of the history of human dietary carbohydrate is necessary.

Carbohydrates of some variety have long been an important component of the human diet.[2] Carbohydrate has been important not only as a nutrient and a source of energy, but also as a politicoeconomic force in the development of Western civilization. Our hunter-gatherer ancestors changed to the domestication of various wild grains for a more reliable food supply. Wheat, rice, maize, various legumes and potato, all provide carbohydrate, mainly as starch. Honey was rare and valuable and its use was restricted to the wealthy. The role of these cereal and leguminous carbohydrates in infant feeding and nutrition in early times is speculative. In more recently studied primitive societies, the estimated timing of breast milk weaning is between two to three years. This period probably marked the point at which carbohydrates became a significant caloric source. Any earlier introduction of such foodstuffs, either by trial to supplement breast milk or by necessity as a result of forced early weaning, probably was accomplished with prior mastication by the mother.

The introduction of sucrose to the diet of Western man occurred slowly over the past two millennia. Sugar cane, initially cultivated in India, soon spread to the rest of the world. In Europe, cane sugar long remained a prized delicacy and a component to neutralize the bitterness of medicines. The introduction of beet sugar, along with the continued availability of traditional cane sources and increased proficiency in production, allowed sucrose to become widely available.

As a result, the consumption of sugar and distribution of dietary calories between simple and more complex carbohydrates (starch) have changed dramatically.[2, 3] World production of refined sucrose has increased from 8,000,000 tons in 1900 to 70,000,000 tons in 1970, a rate of increase unmatched by any other foodstuff. In the more affluent countries consumption of refined sucrose has leveled off. The highest levels—50 to 60 kg per capita per year, or about 18% of total calories—are reported in the United Kingdom, Australia, and Switzerland. U.S. consumption lags slightly at 50 kg per capita per year. Increasing consumption is still seen in countries of the developing world. In general, a relationship exists between income and an increasing consumption of both fat and sugar.[4, 5] This occurs at the expense of decreasing intakes of complex carbohydrates like starch. In the United States, per capita consumption of complex carbohydrates since 1900 has decreased from 500 gm to 380 gm per day, mainly as a result of the decreased use of flour and cereal (300 lb to 142 lb per capita).[2] The apparent use (disappearance into commerical and industrial channels) of refined sugar has increased by one third, from 76.4 to 101 lb per capita per year, principally due to the increased consumption of prepared food products and sweetened beverages. Most of this increase took place prior to 1920 and for the past 50 years refined sugar consumption in the U.S. has been relatively stable.[6]

Consumption of Carbohydrates by the Infant and Child— Current Trends

Carbohydrates of many varieties are consumed throughout the growing years. They serve many functions, as inexpensive and readily available nutrients, and as valuable aids in commercial food processing. Three dietary periods may be loosely defined during which the major sources of dietary carbohydrate are changing: the exclusive feeding of breast milk and/or formula, the introduction and gradual ascendancy of Beikost, and the predominance of home-cooked food associated with a relative decrease in the contribution of milk to total calorie intake.

During early infancy, until the introduction of Beikost, the sole source of carbohydrate is from breast milk and/or commercial milk-based formulas. The relative preponderance of breast or commercial formula feeding during the early newborn period in the United States has been changing.[7-13] In the early 1940s approximately 65% of infants were breast-fed at birth. This figure steadily decreased to approximately 25% by the late 1950s and then remained stationary for the following decade. By the early 1970s the increased popularity of breast-feeding was evi-

TABLE 1. — Carbohydrates in Infant Formula

Formula	Carbohydrate (g/100 ml)	Calorie Distribution*			Carbohydrate
		Protein	Fat	CHO	
Regular					
Enfamil® 20	7.0	9	50	41	Lactose
Similac® 20	7.2	9	48	43	Lactose
SMA®	7.2	9	48	43	Lactose
Soy					
Isomil®	6.8	12	48	40	Sucrose, corn syrup
ProSobee®	6.9	12	48	40	Corn syrup solids
Special Formulas					
Nutramigen®	8.8	13	35	52	Sucrose, modified tapioca starch
Portagen®	7.8	14	41	45	Corn syrup solids, sucrose
Pregestimil®	9.1	11	35	54	Corn syrup solids, modified tapioca starch

Human milk	7.0-9.0	6	56	38	Lactose
Evaporated milk**	5.3	21	49	30	Lactose
Whole cow's milk	4.8	21	49	30	Lactose
Skim milk	5.0	39	5	56	Lactose

*Percentage supplied by
**Diluted 1:1 with water

TABLE 1.—CARBOHYDRATES IN INFANT FORMULAS

FORMULA	CARBOHYDRATE (gm/100 ml)	Protein	Fat	CHO	CARBOHYDRATE
Regular					
Enfamil 20	7.0	9	50	41	Lactose
Similac 20	7.20	9	48	43	Lactose
SMA	7.20	9	48	43	Lactose
Soy					
CHO-free w/12.8%	6.40	11	49	40	12.8% dextrose
Dextrose Isomil	6.80	12	48	40	Sucrose, corn syrup solids
Neo-Mullsoy	6.40	11	49	40	Sucrose
Prosoybee	6.80	15	45	40	Maltose, dextrins
Special Formulas					
Nutriamigen	8.76	13	35	52	Sucrose, tapioca
Portagen	7.74	14	42	44	Dextrose, maltose, sucrose, lactose (15%)
Pregestimil	8.80	13	36	51	Dextrose, tapioca, starch, corn syrup solids
Human milk	7.0–9.0	7	51	42	Lactose
Evaporated milk	5.30	20	51	29	Lactose
Whole cow's milk	4.80	20	51	29	Lactose
Skim milk	4.80	40	5	55	Lactose

*Percentage supplied by.

dent, for approximately 35% of newborns were breast-fed.[14, 15] This increased to 45% according to a recent survey by Martinez.[16]

Breast-feeding subsequent to the neonatal period has also been popularized. By the end of the 1960s only 10% of infants were breast-fed at two months of age.[16] During these years bottle-fed infants received mainly commercially prepared infant formula, as evaporated milk became less popular and the use of whole cow's milk has remained minimal prior to three months.

The carbohydrate content of human milk is approximately 7 to 9 gm per 100 ml,[17] of which 90% is lactose and the remainder a group of poorly understood oligosaccharides (Table 1). Carbohydrate accounts for approximately 42% of total human breast milk calories.[17] Commercially prepared cow's milk-based formula marketed in the United States for the newborn provides 41 to 43% of calories as carbohydrate. Infants that require milk-free formulas with protein from soy isolate or flour consume 39–40% of calories as carbohydrate. Several special purpose formulas contain substantially higher contents of carbohydrate, from 44 to 52%. For comparison, the variety of carbohydrates currently used in commercially prepared formulas are listed in Table 2.

The second period of infant feeding is associated with a progressive decline in lactose as a carbohydrate source. During this period, commercially prepared Beikost dominates the solid food intake. A trend toward the earlier introduction and more rapid diversification of infant solids has been apparent during this century. By 1970 Filer[18] stated that Beikost supplied 31% of calorie intake at three months of age, 38% at six months, 58% at nine months, and 64% at 12 months of age. Recent food intake studies in infants two to 12 months of age, however, indicate that while total calorie intake has remained stable, Beikost accounted for 34% of calories during the three-to-nine-month age period in 1972 and only 26% of calories by 1977.[19] This might be a sign that the trend is reversing.

The average carbohydrate contents for various infant diets are listed in Table 3. With the exception of meats and high meat dinners, all are rich sources of carbohydrate. Substantial public concern about added sweeteners in commercial baby foods prompted the major manufacturers in 1977 to reduce the

TABLE 2.—TYPES OF CARBOHYDRATES USED IN COMMERCIALLY PREPARED INFANT FORMULAS

CARBOHYDRATES	SOURCE	FUNCTION	DIGESTIBILITY
Lactose	Milk	Calories	Excellent
Corn syrup solids	Acid-hydrolized corn starch	Calories	Excellent
Sucrose	Beet/cane	Calories	Excellent
Dextrose		Calories	Excellent
Dextrin-maltose-dextrose	Acid-hydrolyzed corn starch	Calories	Excellent
Arrowroot starch	Tuber of *Maranta arundinecea*	Thickener and in suspension added minerals	Excellent
Cornstarch	Corn	ditto	Excellent
Modified cornstarch	Chemically treated corn starch	ditto	Excellent
Modified tapioca starch	Chemically treated starch root of cassava (manioc) plant		Excellent
Banana powder			Excellent
Carrageenan	Sulfated polysaccharide from red seaweed		None

TABLE 3.—AVERAGE CARBOHYDRATE
CONTENT OF SEVERAL COMMERCIAL
BEIKOST PRODUCTS FOR INFANTS*

FOOD	CARBOHYDRATE (% OF CALORIES)
Strained meats	5
Strained fruits	92
Strained cereals with fruit	83
Strained desserts	88
Strained vegetables	76
Soups and dinners	58
High meat dinners	34
Juices	95
Dry cereals	70

*Based on information published in the past
four years.

amount of added sweeteners in their products. Tart products
such as apricots and peaches require added sugar (sucrose) for
taste, but the maximum has been 9% by weight. Currently,
only 25 of 108 Heinz baby foods contain added sweeteners,
while 125 of 152 Gerber products, and all Beechnut products
except Cera-Meal, have no added sucrose.[20] The majority (65%)
of commercial strained foods for infants contain a sweetener of
numerous modified corn, milo, or tapioca starches. These modified food starches may account for a high percentage of total
calories in many soups and dinners.

The introduction of home-prepared food commences between
six to 18 months of age and signifies the final transition period
from the infant to adult diet.[21] As solid food intake increases
and milk intake remains constant or declines, home foods become the predominant source of calories. From age one the percentage of calories derived from carbohydrate remains relatively constant at 48 to 50% until a decline is seen at the termination of the adolescent growth years (Fig 1).[22]

Specific Carbohydrates in the Pediatric Diet

The developing child is exposed to a wide variety of carbohydrates as the diet proceeds from the exclusive feeding of
breast milk or commercial formula to the standard adult diet.
Specific sugars and their relative contributions to total carbohydrate calories change within this setting. Sugars present in

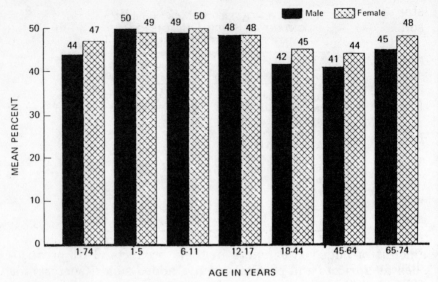

Fig 1.—Mean percent calories from carbohydrates for persons 1–74 years by sex and age: United States, 1971–1974. (Courtesy of Havlik, R.J., et al.: Proceedings of the Conference on the Decline in Coronary Heart Disease Mortality. Bethesda, 1979.)

different foodstuffs are either intentionally added, generated during some stage of processing, or occur naturally in the food. Sugars are polyhydroxyl aldehydes or ketones and their derivatives. Monosaccharides exist in a hemiacetal ring structure. Oligosaccharides are chains containing two to ten monosaccharide units (an arbitrary definition) joined by glycosidic linkage. Polysaccharides are longer, including linear or branched chains of individual monosaccharides. Most polysaccharides contain only one or two kinds of monosaccharides.

MONOSACCHARIDES

Glucose is one of the two most common monosaccharides occurring in nature. It is found in honey, many fruits, vegetables, and legumes. Crystalline glucose was initially developed as an easily assimilated baby food component in response to use by pediatricians. Commercial dextrose syrup is currently produced by the acid-enzyme treatment and the more recent process of α-amylase hydrolysis. Various sugars and sugar dehydration products are generated from glucose during processing and storage of many foods. Dextrose is supplemented in some infant solid foods but is not added to commercial liquid formulas.

Fructose, the second most common monosaccharide found in nature, is present in many of the same foods as glucose. It has several interesting properties. Fructose is sweeter, more soluble, and less cariogenic than sucrose. It improves fruit flavors. Fructose is added to infant solids and recommended for use in reconstituting Carbohydrate-Free (Ross Laboratories), a soy-based formula designed as a lactose-free diet.

OLIGOSACCHARIDES

The important natural oligosaccharides are polymers of three specific monosaccharides, D-glucose, fructose, and galactose. Approximately 40 oligosaccharides are known to occur naturally. Those of significance in infant nutrition include several disaccharides, trisaccharides, and the shorter chain length components as in Polycose (Ross Laboratories), an oligopolysaccharide food supplement.

DISACCHARIDES.—Lactose is the sugar in mammalian milks. It is made up of one glucose and one galactose molecule joined by a β-1,4 glycosidic linkage that must be hydrolyzed by intestinal lactase for absorption. Lactose may be the sole carbohydrate in the newborn infant's diet and remains a major contributor late into the first year of life.

Sucrose is the only common sugar of nutritional importance that is not a reducing substance. It is composed of a molecule of glucose and one of fructose linked together by an α-1,2 glycosidic bond. Hydrolysis may be accomplished by the addition of acid (as in the clinical testing of stools for unabsorbed sucrose by the Clinitest Method) or by the specific action of the enzyme sucrase. Naturally occurring sources of sucrose include fruits, vegetables, legumes, and honey (3.9% by weight). The usual commercial sources are sugar beets and sugar cane. Fructose and sucrose are the sweetest of the commonly used sugars. Sucrose is added to some strained and junior food, as noted above. Because lactose is often contaminated with traces of cow's milk protein, sucrose is used instead in several hypoallergenic formulas.

Maltose is a disaccharide of two glucose molecules joined by an α-1,4 glycosidic linkage. It occurs naturally in several fruits, but the major dietary sources are from starch digestion and food supplemented with corn syrup solids. Maltose is present in infant solid foods and many formulas.

Isomaltose, which consists of two glucose molecules linked by an α-1,6 glycosidic bond, would be formed as an intermediate product of digestion when glycogen or amylopectin is incompletely hydrolyzed to yield a disaccharide containing the branch point. But the sugar does not exist free in nature and is not found in the lumen of the bowel, as it would be hydrolyzed by isomaltase as soon as it is formed.

TRISACCHARIDES.—Maltotriose is a trisaccharide consisting of three glucose units connected by α-1,4 linkage. It occurs naturally in grapes but most commonly as an intermediate product in the hydrolysis of starch. Raffinose is a trisaccharide consisting of glucose, galactose, and fructose with α-linkages. As no α-galactosidase is present in the human intestine, raffinose is probably metabolically inert. Although sucrase or maltase may partially hydrolyze this sugar, most of it is fermented in the distal bowel by bacterial enzymes to yield gas and galactose.

POLYSACCHARIDES

CORN SYRUP SUGARS.—Corn syrup solids are capturing a greater proportion of the sweetener market and are prepared by controlled hydrolysis of corn starch. Hydrolysis of corn starch yields a series of glucose, maltose, and longer length glucosidic saccharides. The relative amounts of the various components depend on the extent of hydrolysis, which usually is expressed as dextrose equivalent (DE). As the extent of hydrolysis increases, the DE increases and the content of larger saccharides decreases. Corn syrup solids in commercial infant formulas have DEs in the range of 30 to 42.[23]

STARCH.—Starch occurs in plant seeds, cereal grains, tubers, fruits, roots, and stem piths. Depending on the source, most native starch contains 17 to 30% amylose; the balance is made up of amylopectin. Some varieties of corn and pea starch may contain up to 75% amylose. Amylose is a linear polymer of glucose units in α-1,4 glycosidic linkage, while amylopectin contains α-1,6 branch points, occurring approximately every 26 glucose units. The number of glucose units varies with different starches and may be different even for a given starch. Potato starch has about 2,000 glucose units in their linear molecule, while the smaller corn starch has only 400 units. Native starches are in the form of crystals, which form granules of different size and shape depending on the plant source.

MODIFIED STARCH.—Due to its supercrystalline structure, starch granules are insoluble in water and irreversibly changed after heating. These properties make native starches undesirable for food processing. To overcome these, native starches are chemically modified. The processes usually employed by the food industry are substitution and cross-linking. Modifying groups are coupled to the hydroxyl groups of the starch through either an ester or ether linkage. According to the food additives regulation of the FDA, food starches may be esterified with acetyl, phosphate, and succinate groups and etherized with the hydroxylpropyl group. Cross-linking prevents disintegration of the granules when they are cooked and preserves the viscosity in acids and after mechanical shearing. Substitution improves the stability and clarity of the starch in the food mixture. The number of modified groups introduced in the processing ranges from 40 hydroxypropylene per 100 glucose residues to one phosphate per 600 glucose residues. In general, substitution is used more frequently than cross-linking.

Digestion of Dietary Carbohydrate

For the majority of newborn infants, the disaccharide lactose may be the only carbohydrate consumed. The principle carbohydrates of the adult diet include natural starch, modified food starches, sucrose, and lactose. Minor dietary sugars including mannose, ribose, glucosamine, fucose, trehalose, galactosamine, and raffinose are of no important nutritional or metabolic consequence. Except for the monosaccharides, most carbohydrates have to be properly broken down into their constituent monosugars before they can be absorbed. Two separate families of carbohydrases (enzymes that hydrolyze carbohydrates) are recognized. One is secreted into the gastrointestinal track lumen and represented by the α-amylases. The other is localized in the brush border of the small intestinal epithelial cells and includes the disaccharidases and trisaccharidases and glucoamylase. Because of the difference in their location, these enzymes carry out two modes of hydrolysis, lumenal and membrane. Major dietary carbohydrates are digested in the proximal jejunum[24] as the majority of the carbohydrases are concentrated in this portion of the small intestine.

LUMENAL DIGESTION

Starch and glycogen are hydrolyzed in the lumen of the gastrointestinal tract by two α-amylases, one from the salivary glands and the other from the pancreas. These enzymes have optimal activity in near neutral medium (pH, 6.9–7.0) similar to the environment in the proximal bowel.[25] Salivary amylase is inactivated by the low pH of gastric juice, yet activity may persist for some time in the central portion of fundic chyme when solids are consumed. Except for early infancy, pancreatic amylase predominates in the small intestine. Its activity is located mainly in the lumen, but some is found on the epithelial surface, probably resulting from adsorption of α-amylase to the mucosal surface.[26] α-Amylase specifically catalyzes the hydrolysis of α-1,4 glycosidic linkages present in natural starch. Thus amylose is hydrolyzed to maltotriose, maltose, and glucose. In amylopectin the α-1,6 bonds in the branch points make the linkage and the surrounding α-1,4 bonds resistant to amylase attack. The result is the production of α-limit dextrins (oligo-1,6-glycosides with three to six glucose units). The hydrolysis of starch with α-amylase alone produces only small quantities of free glucose even after prolonged enzyme activity. Amylase is specific for starches and does not act on sucrose or maltose. A small amount of hydrolase activity for disaccharides and trisaccharides is present in the lumenal content.[27] These free oligosaccharidase activities in the lumen have been shown to increase following the administration of cholecystokinin and secretin. These activities presumably originate from the brush border[28] and are most probably due to shedding of cells into the lumen.

BRUSH-BORDER MEMBRANE DIGESTION

The digestion of sucrose, lactose, and the amylolytic products of starch takes place under the influence of specific brush-border-membrane-bound oligosaccharidases.[29-31] These enzymes are present in the area of the mature upper intestinal villus but are not present in substantial amounts in the crypts. Lactase, a neutral-β-galactosidase, in the brush border catalyzes the hydrolysis of lactose to glucose and galactose. Two separate β-galactosidases, acid β-galactosidase in the lysosome and hetero-β-galactosidase in the cell sap, have been isolated, but they probably play no functional role in lactose digestion. Lactase is the least abundant of the disaccharidases in the intestinal mucosa, which makes the hydrolysis of lactose possibly the rate-limiting step in the digestion and absorption of this sugar, particularly when levels of lactase are further decreased by villus disease or by physiologic hypolactasia in the postweaning period. Maltase (α-1,4-glucosidase) is the most abundant of the disaccharidase activities. At least five separate brush border enzymes possess maltase activity and are usually reported together as maltase. One of these enzymes, glucoamylase, hydrolyzes specifically the nonreducing end of oligosaccharides and shows a higher affinity for 5–9 glucose unit lengths.[32] This is of particular importance because it will also act on starch. Sucrase-isomaltase is a hybrid enzyme with two separable subunits.[33] One subunit is specific for sucrose, catalyzing the hydrolysis of the α-1,2-glycosidic linkage between glucose and fructose. The other subunit has affinity for the α-1,6-linkage of the α-limit dextrins, though the disaccharide isomaltase probably is rarely detected in the human intestine.

Starch Consumption and Digestibility

Besides sucrose, starch is probably the most extensively used carbohydrate in food preparations. In underdeveloped countries, starch may even be the main source of calories for the majority of the population because of its availability and low cost. Consumption of starch in the form of flour and cereals in the United States has shown a decreasing trend since 1900 but is still substantial. It has been calculated to be about 0.5 to 1.0 lb per person per day.[2] More importantly, the use of modified starches is becoming a more common practice. The average daily consumption of modified starches, however, has not been accurately measured. An estimation of an average of 5.7 gm was obtained from the dietary history of 430 infants between one to 14 months of age.[34] On the other hand, based on the levels of 5–6.5% incorporation of modified starches into baby foods, as much as 29 gm might be consumed per infant per day.[35]

The fate of dietary starches has an important impact on nutrition and intestinal function. The adverse effect on nutrition is more likely secondary to impaired intestinal function rather than to biounavailability of the starch. The digestibility of starch is primarily determined by the activity and distribution of α-amylase and the brush-border carbohydrases, specifically maltase and isomaltase and maybe glucoamylase. Other factors that influence starch digestibility include the type and degree of modification and method of preparation. Thus wheat starch has a higher absorption coefficient than potato starch with children from one to two years old.[36] Modified starches with ether linkages are less digestible than those with ester linkages.[37] The ease of hydrolysis of these starches is inversely proportional to the number of substitution groups and cross-links,[38] so that highly modified starch has a very low digestibility.

A most controversial issue is the digestibility of starch in infants. Early investigations monitoring the increase in blood glucose following oral feeding of starches as an indirect measurement of starch digestibility showed negligible digestion and absorption of starch in three-day-old infants.[39] Measurement of undigested starch in fecal excretion after starch feeding in one- to three-month-old infants was inconclusive.[36] However, long-term studies on infants fed starch show that a significant proportion of these infants have weights below the 10th percentile.[40] This suggests a relationship between starch feeding in early infancy and growth failure. Judging from the late appearance of the luminal pancreatic α-amylase (see the following section). It is reasonable to assume that, before four months of age, infants have only a limited capacity to digest starch. Supportive evidence provided by Auricchio et al.[41] demonstrated complete hydrolysis of amylopectin in 1-year-old but not in six-month-old infants. The presence of glucoamylase may, in part, alleviate the inability of these infants to digest starch, but the exact contribution of this enzyme to the overall digestion of starch has not been established. The digestive system of infants younger than four months is therefore considered to be immature with regard to the digestion of starch.

Ontogeny of Salivary and Pancreatic Amylase and Glucoamylase

Although no documentation of the development of salivary amylase in man is available, infants presumably can synthesize and secrete a full complement of salivary α-amylases. The contribution of these salivary amylases to the overall digestion of starch has not been definitively established. In view of the short contact time in the oral cavity and the acid-labile properties of the salivary amylases, the general consensus is that salivary amylases do not play a major role in the entire scheme of starch digestion.

The development of pancreatic amylases during perinatal life is highly controversial. Keene and Hewer[42] reported the presence of α-amylase in 22-week-old fetal pancreas. Wolf and Taussig[43] also demonstrated the presence of pancreatic isoamylase in amniotic fluid at 22 weeks of gestation but failed to distinguish maternal and fetal origins. Auricchio et al.[44] claimed that the pancreas of full-term babies has amylase activity equal to one tenth of that found in adults and older children. More importantly, no amylase was detected in the duodenal content of these newborns. The absence of or very low amylase activities in the duodenal lumen has been confirmed by a number of investigators.[45-47] Newborns, both prematures[47] and full-terms [48] up to one month of age and infants who weigh less than 8 kg,[49] have been investigated and show similar findings. In contrast to the findings of Auricchio, however, Track et al.[50] found no amylase in the pancreatic tissue of fetuses and infants up to three weeks old, while substantial lipase, trypsin, chymotrypsin, and phospholipase were demonstrated in the same specimens.[50] These contrasting findings relate to differences in amylase in the duodenal lumen. The presence of amylase in the pancreas as reported by Auricchio would suggest a failure of amylase secretion, while the absence of amylase in the pancreas as observed by Track would represent the absence of amylase synthesis. A more definitive and exhaustive study of the development of pancreatic amylase during the perinatal period is necessary to make a distinction between these two alternatives. It is, however, safe to conclude that the pancreases of infants during the first three months of life do not secrete any appreciable quantity of amylase into the duodenal lumen.

The discovery of brush-border glucosidase, glucoamylase, adds a new dimension in the study of enzymes involved in starch digestion. By virtue of its ability to hydrolyze starch directly to glucose by the stepwise removal of glucose residues from the nonreducing end, glucoamylase provides an alternative pathway for the conversion of starch to the monosaccharides. Glucoamylase has been shown to be present in newborns[51] and one-month-old infants.[52] Although the role of glucoamylase in starch digestion in infants has not been studied at length, the enzyme is potentially important because of the absence of pancreatic amylase in the duodenal lumen during early infancy.

Ontogeny of Disaccharidase Activities

Intestinal disaccharidase activities have been demonstrated in animals other than mammals and in a variety of primates and other mammals. All nonmammals are deficient in lactase. Mammals usually possess all five disaccharidase activities, lactase, sucrase, isomaltase, maltase, and trehalase. Individual enzymes besides lactase may be absent or possess different biochemical characteristics in certain species. In man, lactase activity may be low in adults or may remain high throughout life.[53] Ethnic differences seem to play a role in adult lactase deficiency.[53]

The unique pattern of disaccharidase development in the human fetus and child should be viewed with respect to the following frames of reference: (1) the formation, migration, and maturation of the epithelial cell from the crypts of Lieberkühn to its loss from the villus tip; (2) the topographic distribution of enzyme activity in the gastrointestinal tract; and (3) the development of enzyme activity from conception to birth and the later acquisition of the adult complement of disaccharidase activities.

EPITHELIAL RENEWAL

Disaccharidase activities are first noted in the brush-border membrane of the mature animal approximately 24 hours after the immature multipotential crypt enterocyte migrates to the lower villus. The cell assumes a more mature columnar shape and develops microvilli. Maximal disaccharidase activity develops during migration through the middle and upper villus regions. This process requires two to three days in rodents.[54-56] In man, epithelial migration time has been estimated to be five to six days in the proximal small intestine and about three days in the ileum. Epithelial renewal after birth is normally regulated by the interplay of several mechanisms.

Enzyme activities in intestinal mucosa are associated with the membrane fraction and appear to be present as structural groups of that membrane.[57, 58] In the rat, the turnover of brush-border proteins is rapid compared to the enterocyte life cycle.[59, 60] In vitro the turnover of the disaccharidases is slower than that of the total mucosal glycoprotein.[61] Turnover seems to be related to the molecular weight of the enzyme; more rapid rates are seen with the larger proteins.[62] Disaccharidase turnover has been shown to be modulated by the action of pancreatic protease within the intestinal lumen.[63, 64] In the well-fed mature experimental animal, a rhythmic fluctuation in enzyme activity is apparent, with increases prior to feeding that relate to the anticipation of a standardized feeding time.[65, 66] The processes of epithelial cell renewal and brush border protein turnover are assumed to be immature in the human fetus and newborn, but these have not been fully explored. The appearance of fetal disaccharidase activity in the intestine correlates well with mucosal differentiation and the definition of villus structure.[67-71] Epithelial renewal in the fetal small intestine is evidenced by the early appearance of disaccharidase activity in amniotic fluid, probably as the result of the loss of villus tip cells. Information on mitotic rates, crypt cell populations, and migration rates are not readily available in the human infant. In the fetal rat, the "proliferation zone" extends the entire length of the villus and is only confined to the crypt after birth.[72] Application of these animal data to the human situation must be made with care.

THE TOPOGRAPHIC DISTRIBUTION OF DISACCHARIDASE ALONG THE INTESTINE

In human adults, the individual disaccharidases have unique patterns of distribution in the small intestine. The activities of lactase, sucrase-isomaltase, and maltase are highest in the proximal and midjejunum.[73, 74] In both the orad and aborad directions, activities decrease, but at varying rates; those in the duodenum are lower than that in the ileum. Sucrase and maltase levels peak near the ligament of Treitz, while lactase continues to rise for another 30 cm in the adult.

The proximal-distal gradient in disaccharidase activities is established during fetal life and persists into adulthood.[75-77] Individual activities appear throughout the intestine; levels in the ileum remain constant and in the proximal intestine they increase.

DISACCHARIDASE ACTIVITIES DURING ONTOGENY

Compared to a number of mammals, man demonstrates a unique developmental pattern of the intestinal disaccharidases. In the rat, calf, pig, lamb, horse, and rabbit, α-glucosidase activity is absent or minimal at birth and develops later, usually near the end of the weaning period.[78-82] In contrast, the term newborn infant possesses well developed α-glucosidase activity (see below). Lactase (β-galactosidase) activity in the animals noted above is high in the newborn period, increases for several weeks following birth, and subsequently declines to adult levels.[83] In contrast, lactase activity in the human fetus increases markedly during the last trimester and, at term, approaches levels seen in the older child and adult with persistence of lactase.

Interest in the presence of intestinal disaccharidases in the human fetus and newborn during the past century has allowed a reasonable characterization of the ontogeny of these enzyme activities. α-Glucosidase activity (sucrase-isomaltase and maltase) is identified in the human fetus during the first trimester of gestation.[77] These activities increase rapidly and reach high levels as early as the 10th to 16th weeks.[75, 77, 84] Subsequently, a slow but detectable rise occurs, so that, by 26 to 34 weeks, sucrase and maltase activities approach 70% of those seen in the full-term infant.[85] Adult levels are present in the normal term infant and remain relatively constant thereafter. Auricchio[76] and Dahlqvist and Lindberg[84] pointed out that not all maltases follow this general pattern of development. Maltase II and III, by the method of Dahlqvist, develop only during the last trimester of gestation; Maltase III develops fully only after birth. By Auricchio's method, Maltase I is the last to develop.

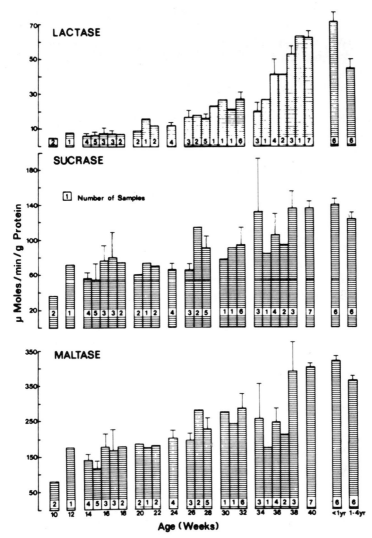

Fig 2.—Developmental pattern of disaccharidase activities in human fetal midjejunum between the 10th to 40th week of gestation. Each column is a mean ± SEM of number of samples given on the columns. (Courtesy of Antonowicz I., Lebenthal E.: *Gastroenterology* 72(6):1299, 1977.)

β-Galactosidase activity (lactase) in man develops mainly during the latter portions of fetal life, shortly before birth (Fig 2). Lactase activity is present but low prior to 12 weeks' gestation.[53, 75, 84] By 26 to 34 weeks of gestation the activity is approximately 30% of that seen in full terms. An increase to 70% of the level found at term is seen between 35 to 38 weeks. Lactase activity in the newborn is similar to that in babies less than one year of age.[85] Thus, lactase develops late, during the immediate preterm period, and reaches a relatively mature level at term in the newborn infant.

Based on the knowledge of the disaccharidase activities during ontogeny, Auricchio et al.[44] calculated the optimal amounts of disaccharides that would be hydrolyzed in vitro by the whole small intestine at various gestational ages. The results indicated that between three to four months of intrauterine life, the capacity of the fetus to hydrolyze disaccharides is minimal. At term, the infant intestine can hydrolyze in 24 hours a mean of 107 gm of maltose, 72 gm sucrose, 46 gm isomaltose, and 60 gm lactose. At eight months of gestation, the fetus can hydrolyze only about 70 gm maltose, 35 gm sucrose, 26 gm isomaltose, and a mere 6 gm of lactose per day. Extrapolation of these data would suggest that prematures born around the eighth month of gestation can use maltose, sucrose, and isomaltose reasonably well, but not lactose. This information may be useful in choosing suitable sugars to include in the diets of premature newborns.

Absorption of Carbohydrates

The type and amount of monosaccharides presented for absorption vary with the changing diet during development. An infant fed exclusively on milk will have approximately equal amounts of glucose and galactose. The average adult diet upon hydrolysis yields monosaccharides of the following composition: 80% glucose, 15% fructose, and 5% galactose.[86] Disaccharides are usually not absorbed intact but may be taken up by the epithelial cells in certain conditions and appear in the serum and urine. Lactosuria and sucrosuria may be seen when the respective disaccharides are given in high concentrations to patients with mucosal damage, such as those with celiac disease and regional enteritis and those with disaccharidase deficiency.

MONOSACCHARIDE TRANSPORT

Glucose is absorbed primarily in the proximal small intestine; only small quantities reach the distal bowel in the healthy individual. In the adult duodenum, glucose is absorbed at the rate of 5 to 20 gm per hour, and in the jejunum, 25 to 40 gm may be absorbed per hour in a 45-cm segment. Absorption occurs against a concentration gradient, is inhibited by conditions that impair cellular metabolism, and demonstrates a substrate and rate relationship similar to the Michaelis-Menton kinetics for a typical enzyme substrate reaction. Thus, glucose absorption appears to be mediated by an energy-dependent enzyme-like mechanism. Sodium is required for at least 50% of carrier-mediated glucose absorption in vivo.[87] A sodium gradient between the lumenal phase (or at least the unstirred water layer) and the intracellular environment appears to be necessary in most circumstances. This suggests a model in which sodium and glucose share a common carrier. Further, the concomitant entrance of sodium during active transport of glucose leads to an increase in intracellular concentration of sodium. In order to maintain a low concentration of sodium in the cell, the energy-dependent basal lateral membrane sodium pump is activated.[59] Thus it appears that glucose transport is coupled to the sodium pump.

Galactose appears to share the active transport system for glucose. The uptake of galactose occurs more rapidly than glucose and is inhibited by glucose, while such inhibition of glucose absorption by galactose does not occur.[88] Multiple forms of sugar-carriers may exist in the intestine, as evidenced by kinetic variations in electrogenic transport that may be induced by diet.[89] In congenital glucose-galactose malabsorption, all absorption against a concentration gradient is absent (see below).

Fructose absorption occurs by a different mechanism than that of glucose and galactose. The absorption of fructose is directly related to the concentration gradient across the cell surface, yet the rate of absorption is too rapid to be explained by simple diffusion alone. No active process can be demonstrated, so a carrier mechanism (facilitated transport) has been proposed. This carrier may also use the transmembrane sodium gradient.[90]

HYDROLASE-RELATED TRANSPORT (HRT)

The hydrolysis of oligosaccharides appears to be closely linked to the active transport processes for component monosaccharides and to a separate transport mechanism termed hydrolase-related transport.[91, 92] Membrane oligosaccharidases behave as vectoral enzymes with respect to the monosaccharide products of carbohydrate hydrolysis, transferring these products across the membrane independent of the carrier systems. This process is independent of sodium. No physiologic significance can be ascribed to the process of HRT, as monosaccharide absorption is not augmented by the addition of the related disaccharide, and the impairment of absorption in congenital glucose-galactose malabsorption is not corrected with the use of related disaccharides (sucrose or maltose).[65, 93]

Ontogeny of Monosaccharide Transport Mechanisms

Active transport of monosaccharides seems to develop fairly early in intrauterine life. An active transport of glucose against a concentration gradient can already be demonstrated in the jejunum and ileum of 11- to 19-week-old fetuses.[94] Changes in potential difference, presumably as a result of glucose transport against a concentration gradient, are found in the small intestine of 11-week-old fetuses following exposure to glucose in vitro. The amount of changes in potential difference implying the magnitude of glucose transport increases with age of the fetus.[95] Active transport of monosaccharide, therefore, is present at the end of the first trimester, but whether the system actually functions at this stage of development is unknown.

Scarce data are available on the transport of monosaccharides both at birth and during early infancy. Indirect measurement of absorption by blood glucose level following a peroral load of glucose showed that infants younger than 38 days reached the maximum serum glucose level at 60 minutes after feeding, while older infants reached the maximum at 30 minutes after feeding. The delayed appearance of maximal blood glucose in younger infants may represent a slower rate of absorption but can also be due to a more sluggish use of glucose.[96, 97] A comparison of results obtained by Younoszai[98] in infants and by Fordtran and Ingelfinger[99] in adults indicated that infants have lower capacity than adults to absorb glucose.[100] Other studies also showed a lower absorption of galactose[101] and xylose[102] by infants as compared to older children and adults. Thus the ability to transport monosaccharides develops early but the adult capacity is not reached until later in postnatal development.

Deficiency in Carbohydrate Absorption—Causes and Effects

The digestion and absorption of individual carbohydrates are relatively specific processes that may be impaired by a wide variety of events. Incomplete hydrolysis of carbohydrates and/or deficient absorption (transport) of component monosaccharides are the basic defects resulting in carbohydrate malabsorption. The association of protracted diarrhea and dietary sugar was described early in this century by Jacobi (1901)[103] and Howland (1921),[104] long before the details of carbohydrate digestion and absorption were defined and the capacities to measure enzyme activities through small intestinal biopsy were developed.

CLINICAL FEATURES AND MECHANISMS

The absorption of dietary carbohydrate is usually rapid and fairly complete in the proximal small intestine. In the newborn, particularly those who are breast-fed and have a higher lactose intake, this may not be true, since they have relatively more reducing substances in their stool than older infants. But there is some dispute as to whether unabsorbed lactose alone accounts for the majority of reducing substances commonly identified in the stools of these infants.

In the intestinal lumen, unabsorbed carbohydrates are osmotically active. A new equilibrium in the lumen is achieved only as a result of the secretion of water and electrolytes by the small intestine and colon. In addition, bacterial degradation alters the majority of carbohydrate prior to its passage into the feces, producing lactic acid, other short-chain organic acids, carbon dioxide and hydrogen gases and additional water. Increases in water and gases lead to volume distention and, with other factors, promote intestinal motility and shorten transit time. The generation of acidic products lowers the luminal pH and impairs the normal reserve absorptive capacity of the distal small intestine and large bowel.

A spectrum of clinical signs and symptoms usually characterizes carbohydrate malabsorption. The classic presentation is a watery, acidic, explosive, and fermentative diarrhea. Associated features may include specific food aversions (sucrose-containing foods, for example), vomiting, abdominal distention, borborygmi, colicky abdominal pain, excessive gas and flatus production, an excoriated diaper rash in infancy, and failure to thrive. In young infants, fluid and electrolyte losses may be quite large; older children may not have diarrhea.

The appearance of symptoms of carbohydrate intolerance is related to several factors associated with the underlying pathologic process, including the nature of enzyme deficiency, i.e., primary or secondary (see below); the age and reserve absorptive capacity of the distal intestine of the child; the severity and duration of mucosal structural damage in the proximal small intestine; and the dietary load of offending substances.

PRIMARY DISORDERS

SUCRASE-ISOMALTASE DEFICIENCY.—Sucrase-isomaltase is the most common disaccharidase deficiency, present in the homozygous state in 0.2% of the North American population and in up to 10% of the Greenland Eskimos. Inheritance is by the autosomal recessive trait.[105] Heterozygotes may have identifiable deficiencies of enzyme activity and be symptomatic when stressed. Loss of enzyme activity has been correlated with a deficiency of enzyme protein from the microvillus membrane.[106] Symptoms usually correlate with the introduction of a substantial quantity of sucrose in the diet. Presentation varies from the absence of symptoms to severe conditions.[107] Tolerance may improve with age; this presumably relates to functional adaptation of the distal bowel. Starch and dextrins appear to be well tolerated. Diagnosis is confirmed by determining disaccharidase activities in intestinal biopsy. The ratio of sucrase to lactase activities is often very useful.

PRIMARY ALACTASIA.—This is an exceedingly rare inborn error of the small intestine in which brush-border lactase (neutral β-galactosidase) is absent. In the few cases that have been reported, boys predominate but no inheritance pattern can be obtained. The specific absence of lactase activity in an otherwise normal biopsy specimen is required to establish the diagnosis. Diagnoses to be distinguished include secondary lactase deficiency (due to existing intestinal damage) and developmental lactose intolerance (see below). Symptoms usually appear in the first few days of life and respond to the elimination of lactose from the diet; tolerance of lactose does not appear to improve with age.

CONGENITAL LACTOSE INTOLERANCE.—At onset in the newborn period, this potentially lethal intolerance is characterized by vomiting, failure to thrive, dehydration, lactosuria, aminoaciduria, renal tubular acidosis, and liver dysfunction with bleeding.[108, 109] Minimal diarrhea, eventual recovery, and measurable lactase activity in small intestinal biopsy specimens distinguish this entity from congenital alactasia. Symptoms often abate by six to 18 months of age.

PRIMARY TREHALASE DEFICIENCY.—Trehalose is a sugar occurring only in lower plants, mushrooms, insects and some worms. Clinical intolerance has been described in two families,[110] and isolated absence of the brush-border enzyme trehalase, which catalyzes the hydrolysis of trehalose to form 2 D-glucose, has been demonstrated.

CONGENITAL GLUCOSE-GALACTOSE MALABSORPTION.—This uncommon autosomal recessive condition is characterized by an inability to accumulate glucose or galactose against a concentration gradient. A reduced number of binding sites for the active transport of glucose and galactose has been postulated, for the affinity of the existing binding sites for carbohydrates is normal. Watery diarrhea occurs in the newborn period; this condition is controlled by the exclusion of both galactose and glucose and substrate carbohydrates containing these monosaccharides from the diet.[111-113] Symptoms are less severe with advancing age for unknown reasons. No similar defect has been reported for the facilitated absorption process for fructose.

LATE-ONSET HYPOLACTASIA.—As with mammals in general, intestinal brush-border lactase activity and clinical intolerance of lactose diminish markedly in man after the weaning period, from three to six years of age.[25, 114, 115] It has been hypothesized that in societies that traditionally domesticated and herded milk-producing animals, persistence of lactase activity into adulthood had selective advantage.[116, 117] Only 10–20% of lactose-tolerant populations, such as those originating from northern Europe, are partially lactase-deficient, while the majority (80–90%) of the world's populations are lactose intolerant. This mutation or polymorphism, which results in persistent lactase activity, does not demonstrate a clear inheritance pattern, but 30–50% of the offspring of adults with acquired hypolactasia are also deficient and demonstrate clinical intolerance.

Of the three separate intestinal lactase activities, only the brush-border lactase (neutral β-galactosidase) is low and rarely is totally absent.[118] The spectrum of clinical severity among older patients with acquired hypolactasia relates to both residual enzyme activities and the existence of compensatory mechanisms. Intestinal lactase is probably not inducible by the feeding of lactose or diminished by a diet low in lactose.[119]

Acquired lactose intolerance usually is apparent by three to seven years of age. Many lactase deficient subjects spontaneously refrain from consuming larger amounts of lactose. Some dispute exists as to whether this developmental diminution of activity may be accelerated by the occurrence of severe mucosal disease and/or protracted malnutrition at younger ages.

SECONDARY DISACCHARIDASE DEFICIENCY.—In diseases associated with injury to the small intestinal mucosa, all of the disaccharidase activities are depressed.[120] Lactase activity appears to be the most sensitive to injury, for it is the first disaccharidase activity to decrease and the slowest to recover. A wide variety of diseases are associated with secondary reduced disaccharidase activity, including celiac sprue,[120] tropical sprue,[121], intractable diarrhea of infancy,[122, 123] and acute viral gastroenteritis.[122] Drugs that affect the mucosa, particularly neomycin,[124] kanamycin, methotrexate,[125] and colchicine,[126] also lower disaccharidase activities. Relative deficiency of multiple enzymes may occur in the short bowel syndrome,[126] after gastric surgery,[127] in starvation,[128] and with protein-calorie malnutrition.[129] Occasionally, secondary disaccharidase deficiencies, especially low lactase activity, will persist after the clinical remission of many of these disorders.[130] In acute gastroenteritis, transient lactase deficiency may persist for up to four months or longer in some situations. In early studies of lactase deficiency, a number of disease entities, including duodenal ulcer,[130] irritable colon syndrome,[131] ulcerative colitis,[132, 133] viral hepatitis,[134] and others, were reported to be associated with a deficiency of lactase activity. Critical evaluations of the racial-ethnic origins and ages of these populations reported in more recent observations suggest that these associations may have been artifactual. In patients with severe architectural disarray of the intestinal villus, impairment of monosaccharide transport may also be encountered. Treatment is accomplished by the removal of appropriate sugars and their products from the diet.

DIAGNOSTIC TESTS FOR CARBOHYDRATE INTOLERANCE

Several simple screening tests are informative in the evaluation of carbohydrate intolerance. Oral challenge through a tolerance test may reproduce abdominal symptomatology. The stools produced during regular feeding or upon challenge may be tested for reducing substances. The presence of 0.5 mg/100 ml or greater of reducing substance, particularly after the newborn period, is considered to be abnormal. Although less reliable, a stool pH of less than 6.0 is suggestive of carbohydrate intolerance. This pH test is not valid in patients who receive antibiotics, since the flora responsible for organic acid formation may be eliminated. Higher pH in the stool does not exclude the diagnosis, nor does the presence of an acid stool alone necessarily establish a diagnosis of carbohydrate intolerance. The presence of carbohydrates in the urine is often noted, but is usually not of diagnostic value.

Oral tolerance testing separately with glucose, sucrose, and lactose are traditional methods for establishing the diagnosis for specific carbohydrates intolerance. These tests offer a semi-quantitative clinical assessment of the degree of intolerance. After overnight fasting the tests are performed by oral feeding of a 10% carbohydrate solution at a dose of 2 gm/kg of body weight. Blood glucose is then measured immediately and 15, 30, 90, and 120 minutes after feeding. A rise in the venous blood glucose of less than 20 mg/100 ml is generally considered abnormal. Clinical symptoms and stool examination should accompany the assessment of a tolerance test. Variables that affect the oral tolerance test include occasional emesis and variation in gastric emptying time and the rate of clearance of glucose from the blood. Omission of the 15-minute glucose determination may result in a falsely negative test, since an early rise may be missed. In order to establish positive results, tolerance tests of the component sugars are also required when one is considering the absorption of a polysaccharide. Clinically, tolerance tests have been satisfactory. For example, less than 1% of lactose tolerance tests are falsely positive in patients with normal lactase activity, while 7% of them are falsely negative in lactase-deficient patients.[135]

Modifications of the lactose tolerance test include the barium-lactose roentgenographic study,[136, 137] analysis of breath hydrogen after carbohydrate feeding,[138, 139] and analysis of labeled CO_2 in the breath after administration of ^{14}C-labeled carbohydrates. A small bowel series after the ingestion of a carbohydrate-barium meal in a child, for example, with lactase deficiency, will show dilution of barium and dilation of intestinal loops.[136, 137] The breath hydrogen test is performed after an overnight fast, with an oral carbohydrate load of 2 gm/kg of body weight, given as an isotonic solution. Breath hydrogen is determined then and two hours afterward by gas liquid chromatography.[138, 139] The exhaled hydrogen is derived from fermentable substrate that reaches the colon. Values greater than 0.2 ml per minute of breath hydrogen are taken as indications of carbohydrate intolerance.

A more recent direct test for disaccharidase deficiency is the determination of intestinal enzyme activity after small intestinal biopsy.

Excessive Carbohydrate Intake—the Genesis of Disease?

It has always been controversial whether excessive consumption of carbohydrate, specifically sucrose, is harmful to the growing child or adolescent. The definition of excessive versus moderate levels of consumption is difficult to formulate. Concerns are increasingly raised in the public arena based on perceptions, not necessarily valid, of ever-increasing levels of individual consumption and the inherent value of "natural foods" in contrast to processed or refined food (presumably not "natural"). The consumption of "excessive amounts" of carbohydrate, specifically sugars, has been implicated as playing an etiologic or permissive role in association with dental disease (caries and periodontal disease), obesity, alterations in blood lipids, and increasing risk of cardiovascular disease in adult life, disturbances in childhood behavior, chronic nonspecific diarrhea, recurrent abdominal pain of childhood, abnormalities in glucose metabolism and diabetes mellitus, alterations of subsequent adult taste preferences, and many other problems. Only the first three topics will be reviewed in this section.

DENTAL DISEASE

Perhaps the only area in which the pathologic potential of sugar has been demonstrated with certainty is in acquired dental disease. Dental disease includes both dental caries and periodontal disease, both virtually universal in occurrence. Dental caries, most prevalent in childhood, is defined as destruction of enamel, dentine, and cementum, requiring the presence of a susceptible tooth, certain bacteria, and dietary factors. Cariogenic bacteria, particularly *Streptococcus mutans* and some lactobacilli and actinomycetes, colonize and accumulate in dental plaque formed in uncleansed areas of the teeth. When ingested, low molecular weight, fermentable carbohydrates (sucrose, fructose, and glucose) diffuse at different rates into plaque and are metabolized at various rates to acid. The production of acids lowers the microenvironmental pH to 4.5 to 5.0 within minutes after ingestion and lasts for 10 to 30 minutes. This localization of acidity increases the solubility of the enamel within the immediate area of the plaque. Periodontal progressive inflammation of tissues surrounding the teeth is initiated through the presence of plaque. This process is not usually clinically evident until adulthood but its precursors are probably established in childhood.

Though some conflicting results have been published, the overwhelming weight of evidence from studies of primitive societies in transition, groups subjected to deprivation associated with war, institutionalized children, children with hereditary fructose intolerance (or restricted diets), school-aged populations, and experiments on animals point to a strong correlation of carbohydrate ingestion and caries.[6] Factors of importance include the frequency of intake, amount consumed, and physical and chemical properties of the carbohydrate. The latter specifically refers to oral digestibility and how readily the carbohydrate diffuses into plaques and forms acids.

Protective measures of use against dental disease include

control of diet, prevention or removal of plaque, and increasing the resistance of the teeth.[140] Specifically, dietary counseling by the physician might include a reduction of the intake of cariogenic carbohydrates and the use of protective natural foods (milk and cheese).

OBESITY

It has been suggested that obesity acquired during infancy and most certainly during the school-age and adolescent years persists into adult life.

The specific role of excessive carbohydrate in the genesis of obesity remains unknown. Generically, it may be stated that an excess of sugar or starch should be more fattening than a calorically equivalent amount of any other nutrient. In fact, weight for weight, carbohydrate contains fewer calories than fat. Though overindulgence in carbohydrates has been postulated as a cause of obesity,[141] and obese adults have been shown to consume fats and carbohydrates[142-144] to a greater degree than those with normal weight, there appears to be no measurable parameter of taste for carbohydrate (i.e., threshold, perceptions of sweetness intensity, etc.) that specifically separates the obese from the nonobese.[145] Indeed, few studies of actual daily intakes are available and several actually report lower intakes of carbohydrates for the obese adolescent[143] and adult.[146] Studies of the development of infant taste document the early appearance of sweet differentiation and preference but fail to reliably separate obese from nonobese infants. The role of carbohydrate in obesity therefore remains undetermined.

CORONARY HEART DISEASE

A great deal of interest is currently focused on the etiology and pathogenesis of atherosclerosis, a form of arteriosclerosis, complicated by coronary heart disease (CHD).[147] Atherosclerosis begins during adolescence. Although the disease is related to the process of aging, it is quite variable in its extent within a population, and its etiology appears to relate to a number of environmental and genetic factors.[148] Of principal importance among environmental factors is diet and, more specifically, the total content of calories, cholesterol, saturated fatty acids, and polyunsaturated fatty acids one consumes. All these determine the total serum cholesterol, a risk factor for CHD.[149-152]

Sugar (sucrose) allegedly plays an etiologic role in CHD, particularly through modulation of plasma lipids.[153-158] The principle arguments, as summarized by Stare,[6] include correlations of sugar consumption with the rates of coronary mortality in some countries, similar increases in the consumption of sugar and the incidence of CHD, high levels of sugar consumption in men with CHD, and sugar-induced elevation in serum lipids. In general, the epidemiologic associations noted in these arguments have not been substantiated. However, it has been shown in some hyperlipidemic adults that sugar (sucrose) is associated with higher fasting lipid levels, particularly those of the triglycerides, than starch. In contrast, no such effect is apparent in normolipemic men in energy balance.[6]

Several studies have evaluated the relationship of carbohydrate and sucrose intake on serum lipids in childhood. Tamir et al.[159] studied six healthy infants aged four to 11 months. They were fed carbohydrate-rich food for five days. A transient increase in serum triglycerides was seen and there were no constant changes in total serum cholesterol or phospholipids. This study and others in infants suggest there may be a direct association between the amount of saturated fat intake and the level of serum cholesterol. An inverse relationship appears to exist between the polyunsaturated/saturated fatty acid ratio of the diet and serum cholesterol. No other association with dietary constituents is apparent for serum level of cholesterol. Beyond infancy, there appears to be no association of serum cholesterol and intake of nutrients, including saturated fatty acids.[160]

Studies of children and adolescents again failed to relate sucrose intake to significant changes in serum lipids. In the Rochester Study of 103 healthy children six to 16 years of age, Weidman et al.[161] found no correlation of dietary variable to serum cholesterol. The Bogalusa Heart Study of 185 children aged ten failed to relate dietary components to risk factor variables for CHD.[162] In addition, children with middle and high serum cholesterols showed lower intakes of carbohydrates and sucrose. On the other hand, in the Princeton School District Study of children six to 19 years of age, Morrison et al.[163] found that plasma cholesterol was inversely and plasma triglyceride level positively correlated with dietary sucrose. Plasma LDL-cholesterol and HDL-cholesterol levels fell with increasing calorie and sucrose intakes. The coefficient of correlation was significant but of absolute low magnitude.

Dietary Fiber and Prevention of Gastrointestinal Disease

A deficiency of dietary fiber in the adult diets of Western nations has been causally implicated in the increased prevalence of several "diseases of civilization," including constipation, diverticulosis, gallstones, obesity, ischemic heart disease, intestinal polyps, hiatal hernia, and colonic cancer. The increasing consumption of inexpensive refined carbohydrate and the availability of convenient foods has resulted in lower intakes of dietary bulk. A parallel concern has not been voiced about the diets of the young. Little information is available concerning the fiber intake of the infant or toddler or the unique physiologic responses of the young to the intake of fiber.

Dietary fiber is best defined as the residue of plant cells resistant to digestion in the human intestinal tract. Included are complex carbohydrates (cellulose, hemicellulose, gums, and pectin) and the noncarbohydrate lignin. Published data on fiber are often expressed as crude fiber (the insoluble residue of acid and alkaline hydrolysis). Actual dietary fiber is often three to four times the weight of crude fiber content of foods, for significant destruction of cellulose, hemicellulose, and lignin occurs during the determination of crude fiber content.

The physiologic effects of fiber consumption appear to relate to its chemical properties and to the osmotic effects of unabsorbed carbohydrate in the distal bowel. Fiber appears to bind several minerals and trace elements, including zinc and copper, and to affect the efficiency of absorption of several nutrients. Increased caloric loss in the form of fecal fat parallels fiber intake.[164] Fiber acts as a cation exchanger for many minerals and trace elements. Lignin binds secondary bile acids.[165] Fiber acts to decrease insulin response and blood glucose concentration during glucose tolerance testing.[166] Sequelae of these actions include decreased intestinal transit time, increased stool bulk, and perhaps a reduction in serum cholesterol and postprandial hyperglycemia.

Dietary sources of fiber include vegetables, fruits, and brans. The former two contain more fiber per calorie than other foods. The composition of fiber in different foods varies. Though little data is available, the infant and toddler who consume commercial or homemade solid foods appear to be consuming relatively large portions of fiber, perhaps in excess of that related to their increased calorie consumption. This fiber appears to be well tolerated but the chemistry and physiology of dietary fiber in the young remain relatively unstudied.

Summary

Carbohydrates play important roles in pediatric nutrition, not only as a source of calories but also as a potential cause of disease. The spectrum of carbohydrates in the pediatric diet changes with the growth of the child. The predominant lactose diet in the first three to six months of life is gradually shifted to that of a combination of various sugars and more complex carbohydrates such as starches and glycogen. Such transitions normally have no adverse effect on the healthy child. However, an early introduction of starches before three months of age may have a detrimental effect on the growing infant. The essential absence of pancreatic α-amylase in these infants would leave the starches at best partially digested. Undigested starches in the intestinal lumen have been implicated as a cause of iatrogenic diarrhea and malabsorption of other nutrients. This results in overall impairment of growth of the infant. The use of modified starches in baby food presents additional concerns, since the digestibility of these modified starches has not been studied in length. The increasing consumption of sucrose has been associated with increasing incidences of dental disease, obesity, and heart disease. But the exact role of refined sugars, especially their overconsumption during childhood, in the etiology and predisposition to these dysfunctions has not been elucidated. Carefully controlled studies on these aspects would be important in understanding the interrelationship between sucrose consumption, physical development, and disease, so that proper measures can be instituted to minimize the risk.

The general mechanism of carbohydrate digestion and absorption and their development have been worked out in reasonable detail. The control of the synthesis, assembly, and placement of various carbohydrates and transport entities in the mature intestinal epithelial cells is still forthcoming. Until we have more information on the molecular level, the exact cause for defects such as disaccharide intolerance and malabsorption remain unexplained. Such information would perhaps permit the manipulation of the controlling factors, be they environmental or hormonal, at a precise time during ontogeny of the child to achieve a therapeutic goal. At present, we are left with only one alternative: exclusion of the offending sugar from the diet of the deficient patient.

REFERENCES

1. Greaves J.P., Hollingsworth D.F.: Changes in the pattern of carbohydrate consumption in Britain. *Proc. Nutr. Soc.* 23:136, 1964.
2. Sipple H.L., et al. (eds): *Sugars in Nutrition.* New York: Academic Press, 1974, p 3.
3. Food and Agriculture Organization of the United Nations: *The State of Food and Agriculture.* Rome: Food and Agriculture Organization of the United Nations, 1971.
4. McGandy R.B., Hegsted D.M., Stare F.J.: Dietary fats, carbohydrates, and atherosclerotic vascular disease. *N. Engl. J. Med.* 277:186, 1967.
5. Perisse J., Sizaret F., Francois P.: Sugars and nutrition: The effect of income on the structure of the diet. *Nutr. News.* 1:7, 1969.
6. Stare F.J.: Sugar in the diet of man. *World Rev. Nutr. Diet* 22:237, 1975.
7. Bain K.: The incidence of breast feeding in hospitals in the United States. *Pediatrics* 2:313, 1948.
8. Jackson E.B., Wildin L.C., Auerbach H.: Statistical report on incidence and duration of breast feeding in relation to personal-social and hospital maternity factors. *Pediatrics* 17:700, 1956.
9. Meyer H.F.: Breast feeding in the United States: Extent and possible trend; a survey of 1,904 hospitals with two and a quarter million births in 1956. *Pediatrics* 22:116, 1958.
10. Meyer H.F.: Breast feeding in the United States: Report of a 1966 national survey with comparable 1946 and 1956 data. *Clin. Pediatr.* 7:798, 1968.
11. Salber E.J., Stitt P.G., Babott J.G.: Patterns of breast feeding: I. Factors effecting the frequency of breast feeding in the newborn period. *N. Engl. J. Med.* 259:707, 1958.
12. Robertson W.O.: Breast feeding practices: Some implications of regional variations. *Am. J. Pub. Health* 51:1035, 1961.
13. Salber E.J., Feinleib M.: Breast-feeding in Boston. *Pediatrics* 37:299, 1966.
14. Public Health Service: National survey of family growth: Trends in breast feeding among American mothers. Series 23, No. 3, DHEW Pub. No. (PHS) 79–1979. Washington, D.C.: U.S. Govt. Printing Office, 1979.
15. Advanced Data: National Center for Health Statistics. U.S. Dept. of HEW, Public Health Service Office of Research, Statistics, and Technology, no. 59, March 28, 1980.
16. Martinez G.A., Nalezienski J.P.: The recent trend in breast-feeding. *Pediatrics* 64 (5):686, 1979.
17. Jensen R.L., Thomas L.N., Bergmann K.E., et al.: Composition of milk of Iowa City women. Unpublished data, 1972.

18. Filer L.J. Jr.: Citation of unpublished data of Gilbert A. Martinez, Ross Laboratories, 1970, in Fomon S.J., et al. (eds): *Practices of Low-Income Families in Feeding Infants and Small Children with Particular Attention to Cultural Subgroups.* DGEW/HSMHA. Publ. No. 725605. Washington, D.C.: Maternal & Child Health Services, 1972.
19. Purvis G.A.: Nutritional values, carbohydrate content of infant foods and beverages. Iowa City: Symposium on Dental Nutrition, 1978.
20. Anonymous: Food for thought. *Heinz Baby Food Newsletter* 1 (1)(No date).
21. Anonymous: Personal correspondence. Heinz U.S.A., Division of H.J. Heinz Company.
22. Havlik R.J., et al.: Proceedings of the Conference on the Decline in Coronary Heart Disease Mortality. Bethesda, Maryland, 1979.
23. Fomon S.J.: *Infant Nutrition,* ed 2. Philadelphia: W.B. Saunders Co., 1974.
24. Johansson C.: Studies of gastrointestinal interactions: VII. Characteristics of the absorption pattern of sugar, fat and protein from composite meals in man. A quantitative study. *Scand. J. Gastroenterol.* 10(1):33, 1975.
25. McMichael H.B.: Absorption of carbohydrates, in McColl I., et al. (eds): *Intestinal Absorption in Man.* London: Academic Press, 1975, pp 99–141.
26. Ugolev A.M.: Membrane (contact) digestion. *Physiol. Rev.* 45:555, 1965.
27. Dyck W.P., Bonnet D., Lasator J., et al.: Hormonal stimulation of intestinal disaccharidase release in the dog. *Gastroenterology* 66:533, 1974.
28. Gibson J.A., Sladen G.E., Dawson A.M.: Protein absorption and ammonia production: The effects of dietary protein and removal of the colon. *Br. J. Nutr.* 35(1):61, 1976.
29. Maestracci D., Preiser H., Hedges T., et al.: Enzymes of the human intestinal brush border membrane: Identification after gel electrophoretic separation. *Biochim. Biophys. Acta* 382(2):147, 1975.
30. Schmitz J., Preiser H., Maestracci D., et al.: Purification of the human intestinal brush border membrane. *Biochim. Biophys. Acta* 323:98, 1973.
31. Welsh J.D., Preiser H., Woodley J.F., et al.: An enriched microvillus membrane preparation from frozen specimens of human small intestine. *Gastroenterology* 62:572, 1972.
32. Kelly J.J., Alpers D.H.: Properties of human intestinal glucoamylase. *Biochim. Biophys. Acta* 315:113, 1973.
33. Coklin K.A., Yamashiro K.M., Gray G.M.: Human intestinal sucrase-isomaltase: Identification of free sucrase and isomaltase and cleavage of the hybrid into active distinct subunits. *J. Biol. Chem.* 250(15):5735, 1975.
34. Filer L.J. Jr.: Modified food starches for use in infant foods. *Nutr. Rev.* 29:55, 1971.
35. Lebenthal E.: Use of modified food starches in infant nutrition. *Am. J. Dis. Child.* 132:850, 1978.
36. DeVizia B., Ciccimarra F., DeCicco N., et al.: Digestibilty of starches in infants and children. *J. Pediatr.* 86:50, 1975.
37. Conway R.L., Hood L.F.: Pancreatic α-amylase hydrolysis products of modified and unmodified tapioca starches. *Die Starke* 28:341, 1976.
38. Banks W., Greenwood C.T., Mair D.D.: Studies on hydroxyethyl starch. *DieStarke* 24:181, 1972.
39. Anderson T.A., Fomon S.J., Filer L.J.: Carbohydrate tolerance studies with 3 day old infants. *J. Lab. Clin. Med.* 79:31, 1972.
40. Committee on Nutrition: Safety and suitability of modified starches for use in baby food: The subcommittee on the evaluation of the safety of modified starches in infant foods. Houston: American Academy of Pediatrics, 1977.
41. Auricchio S., Della Pietra D., Vegnente A.: Studies on intestinal digestion of starches in man: II. Intestinal hydrolysis of amylopectin in infants and children. *Pediatrics* 39:853, 1967.

42. Keene M.F.L., Hewer E.E.: Digestive enzymes of the human fetus. *Lancet* 1:766, 1929.
43. Wolf R.O., Taussig L.M.: Human amniotic fluid isoamylases. *Obstet. Gynecol.* 41:337, 1973.
44. Auricchio S., Rubio A., Murset G.: Intestinal glycosidase activities with human embryo, foetus and newborn. *Pediatrics* 35:944, 1965.
45. Klumpp T.G., Neale A.V.: The gastric and duodenal contents of normal infants and children. *Am. J. Dis. Child.* 40:1215, 1930.
46. Shwachman H., Leubner H.: Mucoviscidosis. *Adv. Pediatr.* 7:249, 1955.
47. Zoppi G., Andreotti G., Pajno-Ferrara F., et al.: Exocrine pancreas function in premature and full term neonates. *Pediatr. Res.* 6:880, 1972.
48. Lebenthal E., Lee P.C.: Development of functional response in human exocrine pancreas. *Pediatrics.* 66:556, 1980.
49. Delachaume-Salem E., Sarles H.:Évolution en fonction de l'age de la sécrétion pancréatique humaine normale. *Biol. Gastroenterol.* (Paris)2:135, 1970.
50. Track N.S., Cretzfeldt C., Bokemann M.: Enzymatic functional and structural development of the exocrine pancreas: II. The human pancreas. *Comp. Biochem. Physiol.* 51A:95, 1975.
51. Eggermont E.: Hydrolysis of the naturally occurring α-glucosides by the human intestinal mucosa. *Eur. J. Biochem.* 9:483, 1969.
52. Lebenthal E., Lee P.C.: Glucoamylase and disaccharidase activities in normal subjects and in patients with mucosa injury of the small intestine. *J. Pediatr.* 97:389, 1980.
53. Lebenthal E.: Lactose intolerance, in Lebenthal E. (ed): *Digestive Disease in Children.* New York: Grune & Stratton, 1978, pp 367–388.
54. Leblond C.P., Walker B.E.: Renewal of cell populations. *Physiol. Rev.* 36:255, 1956.
55. Messier B., Leblond C.P.: Cell proliferation and migration as revealed by radioautography after injection of thymidine H₃ into male rats and mice. *Am. J. Anat.* 106:247, 1960.
56. Cheng H., Leblond C.P.: Origin, differentiation and renewal of the four main epithelial cell types in the mouse small intestine: I. Columnar cell. *Am. J. Anat.* 141(4):461, 1974.
57. Eichholz A.: Structural and functional organization of the brush border of intestinal epithelial cells: 3. Enzymic activities and chemical composition of various fractions of tris-disrupted brush borders. *Biochim. Biophys. Acta* 135:475, 1967.
58. Eichholz A.: Studies on the organization of the brush border in intestinal epithelial cells: V. Subfractionation of enzymatic activities of the microvillus membrane. *Biochim. Biophys. Acta* 163:101, 1968.
59. Crane R.K., Holmes R.: Protein turnover in the digestive-absorptive surface (brush border membrane) of the rat small intestine. *J. Physiol. (Lond.)* 197:79, 1968.
60. James W.P., Alpers D.H., Gerber J.E., et al.: The turnover of disaccharidases and brush border proteins in rat intestine. *Biochim. Biophys. Acta* 230:194, 1971.
61. Kedinger M., Hauri H.P., Haffen J., et al.: Turnover studies of human intestinal brush border membrane glycoprotein in organ culture. *Enzyme* 24:96, 1979.
62. Alpers D.H.: The relation of size to the relative rates of degradation on intestinal brush border proteins. *J. Clin. Invest.* 51:2621, 1972.
63. Alpers D.H., Tedesco F.J.: The possible role of pancreatic proteases in the turnover of intestinal brush border proteins. *Biochim. Biophys. Acta* 401:28, 1975.
64. Caspary W.F., Winckler K., Lankisch P.G., et al.: Influence of exocrine and endocrine pancreatic function on intestinal brush border enzymatic activities. *Gut* 16:89, 1975.
65. Crane R.K.: Digestion and absorption: Water-soluble organics. *Int. Rev. Physiol.* 12:325, 1977.

66. Saito M., Murakami E., Suda M.: Circadian rhythms in disaccharidases of rat small intestine and its relation to food intake. *Biochim. Biophys. Acta* 421:177, 1976.
67. Antonowicz I., Milunsky A., Lebenthal E., et al.: Disaccharidase and lysosomal enzyme activities in amniotic fluid, intestinal mucosa and meconium: Correlation between morphology and disaccharidase activities in human fetal small intestine. *Biol. Neonate* 32:280, 1977.
68. Caspary W.F., Winckler K., Creutzfeldt W.: Intestinal brush border enzyme activity in juvenile and maturity onset diabetes mellitus. *Diabetologia* 10(4):353, 1974.
69. Alpers D.H., Isselbacher K.J.: Disaccharidase deficiency. *Adv. Metab. Disord.* 4:75, 1970.
70. Nishida T., Saito M., Suda M.: Parallel between circadian rhythms of intestinal disaccharidases and food intake of rats under constant lighting conditions. *Gastroenterology* 74(2, pt 1):224, 1978.
71. Gracey M., Houghton M., Thomas J.: Deoxycholate depresses small-intestinal enzyme activity. *Gut* 16(1):53, 1975.
72. Hermos J.A., Mathan M., Trier J.S.,: DNA synthesis and proliferation by villous epithelial cells in fetal rats. *J. Cell Biol.* 50:255, 1971.
73. Newcomer A.D., McGill D.B.: Distribution of disaccharidase activity in the small bowel of normal and lactose-deficient subjects. *Gastroenterology* 51(4):481, 1966.
74. Hansen H.T., Drube H.C., Klein U.E., et al.: Untersuchungen über Muster und Verteilung von Enzymen in der Schleimhaut des Gastrointestinaltraktes:I. Über den normalen Disaccharidasen-Gehalt in Duodenum von Erwachseney. *Gastroenterologia (Basel)* 106:345, 1966.
75. Antonowicz I., Chang S.K., Grand R.J.: Development and distribution of lysosomal enzymes and disaccharidases in human fetal intestine. *Gastroenterology* 67:51, 1974.
76. Auricchio S., Ciccimarra F., Vegnente A., et al.: Enzymatic activity hydrolyzing-glutamyl-naphthylamide in human intestine during adult and fetal life. *Pediatr. Res.* 7:95, 1973.
77. Sheehy T.W., Anderson P.R.: Fetal disaccharidases. *Am. J. Dis. Child* 121:464, 1971.
78. Rubino A., Zimbalatti F., Auricchio S.: Intestinal disaccharidase activities in adult and suckling rats. *Biochim. Biophys. Acta* 92:305, 1964.
79. Dahlqvist A.: Intestinal carbohydrase of a new-born pig. *Nature (Lond.)* 190:31, 1961.
80. Huber J.T., Jacobson N.L., Allen R.S., et al.: *J. Dairy Sci.* 44:1494, 1961.
81. Tutton R.J., Helme R.D.: The influence of adrenoreceptor activity on crypt cell proliferation in the rat jejunum. *Cell Tissue Kinet.* 7:125, 1974.
82. Roberts M.C., Hill F.W., Kidder D.E.: The development and distribution of small intestinal disaccharidases in the horse. *Res. Vet. Sci.* 17(1):42, 1974.
83. Koldovsky O., Sunshine P., Kretchmer N.: The digestion of carbohydrates during postnatal development. *Gastroenterology* 50:596, 1966.
84. Dahlqvist A., Lindberg T.: Development of the intestinal disaccharidase and alkaline phosphatase activities in the human foetus. *Clin. Sci.* 30:517, 1966.
85. Antonowicz I., Lebenthal E.: Developmental pattern of small intestinal enterokinase and disaccharidase activities in the human fetus. *Gastroenterology* 72:(6):1299, 1977.
86. Hellier M.D., Holdsworth C.D.: Digestion and absorption of proteins, in McColl I., et al. (eds): *Intestinal Absorption in Man.* London: Academic Press, 1975.
87. Biederdorf F.A., Morawski S., Fordtran J.S.: Effect of sodium, mannitol, and magnesium on glucose, galactose, 3-0-methylglucose, and fructose absorption in the human ileum. *Gastroenterology* 68:58, 1975.
88. Holdsworth C.D.: The absorption of monosaccharides in man. M.D. Thesis, University of Leeds, 1964.

89. Debnam E.S., Levin R.J.: Influence of specific dietary sugars on the jejunal mechanisms for glucose, galactose, and α-methylglucoside absorption: Evidence for multiple sugar carriers. *Gut* 17:92, 1976.
90. Gracey M., Burke V., Oshin A.: Active intestinal transport of D-fructose. *Biochim. Biophys. Acta* 266:397, 1972.
91. Malathi P., Ramaswamy K., Malathi P., et al.: Studies on the transport of glucose from disaccharides by hamster small intestine in vitro: I. Evidence of a disaccharidase-related transport system. *Biochim. Biophys. Acta* 307:613, 1973.
92. Ramaswamy K., Maltathi P., Caspary W.F., et al.: Studies on the transport of glucose from disaccharides by hamster small intestine in vitro: II. Characteristics of the disaccharidase-related transport system. *Biochim. Biophys. Acta* 345:39, 1974.
93. Sandle G.I., Lobley R.W., Holmes R.: Effect of maltose on the absorption of glucose in the jejunum of man. *Gut* 18:A944, 1977.
94. Koldovsky O., Heingova A., Jerosova V., et al.: Transport of glucose against a concentration gradient in everted sacs of jejunum and ileum of human fetus. *Gastroenterology* 48:185, 1965.
95. Levin R.J., Koldovsky O., Hoskova J., et al.: Electrical activity across human foetal small intestine associated with absorption process. *Gut* 9:206, 1968.
96. Pildes R.S., Hart R.J., Warren R., Cornblath M.: Plasma insulin response during oral glucose tolerance tests in newborns of normal and gestational diabetic mothers. *Pediatrics* 44:76, 1969.
97. Bohiner S.W., Beard A.G., Panos T.C.: Impairment of intestinal hydrolysis of lactose in newborn infants. *Pediatrics* 38:542, 1965.
98. Younoszai M.K.: Jejunal absorption of hexose in infants and adults. *J. Pediatr.* 85:446, 1974.
99. Fordtran J.S., Ingelfinger E.J.: Absorption of water, electrolytes and sugars from the human gut, in Code C.F. (ed): *Handbook of Physiology.* Washington, D.C.: American Physiological Society, vol. 3 and 6, pp 1457–1490.
100. Koldovsky O.: Digestion and absorption, in Stove V. (ed): *Perinatal Physiology.* New York: Plenum Publishing Corp., 1977.
101. Hawkins K.: Pediatric xylose absorption test measurements in blood preferable to measurement in urine. *Clin. Chem.* 16:749, 1970.
102. Beyreiss K., Rautenbach M., Willgerodt H., et al.: Besonde Lecten der Resorpton und das stoffwechsels von Kohlerhydraten bei Frah und Neugeboreneir. *Wiess. I. Friedrich Schuller Univ. Jena Math. Natarwiss. Reihe* 21:683, 1972.
103. Jacobi A.: Milk-sugar in infant feeding. *Trans. Am. Pediatr. Soc.* 13:150, 1901.
104. Howland J.: Prolonged intolerance to carbohydrates. *Trans. Am. Pediatr. Soc.* 38:393, 1921.
105. Townley R.R.: Disaccharidase deficiency in infancy and childhood. *Pediatrics* 38:127, 1966.
106. Gray G.M., Conklin K.A., Townley R.R.: Sucrose-isomaltase deficiency: Absence of an inactive enzyme variant. *N. Engl. J. Med.* 294 (14):750, 1976.
107. Kerry K.R., Townley R.R.: Genetic aspects of intestinal sucrase isomaltase deficiency. *Aust. Paediatr. J.* 1:223, 1965.
108. Holzel A.: Defects of sugar absorption: Sugar malabsorption and sugar intolerance in childhood. *Proc. R. Soc. Lond. (Med.)* 61:1095, 1968.
109. Darling S., Mortensen O., Sondergaard G.: Lactosuria and amino-aciduria in infancy: A new inborn error of metabolism? *Acta Paediatr. Scand.* 49:281, 1960.
110. Madzarovova-Nohejlova J.: Trchalase deficiency in a family. *Gastroenterology* 65:130, 1973.
111. Asp N.G., Dahlqvist A.: Intestinal β-galactosidases in adult low lactase activity and in congenital lactase deficiency. *Enzyme* 18:84, 1974.
112. Asp N.G., Dahlqvist A., Kuitunen P., et al.: Complete deficiency of brush-border lactase in congenital lactose malabsorption. *Lancet* 2:329, 1973.

113. Levin B., Abraham J.M., Burgess E.A., et al.: Congenital lactose malabsorption. *Arch. Dis. Child.* 45:173, 1970.
114. Dawson A.M.: The absorption of disaccharides, in Card W.I., et al. (eds): Modern Trends in Gastroenterology, London: Butterworths, 1970, vol 4, pp 105–124.
115. Neal G.: Disaccharidase deficiencies. *J. Clin. Pathol.* 5:22, 1971.
116. Simoons F.J.: Progress report: New light on ethnic differences in adult lactose intolerance. *Am. J. Dig. Dis.* 18:595, 1973.
117. Simoons F.J.: Primary adult lactose intolerance and the milking habit: A problem in biological and cultural interrelations. II. A culture historical hypothesis. *Am. J. Dig. Dis.* 15:695, 1970.
118. Lebenthal E., Tsuboi K., Kretchmer N.: Characterization of human intestinal lactase and hetero-β-galactosidases in infants and adults. *Gastroenterology* 67:1107, 1974.
119. Lebenthal E., Sunshine P., Kretchmer N.: Effect of carbohydrate and corticosteroids on activity of α-glucosidases in intestine of the infant rat. *J. Clin. Invest.* 34:38, 1972.
120. Plotkin G.R., Isselbacher K.J.: Secondary disaccharidase deficiency in adult celiac disease and other malabsorption states. *N. Engl. J. Med.* 271:1033, 1964.
121. Gray G.M., Walter W.M. Jr., Colver E.H.: Persistent deficiency of intestinal lactase in apparently cured tropical sprue. *Gastroenterology* 54:552, 1968.
122. Sunshine P., Kretchmer N.: Studies of small intestine during development: III. Infantile diarrhea associated with intolerance to disaccharides. *Pediatrics* 34:38, 1964.
123. Lebenthal E., Antonowicz I., Shwachman H.: The interrelationship of enterokinase and trypsin activities in intractable diarrhea of infancy, celiac disease and intravenous alimentation. *Pediatrics* 56(4):585, 1975.
124. Paes I.C., Searl P., Rubert M.W., et al.: Intestinal lactase deficiency and saccharide malabsorption during oral neomycin administration. *Gastroenterology* 53:49, 1967.
125. Branski D., Lebenthal E., Freeman A.I., et al.: Effect of leukemia and methotrexate on digestive enzymes in the jejunum of mice. *Digestion.* In press.
126. Herbst J.J., Sunshine P.: Postnatal development of the small intestine of the rat: Changes in mucosal morphology at weaning. *Pediatr. Res.* 3:27, 1969.
127. Welsh J.D., Shaw R.W., Walker A.: Isolated lactase deficiency producing postgastrectomy milk intolerance. *Ann. Intern. Med.* 64:1253, 1966.
128. McNeill L.K., Hamilton J.R.: The effect of fasting on disaccharidase activity in the rat small intestine. *Pediatrics* 47:65, 1971.
129. Cook G.C., Lee F.D.: The jejunum after kwashiorkor. *Lancet* 2:1263, 1966.
130. Lebenthal E.: Small intestinal disaccharidase deficiencies. *Pediatr. Clin. North Am.* 22(4):757, 1975.
131. Weser E., Rubin W., Ross L., et al.: Lactase deficiency in patients with the "irritable-colon syndrome." *N. Engl. J. Med.* 273:1070, 1965.
132. Anderson A.F.R.: Ulcerative colitis an allergic phenomenon. *Am. J. Dig. Dis.* 9:91, 1942.
133. Frazer A.C., Hood C., Montgomery R.D., et al.: Carbohydrate intolerance in ulcerative colitis. *Lancet* 1:503, 1966.
134. Chalfin D., Holt P.R.: Lactase deficiency in ulcerative colitis, regional enteritis and viral hepatitis. *Am. J. Dig. Dis.* 12:81, 1967.
135. Welsh J.D.: Isolated lactase deficiency in humans: Report on 100 patients. *Medicine (Baltimore)* 49:257, 1970.
136. Preger L., Amberg J.R.: Sweet diarrhea: Roentgen diagnosis of disaccharidase deficiency. *Am. J. Roentgenol.* 101:287, 1967.
137. Rosenquist C.J., Heaton J.W., Friedland G.W., et al.: Assessment of a radiographic method for diagnosis of intestinal lactase deficiency: A prospective study. *Invest. Radiol.* 6:40, 1971.

138. Newcomer A.D., McGill D.B., Thomas P.J., et al.: Prospective comparison of indirect methods for detecting lactase deficiency. *N. Engl. J. Med.* 293(24):1232, 1975.
139. Newcomer A.D., Thomas P.J., McGill D.B., et al.: Lactase deficiency: A common genetic trait of the American Indian. *Gastroenterology* 72(2):234, 1977.
140. Johnson N.W.: Aetiology of dental disease and theoretical aspects of dietary control. *J. Hum. Nutr.* 33:98, 1979.
141. Nordsiek F.W.: The sweet tooth. *Am. Sci.* 60:41, 1972.
142. Nisbett R.E.: Hunger, obesity, and the ventromedial hyperthalamus. *Psychol. Rev.* 79:433, 1972.
143. Nisbett R.E.: Taste, deprivation, and weight determinants of eating behavior. *J. Pers. Soc. Psychol.* 10:107, 1968.
144. Price J.M., Grinker J.: Effect of degree of obesity, food deprivation, and palatability on eating behavior of humans. *J. Comp. Physiol. Psychol.* 85:265, 1973.
145. Grinker J.: Obesity and sweet taste. *Am. J. Clin. Nutr.* 31(6):1078, 1978.
146. Keene H.: The incomplete story of obesity and diabetes, in Howard A. (ed): *Recent Advances in Obesity Research: Proceedings of the First International Congress on Obesity.* London, 1975, pp 116–127.
147. Keys A.: The diet and plasma lipids in the etiology of coronary heart disease, in Russek, et al.: *Coronary Heart Disease,* Philadelphia: 1971, pp 59–75.
148. Hatch F.T.: Interactions between nutrition and heredity in coronary heart disease. *Am. J. Clin. Nutr.* 27:80, 1974.
149. Inter-Society Commission for Heart Disease Resources Report: Primary prevention of the atherosclerotic diseases. *Circulation* 42:1, 1970.
150. The American Heart Association: The national diet—Heart study, final report. *Circulation* 37(suppl 1): 1, 1968.
151. Connor W.E., Connor S.L.: The key role of nutritional factors in the prevention of coronary heart disease. *Prev. Med.* 1:49, 1972.
152. Glueck C.J., McGill H.C. Jr., Shank R.E., et al.: Value and safety of diet modification to control hyperlipidemia in childhood and adolescence: A statement for physicians. Ad Hoc Committee of the Steering Committee for Medical and Community Program of the American Heart Association. *Circulation* 58(2):381A, 1978.
153. Cohen A.M.: Fats and carbohydrates as factors in atherosclerosis and diabetes in Yemenite Jews. *Am. Heart. J.* 65:291, 1963.
154. Yudkin J.: Diet and coronary thrombosis: Hypothesis and fact. *Lancet* 2:155, 1957.
155. Yudkin J.: Nutrition and palatability with special reference to obesity, myocardial infarction, and other diseases of civilization. *Lancet* 1:1335, 1963.
156. Yudkin J.: Dietary fat and dietary sugar in relation to ischaemic heart disease and diabetes. *Lancet* 2:4, 1964.
157. Yudkin J.: Dietetic aspects of atherosclerosis. *Angiology* 17:127, 1966.
158. Yudkin J.: Evolutionary and historical changes in dietary carbohydrates. *Am. J. Clin. Nutr.* 20:108, 1967.
159. Tamir I., Epstein D., Heldenberg D., et al.: Serum lipids during short-term high glucose and high sucrose feeding in infants. *Pediatrics* 50:84, 1972.
160. Andersen G.E., Lifschitz E., Friis-Hansen B.: Dietary habits and serum lipids during first four years of life. *Acta Paediatr. Scand.* 68:165, 1979.
161. Weidman W.H., Elveback L.R., Nelson R.A., et al.: Nutrient intake and serum cholesterol level in normal children 6 to 16 years of age. *Pediatrics* 61(3):354, 1978.
162. Frank G.C., Berenson G.S., Webber L.S.: Dietary studies and the relationship of diet to cardiovascular disease risk factor variables in 10-year-old children—The Bogalusa Heart Study. *Am. J. Clin. Nutr.* 31(2):328, 1978.

163. Morrison J.A., Larsen R., Glatfelter L., et al.: Interrelationships between nutrient intake and plasma lipids and lipoproteins in school children aged 6 to 19: The Princeton School District study. *Pediatrics* 65:727, 1980.
164. Southgate D.A., Durnin J.V.: Calorie conversion factors: An experimental reassessment of the factors used in the calculation of the energy value of human diets. *Br. J. Nutr.* 24:517, 1970.
165. Eastwood M.A., Hamilton D.: Studies on the absorption of bile salts to non-absorbed components of diet. Biochim. Biophys. Acta 152:165, 1968.
166. Jenkins D.J., Wolever T.M., Leeds A.R., et al.: Dietary fibres, fibre analogues, and glucose tolerance: Importance of viscosity. *Br. Med. J.* 1:1392, 1978.

Infant Botulism

LAWRENCE W. BROWN, M.D.

Section of Child Neurology
St. Christopher's Hospital for Children
Temple University School of Medicine
Philadelphia, Pennsylvania

BOTULISM is an acute disruption of neuromuscular transmission produced by a powerful toxin elaborated by the anaerobic spore-forming *Clostridium botulinum*. Until recently, most recognized cases of botulinogenic disease were caused by ingestion of preformed toxin in contaminated food.[10] Rarely, introduction of botulinal organisms into traumatized skin wounds has led to bacterial growth and production of the toxin.[29] Infant botulism is a newly-described disorder in which intraintestinal growth of the organisms and systemic absorption of the toxin they produce result in a clinical syndrome of weakness, hypotonia, and respiratory depression.[2, 36]

The source of these organisms is frequently unclear, but botulinogenic spores are widely distributed in nature. Infant botulism is not a new disease, but rather is a newly recognized manifestation of a familiar disorder.[5] Since the first description of infant botulism in 1976,[33] there have been over 200 confirmed cases throughout the United States as well as individual reports from England and Australia.[43, 38] The incidence of infant botulism is uncertain, probably due to the lack of an adequate level of suspicion and recognition. Clinical support of the diagnosis rests on electrophysiologic studies not frequently employed in sick infants. Definitive diagnosis requires a sophisticated microbiology laboratory capable of clostridia identification.

Paralytic disease following consumption of contaminated

0065-3101/81/0028-141-157-$03.75

food has been recognized since the days of the Roman Empire. In fact, the name botulism derives from the Latin word for sausage. In 1895, Van Ermengen isolated a spore-forming anaerobe following an outbreak of food poisoning that caused three deaths. The organism he labeled *Bacillus botulinum* was isolated from the spleen of one victim and from contaminated ham.[45] In the ensuing years, botulism became recognized as a leading cause of food poisoning. The Center for Disease Control documented almost 1,800 cases of such poisoning in the 75-year period between 1899 and 1973 with a mortality rate of over 50%.[10] Major offending food sources included vegetables, fish products, and preserved fruits. Condiments, including honey, accounted for only 8% of these cases.

Clinical Features

The typical clinical syndrome of infant botulism is characterized by variable constipation followed by progressive weakness, hypotonia, cranial nerve dysfunction and hyporeflexia,[25] as shown in Table 1. Constipation (frequency of stools less than every 48 hours) is found in almost every instance, and it may precede the neuromuscular syndrome by as long as three

TABLE 1.—SIGNS AND SYMPTOMS IN
HOSPITALIZED PEDIATRIC PATIENTS

Autonomic dysfunction
  Constipation
  Neurogenic bladder
  Hypertension
Hypotonia and weakness
  Decreased resistance to passive motion
  Lack of spontaneous motor activity
  Motor response to noxious stimuli diminished
  Poor head control
Cranial nerve dysfunction
  Decreased suck and swallow ability
  Weak cry
  Facial diplegia
  External ophthalmoplegia
  Sluggishly reactive pupils
Absent or diminished deep tendon reflexes
Respiratory insufficiency
  Associated with progressive weakness and cranial
    nerve dysfunction
  Provoked by postural manipulation for procedures

weeks. Once apparent, weakness usually progresses rapidly within one to three days. The first signs of generalized weakness are a paucity of spontaneous movements and diminished response to noxious stimuli. Hypotonia refers only to decreased resistance to passive movement, and parallels the weakness. Cranial nerve dysfunction almost always includes diminished gag reflex and poor sucking ability. Other motor cranial nerve involvement may include facial weakness, ptosis, extraocular palsies, and sluggish pupillary light response. Deep tendon reflexes may be present initially, but tend to diminish or disappear within several days.

The preceding clinical description is characteristic of hospitalized infants eventually documented to have botulinogenic infection. The clinical spectrum of the disease, however, includes mild neuromuscular involvement, constipation without recognized weakness, and fulminant neuromuscular failure leading to sudden death. Two infants evaluated as outpatients for "failure to thrive" and poor sucking abilities were later shown to have infant botulism.[1] Two others with only constipation had stool specimens with botulinogenic growth, one of whom had evidence of botulinal toxin production.[1] The relationship between infant botulism and the sudden infant death syndrome (SIDS) is intriguing, and a discussion can be found later in this chapter.

Differential Diagnosis

The typical clinical sequence of constipation followed by weakness, hyporeflexia, and cranial nerve dysfunction in infants under one year of age strongly suggests the diagnosis of infant botulism (Table 2). The nonspecificity of these signs also suggests an extensive differential diagnosis that includes sepsis with or without meningitis.[8] This is the most common initial impression in these acutely ill infants. Alertness despite profound weakness is characteristic of infant botulism, but unusual in sepsis or meningitis. Multiple cranial nerve dysfunction and areflexia are also unusual in common infectious states.

Other possible etiologies for reversible neuromuscular weakness without other specific features include alterations in monovalent or divalent cation homeostasis (sodium, potassium, cal-

TABLE 2.—DIFFERENTIAL DIAGNOSIS OF INFANT
BOTULISM

Systemic
  Sepsis/meningitis
  Electrolyte/mineral imbalance
  Metabolic encephalopathy
  Reye's syndrome
  Intoxication—organophosphates, heavy metals
  Hypothyroidism
  Subacute necrotizing encephalomyelitis
  Organic acidurias
Neuromuscular
  Poliomyelitis
  Infantile spinal muscular atrophy
  Acute polyneuropathy—Guillain-Barré syndrome,
    diphtheria
  Tick paralysis
  Congenital myasthenia gravis
  Muscular dystrophy—"congenital," myotonic dystrophy
  Congenital myopathy

cium, magnesium). Weakness and hypotonia in this age group
may represent the only manifestations of uremic or hepatic encephalopathy, but these may be rapidly excluded by appropriate laboratory studies. Profound weakness, hypotonia, and cranial nerve dysfunction may be seen in disorders of amino acid
metabolism. Reye's syndrome occurs rarely in infancy and can
be distinguished by hypoglycemia, hepatomegaly, hyperammo-
nemia, seizures, and a history of preceding infection.[23] Intoxication by heavy metals such as lead or arsenic can present with
encephalopathy, but cranial nerve dysfunction is rare. Organophosphate poisoning at this age has been reported, but the
characteristic findings of salivation, lacrimation, diaphoresis,
fasciculations, miosis, and seizures are not seen in infant botulism. Hypothyroidism is sometimes considered because of the
constellation of weakness and constipation, but dry skin, coarse
hair, umbilical hernia, and hoarse cry are unique to the endo-
crinopathy. Subacute necrotizing encephalomyelitis (Leigh's
disease) is a chronic progressive disease also characterized by
hypotonia, weakness, and ophthalmoplegia. However, lactic
acidosis, convulsions, blindness, and hearing loss are not found
with infant botulism.[35] Other organic acidoses may present
with hypotonia and require identification of the metabolic defect.

One must consider not only systemic illness but also diseases of the spinal cord, nerve, neuromuscular junction, and muscle in the differential diagnosis. Poliomyelitis may present with bulbar signs, somatic weakness, and areflexia. However, the weakness of poliomyelitis is often asymmetric and follows aseptic meningitis. A normal lumbar puncture without pleocytosis strongly leads away from a diagnosis of poliomyelitis. Infantile spinal muscular atrophy (Werdnig-Hoffmann disease) may occasionally appear acute in onset.[34] Hypotonia, weakness are-flexia, and tongue fasciculations are common features, but extraocular palsies, poorly reactive pupils, and ptosis are rare. Acute polyneuropathy (Guillain-Barré syndrome) is rare in the first year of life, but the clinical syndrome of progressive weakness and bulbar involvement may be indistinguishable from infant botulism.[9] Supporting the diagnosis of acute polyneuropathy are a preceding illness, symmetric weakness starting in the lower extremities, elevation of cerebrospinal protein concentration, and electrophysiologic findings demonstrating abnormalities of peripheral nerve. It is ironic to note that within a year of the era of fecal analysis for botulism, a series of nine infants were described with "idiopathic reversible acute polyneuropathy and cranial nerve dysfunction," primarily on the basis of exclusion of other likely diagnoses.[21] The histories and clinical course of these infants suggest infant botulism; several even demonstrate antecedent constipation.

Other toxic polyneuropathies include diphtheria and tick paralysis. Diphtheritic polyneuropathy follows a pharyngeal infection, and cranial nerve involvement usually precedes generalized muscular weakness. Even chronic polyneuropathies may present with hypotonia and acute respiratory distress.[31] Tick paralysis can persist only as long as the pregnant arthropod elaborates neurotoxin, and failure to locate the tick excludes the diagnosis. Familial infantile myasthenia gravis may present with sudden death.[15] Congenital myasthenia gravis in the absence of maternal disease and occurring beyond the immediate newborn period is a rare disease that may be difficult to distinguish from botulism.[20] One distinctive finding in congenital myasthenia is diurnal variability of weakness, swallowing dysfunction, and ptosis. The marked improvement in weakness following administration of edrophonium chloride or neostigmine and the abnormal decremental response to slow rate of repetitive nerve stimulation are characteristic of infantile myasthenia. As with infantile spinal muscular atrophy, congenital myopathies, myotonic dystrophy, and congenital dystrophy generally present with static weakness, hypotonia, and lack of bulbar involvement.

Laboratory Diagnosis

Electrodiagnostic abnormalities are the only relatively specific findings in infant botulism, short of bacteriologic isolation. Routine studies, including a hemogram, tests for electrolytes, calcium, magnesium, blood urea nitrogen, and hepatic enzymes, lumbar puncture, and a chest x-ray, are usually normal, but may be altered by secondary dehydration or pneumonitis. Special studies performed on infants suspected of botulism should include edrophonium chloride or neostigmine testing for myasthenia gravis, screening tests for heavy metals and organophosphate poisoning when clinically suspected, and electrodiagnostic tests. Needle electromyography in botulism usually demonstrates brief small-amplitude, abundant motor unit potentials.[2, 18] This is a pattern rarely seen in other infantile con-

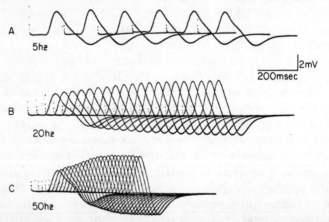

Fig 1.—"Staircase phenomenon" demonstrating marked augmentation of evoked muscle action potential at supratetanic rates of stimulation. In normal infants there is no change in amplitude of response at low or high rates of stimulation. In myasthenia gravis, there is a decremental response with subtetanic repetitive stimulation. A, In the affected infant no change in amplitude is noted at subtetanic rates. B, Supratetanic rates of repetitive nerve stimulation produce an 87% augmentation at 20 Hz. C, 171% increase is produced at 50 Hz.

ditions. The most characteristic electrophysiologic abnormality in botulism is the staircase phenomenon (Fig 1), a marked augmentation of the amplitude of evoked muscle action potential with supratetanic rates of nerve stimulation.[11] Other disorders that produce a similar incremental response include the Eaton-Lambert syndrome, antibiotic toxicity, and snakebite poisoning. Infants with botulism have a normal response at stimulation rates of two to five cycles per second (as seen when they are given the Jolly test), unlike the decremental response seen in myasthenia gravis. The normal motor and sensory conduction velocities help to exclude the Guillain-Barré syndrome and other syndromes of acute polyneuritis.

Confirmation of the clinical diagnosis of infant botulism requires isolation of the organism or demonstration of specific toxin in stool samples. Only rarely is the serum positive for organisms or toxin, in contrast to the "adult" botulism syndromes. Prolonged constipation may make adequate stool collection exceedingly difficult and saline enemas may facilitate the collection of an adequate specimen. Despite clinical improvement, isolation of toxin and organisms may persist for weeks to months.

Epidemiology of Infant Botulism

Botulinogenic spores are widely distributed in soil throughout the world. In the United States, type A organisms are found predominantly west of the Mississippi River, and type B organisms east of it.[40] Outbreaks of foodborne and wound botulism generally reflect this distribution of the spores in the soil. Most botulinogenic outbreaks in Europe have been type B. Type E is most common in Japan.

California has always reported the highest number of U.S. cases of foodborne and infant botulism. This may reflect longstanding physician interest and better botulism surveillance. Supporting this hypothesis is a relative decline in California from 80% of all U.S. cases of infant botulism in 1976 to 32% in 1978, as the disease gained widespread attention in the scientific literature and lay press. It is interesting to note that despite overwhelming soil predominance of type A organisms in California, 40% of that state's cases of infant botulism have been caused by Type B.[4] Other major sites of infant botulism include Utah and the Philadelphia area. Together with California, these areas account for over 75% of confirmed cases.

The age at onset of symptoms has ranged from three weeks to eight months. All but two patients had the onset of symptoms under six months of age. No cases have occurred in family or neighborhood clusters. Honey is the only food source strongly correlated with infant botulism.[4] Preliminary data suggests a protective role of breast-feeding, since all patients with a botulism-related SIDS were bottle-fed.[3] In addition, the age of onset of disease in breast-fed hospital patients was later than that of bottle-fed infants.

Honey is a common source of *C. botulinum* spores, but not of preformed botulinal toxin.[7] Approximately 10% of raw samples obtained throughout the United States contain botulinogenic spores. In a California study, five infants with botulism had eaten honey from which botulinogenic organisms and toxin of identical type (A or B) were subsequently isolated.[4] Prior exposure to honey was significantly greater in victims of type B infant botulism than in age-matched controls. The lack of exposure to honey with type A botulism in this sample suggests other sources of pore exposure. Indeed, botulinogenic spores concordant with disease type have been isolated in soil samples and household dust from the home environment of other affected infants. In the vast majority of patients, however, no source has been identified for preformed toxin or spores.

Management

Current management of infant botulism consists of supportive respiratory and nutritional care. The limited mortality in patients hospitalized with infant botulism has been caused by pulmonary complications. Such hazards include aspiration pneumonia, respiratory arrest secondary to manipulation for lumbar puncture, and complications of ventilatory failure caused by paralysis of the muscles of respiration. To prevent these potentially avoidable deaths, it has been recommended that every child with the suspected diagnosis of infant botulism should be admitted to a center where intensive respiratory support is available. Prolonged need for mechanical ventilation may lead to tracheostomy in the severely affected patient.

Nutritional support may include various measures such as

intravenous, nasogastric, or nasojejunal feeding, and hyperalimentation. Oral feeding should be avoided until swallowing function and protective cough and gag reflexes have recovered enough to prevent aspiration of food.

Unproved and controversial therapies for infant botulism include purgatives and enemas, as well as administration of specific antitoxins, antibiotics, and drugs that affect neuromuscular function. It has been argued that laxatives, cathartics, or enemas may decrease the concentration of intraintestinal organisms and toxin. In one anecdotal report, administration of laxative increased excretion of botulinogenic toxin eightfold, and the patient showed a simultaneous clinical improvement.[32] However, it should be noted that many of these infants are obstipated and may not respond to usual cathartic techniques. These sick infants are generally in a precarious metabolic balance, and fluid or electrolyte disturbance may result from injudicious or repeated purgation.

The indications for antibiotics in the management of infant botulism are unclear. Some infants with botulism are initially treated with antibiotics for possible sepsis; others receive therapy for aspiration pneumonia or other complications. There appears to be no protective influence of penicillin administered either orally or parenterally.[27] There has been no difference in clinical course or eradication of intestinal organisms or toxin. While penicillin is clostridiocidal, some observers have suggested that it may be unsafe, because lysis of the organisms would make more toxin available for absorption.[25] The effect of penicillin and other antimicrobial agents on the intestinal flora of infants with (or without) botulism is unknown. It is possible that an unpredictable alteration of the gut flora may actually favor growth of botulinal organisms. The use of aminoglycosides in the treatment of suspected sepsis may lead to unfortunate consequences in infant botulism. Gentamycin and related antibiotics can produce neuromuscular blockade and may potentiate the clinical syndrome of infant botulism.[27]

Botulinogenic antitoxin has been widely recommended in food-borne botulism, but complications of specific antitoxin may exceed potential benefit in infant botulism. The vast majority of infants diagnosed to date have completely recovered without such therapy. Only two infants have received multivalent botulinogenic antitoxin, a four-month-old infant who had no dramatic improvement following administration of antitoxin and another infant who suffered immediate anaphylaxis despite pretreatment with epinephrine.[25] The argument for antitoxin in infant botulism is theoretically less sound than it is in food-borne botulism. Antitoxin neutralizes only circulating botulinogenic toxin, but measurable serum toxin has been reported in only one patient with infant botulism. In the other patients, it is assumed that the toxin is released in very low concentration below the limits of current assays. Absorbed toxin is rapidly and irreversibly bound at the neuromuscular junction and neutralization by antitoxin is therefore no longer possible.[39] Human botulinogenic hyperimmune serum is still being developed and is not yet clinically available.[26] This preparation should be free of the risks of equine-derived antitoxin. Intragastric equine antitoxin is a potential but untried route of administration. Enteric neutralization of toxin could occur at the site of production, and the risk of anaphylaxis should be negligible if antitoxin is not absorbed systematically. However, the absorption of this macromolecule has never been studied in infants. Drugs that alter neuromuscular transmission have been tried in "adult" botulism with variable success. Guanidine and germine facilitate the release of acetylcholine from nerve terminals and have produced clinical improvement in uncontrolled series of patients.[12–14] Neither drug has fulfilled its initial promise. Recent preliminary reports suggest a role for 4-aminopyridine, a drug with a similar mechanism of action.[28] Since the pharmacology of these drugs in the infant is unknown, most clinical investigators have been hesitant to employ potentially toxic agents in a disease that can be successfully treated with supportive therapy only.

Sudden Infant Death Syndrome

There is no pathoanatomical feature diagnostic of botulism. Indeed, autopsy shows no obvious explanation for the neuromuscular failure in patients with clinically recognized botulism. The age distributions of infant botulism and SIDS overlap closely; peak incidence is between two and four months of age, and less than 10% of cases occur when patients are older than six months of age. Studies from California and Washington have confirmed evidence of botulism in cases otherwise typical of the sudden infant death syndrome (SIDS). Therefore, attempts have been made to link these two disorders.

In a retrospective review of 211 cases of SIDS in California, Arnon et al.[3] reported isolation of botulinogenic organisms or toxin in 4.3%. In two of the nine infants, organisms and toxin were isolated from small intestinal samples but not from feces. A prospective study from Washington demonstrated isolation of botulinogenic organisms without toxin in one of 30 consecutive cases of SIDS.[32] None of these infants had constipation, weakness, or cranial nerve signs. There is one interesting difference between the reported cases of SIDS-botulism and the more typical hospitalized patients. Nine of ten infants were caused by botulism type A, whereas type A comprised only 63% of the first 80 cases west of the Mississippi and only 20% of the five honey-associated cases in California.[4] There is epidemiologic evidence that type A is a more lethal disease. Between 1959 and 1973, the fatality rate from type A foodborne botulism was twice that of type B (32% versus 16%).[10] Botulism has not been found in a small series of SIDS cases in the Philadelphia area, where type B predominates in soil and less than 10% of infant botulism cases were type A. (Brown, L.: Unpublished data.)

Evidence for infant botulism in the SIDS is lacking in several other large population studies. When stool homogenates taken from 116 cadavers were injected into mice, there was no paralysis or unusual mortality. This suggests absence of botulinogenic (or other) toxin.[44] A careful review of terminal symptoms preceding sudden death did not reveal any infant with constipation in a multicenter study of 145 unexpected infant deaths in England.[41]

It appears unlikely that botulism accounts for a large proportion of deaths due to the SIDS even in areas of the world where type A spores are endemic in the soil. However, other considerations alter the estimate of the true incidence. There are technical and logistical difficulties in isolating organisms from appropriate sites (i.e., stool, ileum, liver, spleen). Also, there is the possibility of postmortem inactivation of botulinogenic growth and toxin production by competing anaerobic flora. More sensitive methods for isolating toxin, especially synaptically fixed toxin, should make the diagnosis of SIDS-related botulism more accurate.

Rapid progression of weakness from mild hypotonia to respiratory failure in hospitalized patients with infant botulism may occur over several hours, although the typical history extends over several days. It is reasonable to assume that fulminant cases of infant botulism may occur in which rapid absorption of significant quantities of toxin leads to sudden paralysis of palatal and intercostal musculature. Contributing factors might be increased gastrointestinal absorption of macromolecules in infants, anatomical features of the infant airway, and the higher risk of obstructive apnea during sleep in infants.

Pathophysiology

Infant botulism is produced by intraintestinal germination of spores of *C. botulinum* ingested orally. For unknown reasons, only infants under one year of age appear to have multiplication of organisms in their gastrointestinal tract. Current speculations include an altered bacterial ecology of the infant gut that allows for growth of *C. botulinum,* developmental immunoincompetence, and physiologic deficiency of clostridium-inhibiting bile acids found in older individuals.[22] There is limited experimental support for the role of the infant's intestinal flora. Sugiyama and co-workers[30, 42] have been able to demonstrate intraintestinal germination of spores (with measurable toxin production) only in infant mice and rats under standard laboratory conditions and adult animals raised in a germ-free environment. Studies on man during the 1920s did not demonstrate growth of organisms or toxin production in adults who ingested viable spores, but there were no contemporary reports on infants or children.[17]

Whether botulinogenic toxin is ingested in contaminated food or elaborated by growing organisms in wounds or the intestinal tract, there is the same disruption of orderly synaptic transmission at cholinergic terminals that leads to the clinical expression of disease. This presynaptic disruption affects only the peripheral nervous system, since the blood-brain barrier protects cerebral transmitter release. The toxin will bind to all ganglionic and postganglionic parasympathetic synapses as well as neuromuscular junctions.[39] In the parasympathetic nervous system both preganglionic and postganglionic fibers are involved early, which results in severe autonomic dysfunction.

Adults with foodborne botulism demonstrate blurred vision, dry mouth, and swallowing dysfunction as common early manifestations. The later involvement of neuromuscular junctions ("descending paralysis") is a clinical feature that distinguishes the Guillain-Barré syndrome from infant botulism.

An explanation for the pattern of progressive muscular involvement and resolution is supported by the concept of "margin of safety."[45] Experimentally, the most sensitive skeletal muscle requires blockade of 75% of neuromuscular receptors before any loss of contractibility can be demonstrated. Diaphragmatic muscle has a greater margin of safety, and almost 95% of receptors must be blocked before loss of contractility to individual stimulation can be shown. Increased rates of stimulation produce loss of normal contractility with less receptor occlusion.

Sucking and swallowing, crying, and maintenance of head control are motor functions that require frequent and repetitive neuromuscular transmission. These functions are involved early in infant botulism, sometimes before the appearance of peripheral weakness, and certainly before respiratory failure. When a severely affected infant starts to improve, adequate ventilation is achieved long before effective sucking. While infants will usually be sent home following return of protective gag and swallow reflexes, it may take more time before they no longer require nasogastric feeding. Weeks more may be necessary before normal tone and strength are reestablished. Furthermore, the concept of margin of safety may explain the mechanism of respiratory failure following minor stress. Although an affected infant may appear stable, poor head positioning leading to mild upper airway obstruction or the flexion position for a lumbar puncture leading to impaired intercostal breathing can precipitate respiratory arrest.

As stated above, constipation is the first sign of botulism in infants. This local process is caused by parasympathetic paralysis in autonomic plexi of the intestinal wall. The decreased bowel motility this causes undoubtedly favors further spread of botulinogenic infection.

Mounting pharmacologic and electron microscopic evidence have given rise to an elegant hypothesis that describes the interaction of toxin and cholinergic nerve terminal.[16, 17] Botulinogenic toxin first binds to a receptor on the surface of the pre-

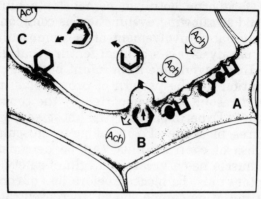

Fig 2.—Proposed model for action of botulinal toxin. **A,** Initial binding step of toxin to an external surface receptor on membrane of presynaptic nerve ending. **B,** Part of the toxin molecule passes into cytoplasm of nerve, possibly by "reverse exocytosis" linked to release of vesicles of acetylcholine. **C,** Intracellular toxin binds to internal membrane receptor within the nerve terminal, blocking further release of acetylcholine.

synaptic nerve membrane (Fig 2). The toxin or some part of it then crosses into the presynaptic terminal bouton and combines with another internal receptor. The toxin interferes with acetylcholine release, and electron microscopic studies have shown a "log jam" of vesicles at nerve terminal release sites.[24] Although the presynaptic nerve can still propagate an impulse, there is no release of acetylcholine. Most investigators believe that the toxin combines with the internal membrane of the terminal bouton to change membrane structure or function. Alternative explanations invoking disturbances of calcium availability, vesicle formation, or mitochondrial activity are either not supported by the available data or mathematically unfeasible. Botulinogenic toxin is the most potent poison known to man: it has been estimated that a lethal dose is only 10^{-9} mg/kg of body weight.[6] Therefore, the small number of molecules of toxin needed to produce neuromuscular blockade would lead one to look for a specific effect at critical locations at the nerve terminal rather than a more diffuse distribution.

Recovery from botulism implies establishment of new anatomical pathways at the synapse, since toxin binding is apparently irreversible. New synaptic sprouting is a slow process that may take many months. The neuromuscular resolution occurs when enough nonoccluded cholinergic junctions are functioning to permit effective transmitter release, which allows the unaffected distal nerve or muscle fibers to function. Even in patients with adult foodborne botulism, recovery in severe cases may take months. In infants in whom ongoing intestinal growth of organisms and production of toxin may still be demonstrated for weeks, rapid recovery cannot be expected. Clinical resolution may occur despite persistent presence of organisms and toxin in the gastrointestinal tract. Intriguing hypotheses include local intestinal neutralization by antitoxin, systemic or local antibody production preventing absorption, changes in enteric flora inhibiting clostridial growth, or developmental changes in bile acid production. Current methods of measurement of botulinogenic toxin and organisms are not sensitive enough to permit detection in serum or at the neuromuscular junction. Even animals recurrently challenged with less than lethal doses of botulinogenic toxin do not develop measurable serum antitoxin. At present, there is no way to further characterize the factors leading to resolution of infant botulism.

BIBLIOGRAPHY

1. Arnon S.S., Chin J.: The clinical spectrum of infant botulism. *Rev. Infect. Dis.* 1:614, 1979.
2. Arnon S.S., Midura T.F., Clay S.A., et al.: Infant botulism: Epidemiologic clinical and laboratory aspects. *J.A.M.A.* 237:1946, 1977.
3. Arnon S.S., Midura T.F., Damus K.D., et al.: Intestinal infection and toxin production by *C. botulinum* as one cause of sudden infant death syndrome. *Lancet* 1:1273, 1978.
4. Arnon S.S., Midura T.F., Damus K.D., et al.: Honey and other environmental risk factors for infant botulism. *J. Pediatr.* 94:331, 1979.
5. Arnon S.S., Werner S.B.: Infant botulism in 1931: Discovery of a misclassified case. *Am. J. Dis. Child.* 133:580, 1979.
6. Bonventre P.F.: Absorption of botulinal toxin from the gastrointestinal tract. *Rev. Infect. Dis.* 1:663, 1979.
7. Brown L.W.: Botulism and the honey connection. *J. Pediatr.* 94:337, 1979.
8. Brown L.W.: Differential diagnosis of infant botulism. *Rev. Infect. Dis.* 1:625, 1979.
9. Carroll J.E., Jedziniak M., Guggenheim M.A.: Guillain-Barré syndrome: Another cause of the "floppy infant." *Am. J. Dis. Child.* 131:699, 1977.
10. Center for Disease Control: *Botulism in the United States, 1899–1977: Handbook for Epidemiologists, Clinicians and Laboratory Workers.* Atlanta, 1979.
11. Cherington M.: Botulism: Electrophysiologic and therapeutic observations, in Desmedt J.E. (ed): *New Developments in Electromyography and Clinical Neurophysiology.* Basel: S. Karger A.G., 1973, vol 1, pp 375–379.
12. Cherington M., Greenburg H.: Botulism and germine. *Neurology* 21:966, 1971.
13. Cherington M., Ryan D.W.: Treatment of botulism with guanidine: Early neurophysiologic studies. *N. Engl. J. Med.* 282:195, 1970.
14. Cherington M., Schultz D.: Effect of guanidine, germine, and steroids in a case of botulism. *Clin. Toxicol.* 11:19, 1977.

15. Conomy J.P., Levinsohn M., Fanaroff A.: Familial infantile myasthenia gravis: A cause of sudden death in young children. *J. Pediatr.* 87:428, 1975.
16. Cull-Candy S.G., Lundh H., Thesleff S.: Effects of botulinum toxin on neuromuscular transmission in the rat. *J. Physiol.* 260:177, 1976.
17. Easton E.J., Meyer K.F.: Occurrence of *B. botulinus* in human and animal excreta. *J. Infect. Dis.* 35:207, 1924.
18. Engel W.K.: Brief small abundant motor action potential: A further critique of electromyographic interpretation. *Neurology* 25:173, 1975.
19. Faich G.A., Graver R.W., Sato S.: Failure of guanidine therapy in botulism A. *N. Engl. J. Med.* 285:713, 1971.
20. Greer M., Schotland D.: Myasthenia gravis in the newborn. *Pediatrics* 26:101, 1960.
21. Grover W.D., Peckham G.J., Berman P.H.: Recovery following cranial nerve dysfunction and muscle weakness in infancy. *Dev. Med. Child Neurol.* 16:163, 1974.
22. Hentges D.J.: The intestinal flora and infant botulism. *Rev. Infect. Dis.* 1:668, 1979.
23. Huttenlocher P.R., Trauner D.A.: Reye's syndrome in infancy. *Pediatrics* 62:84, 1978.
24. Kao I., Drachman D.B., Price D.L.: Botulinum toxin: Mechanism of presynaptic blockade. *Science* 193:1256, 1976.
25. Johnson R.O., Clay S.A., Arnon S.S.: Diagnosis and management of infant botulism. *Am. J. Dis. Child* 133:586, 1979.
26. Lewis G.E., Metzger J.F.: Botulism immune plasma (human). *Lancet* 2:634, 1978.
27. L'Hommedieu C.L., Stough R., Brown L.W., et al.: Potentiation of neuromuscular weakness in infant botulism by aminoglycosides. *J. Pediatr.* 95:1065, 1979.
28. Lundh H., Leander S., Thesleff S.: Antagonism of the paralysis produced by botulinum toxin in the rat: The effect of tetraethylammonium, guanidine and 4-aminopyridine. *J. Neurol. Sci.* 32:29, 1977.
29. Merson M.H., Dowell V.R. Jr.: Epidemiologic, clinical and laboratory aspects of wound botulism. *N. Engl. J. Med.* 289:1005, 1973.
30. Moberg L.J., Sugiyama H.: The rat as an animal model for infant botulism. *Infect. Immunol.* 29:819, 1980.
31. Moss R.B., Siriram S., Kelts A., et al.: Chronic neuropathy presenting as a floppy infant with respiratory distress. *J. Pediatr.* 64:459, 1979.
32. Peterson D.R., Eklund M.W., Chinn N.M.:The sudden infant death syndrome and infant botulism. *Rev. Infect.* 1:630, 1979.
33. Pickett J., Berg B., Chaplin E., et al.: Syndrome of botulism in infancy: Clinical and electrophysiologic study. *N. Engl. J. Med.* 295:770, 1976.
34. Pearn J.H., Wilson J.: Acute Werdnig-Hoffman disease: Acute infantile spinal muscular atrophy. *Arch. Dis. Child.* 48:425, 1973.
35. Pincus J.H.: Subacute necrotizing encephalomyelitis (Leigh's disease): A consideration of clinical features and etiology. *Dev. Med. Child Neurol.* 14:87, 1972.
36. Polin R.A., Brown L.W.: Infant botulism. *Pediatr. Clin. North Am.* 26:345, 1979.
37. Pumplin D.W., Reese T.S.: Action of brown widow spider venom and botulinal toxin on the frog neuromuscular junction examined with the freeze-fracture technique. *J. Physiol.* 273:443, 1977.
38. Shield L.K., Wilkinson R.G., Ritchie M.: Infant botulism in Australia. *Med. J. Aust.* 1:157, 1978.
39. Simpson L.L.: The action of botulinal toxin. *Rev. Infect. Dis.* 1:656, 1979.
40. Smith L.D.S.: *Botulism: The Organism, Its Toxin, the Disease.* Springfield, Ill.: Charles C Thomas, Publisher, 1977.
41. Stanton A.N., Downham M.A.P.S., Oakley J.R., et al.: Terminal symptoms in children dying suddenly and unexpectedly at home. *Br. Med. J.* 2:1249, 1978.
42. Sugiyama H., Mills D.C.: Intraintestinal toxin in infant mice challenged intragastrically with *C. botulinum* spores. *Infect. Immunol.* 21:59, 1978.

43. Turner H.D., Brett E.M., Gilbert R.J., et al.: Infant botulism in England. *Lancet* 1:1277, 1978.
44. Urquhart G.E.D., Grist N.J.: Botulism and sudden infant death. *Lancet* 2:1411, 1976.
45. Van Ermengen E.: A new anaerobic bacillus and its relation to botulism (a reprint). *Rev. Infect. Dis.* 1:701, 1979.
46. Waud B.E., Waud D.R.: The margin of safety: Neuromuscular transmission in the muscle of the diaphragm. *Anesthesiology* 37:417, 1972.

Gastroesophageal Reflux in Children

JOHN J. HERBST, M.D.

AND

WILLIAM F. MEYERS, M.D.

Department of Pediatrics
University of Utah Medical Center
Salt Lake City, Utah

Introduction

THE MAJOR FUNCTIONS OF THE ESOPHAGUS are to transport food and liquids to the stomach and to prevent easy reflux of stomach contents to the esophagus and pharynx. Increased interest in reflux has recently been stimulated in part by the adaptation of several tests of esophageal function for use in children.

Although many terms have been proposed, gastroesophageal reflux (GER) is the preferred one; it clearly denotes pathology without reference to possible causes. The terms, hiatal hernia and partial thoracic stomach refer not to abnormal function, but to an anatomical abnormality that may be present with or without GER.[20, 73] An older term, chalasia, implies an extreme relaxation of the distal esophagus that frequently is not demonstrable.[10] GER must also be differentiated from vomiting, which implies a more active process often associated with neurologic conditions or anatomical or functional intestinal obstructions. In practice, the distinction between reflux and vomiting is often difficult to make in children, and one must rule

NOTE: This chapter was supported in part by a grant from the Thrasher Research Fund and a clinical training grant from the Cystic Fibrosis Foundation.

out other causes of vomiting. In the past, GER was rarely considered as a diagnostic possibility in children. The authors have seen a number of patients treated for reflux who had vomiting caused by such diverse diseases as pyloric stenosis, jejunal stenosis, cystic fibrosis, celiac disease, and brain tumors.

Many questions regarding the diagnosis of reflux, determination of the clinical significance of reflux, best modes of therapy, and the causal relationships of reflux and respiratory symptoms have not been definitely answered. It is hoped that this review of recent developments can provide a rational framework for making clinical decisions that cannot be postponed until the definitive questions have been answered.

History

GER has affected mankind since antiquity. Hiatal hernias have been noted in Egyptian mummies. Rumination, an unusual symptom of reflux, has aroused the interest of a number of historically famous physicians, including Fabricius ab Aquapendente, who is credited with the first description of venous valves. A student of Fallopio, teacher of William Harvey, and physician to Galileo, he performed an autopsy on a ruminator and found two stomachs (a large hiatal hernia?) and thought that this was evidence of a ruminant nature.[44] A mass in the forehead was felt to be a rudimentary horn and to further attest to a bovine nature and explain the symptoms in man. In 1865, Luschka,[74] after whom the lateral foramina of the third ventricle are named, had another such patient. He too thought the large hernia was a kind of ruminant forestomach and caused vomiting. This idea was quickly challenged when others noted similar patients who did not have rumination. Thus began a controversy over the association of reflux and hiatal hernia that is still not resolved. By the Victorian age, GER was thought by some to be a bad habit often learned from a governess.[18] Early in the twentieth century, attention was focused on the unusual mouthing movements; head caps and restraints were designed to immobilize the mouth.[4] Such treatment remained in standard pediatric texts until the 1950s.

X-rays showing evidence of hiatal hernia, reflux, or stricture in children were published in the second decade of this century.[79] Radiography still remains the major laboratory test to confirm the diagnosis. Kanner,[67] the father of child psychiatry, focused on the psychological problems of children with GER. The recommended treatment included constant holding of the children (presumably in an upright position) and frequent feeding. Sedation and thickened feedings were also often recommended, but mortality rates as high as 40% were reported. Only recently has it been recognized that these patients have abnormalities in esophageal function.[16, 24, 54]

The early series of patients with GER usually dealt with the most severe cases, especially patients with strictures secondary to severe esophagitis. In more recent studies emphasis has been placed on patients with milder symptoms and respiratory symptoms caused by aspiration of refluxed material. It is also being recognized that all people, adults and children, normally have reflux to some extent, especially after eating.[34, 66] This concept can explain many of the difficulties in diagnosing GER, for the physician must distinguish normal and pathologic reflux. In recent years, debate has centered about the pathophysiology of reflux, usefulness of different tests in diagnosing reflux, important elements in medical therapy, indication for surgical intervention, and best surgical procedure.

Incidence and Natural History

Estimates of the incidence of GER in children have varied from almost a denial of its existence to simple comments that all children reflux. Carre[24] has estimated an incidence of 1:1,000 live births that he has subsequently revised to approximately 1:300. The problem is one more of recognition than of changing incidence. The frequency with which surgery is performed for GER can serve as an index for recognition of severe cases, especially if one uses cases of congenital diaphragmatic hernia as a denominator. This is a very serious symptomatic congenital problem unlikely to be overlooked. In 1974 surgery for hiatal hernia compared to that of congenital diaphragmatic surgery was almost ten times less frequent in North America (except in Utah) than in Great Britain (Table 1).[48] Shortly thereafter, the incidence in Boston became similar to that in England and Utah as interest in the entity increased.[30] A similar increase in recognition of GER in children has been noted in many centers.

TABLE 1.—
GASTROESOPHAGEAL REFLUX
FREQUENCY OF SURGERY*

England	9:1
Montreal	1:4
Chicago	1:2
Los Angeles	1:5
Memphis	1:7
Boston	1:7
Salt Lake City	10:1

*Adapted from Guttman: *Pediatrics* 50:325, 1972.

Any judgment as to the need of therapy, surgical or medical, must be based on knowledge of the natural history. Careful review of records in a structured medical care system in England suggests that most infants who have GER severe enough to seek medical care have symptoms by two months of age, and that 60% of them have a benign course and are free of symptoms by 18 months of age.[21] An additional 30% have some persistence of symptoms, at least to age four. Five percent develop strictures, and 5% of all patients with reflux will die, usually of inanition and pneumonia, unless adequate treatment is employed. The implications are that most who spit up will improve, usually at about eight to nine months of age, as they assume a more upright position throughout the day, although some will have mild symptoms for at least four years. Extensive therapeutic efforts should be directed at the 10% of patients who would die or develop strictures if untreated, and be of variable intensity for those with benign continuing symptoms. These data also suggest that one can be optimistic about controlling symptoms in an infant whose natural history would suggest that the majority of them would improve regardless of therapy. It would also be reasonable to persist in only partially effective medical care in an eight-month-old infant, since many of these will start to show improvement in the near future. On the other hand, in a four- or six-year-old child, treatment of reflux may be expected to improve symptoms of esophagitis (heartburn) or regurgitation. But here, as in an adult, one is treating the effects of reflux with little hope of stopping reflux itself once medical therapy ceases.

Symptoms

The numerous symptoms of GER may be related directly to reflux of stomach contents into the esophagus, may be an effect of reflux, or may be associated with a group of unusual problems where the pathophysiology is poorly understood (Table 2).

The most common problem is vomiting. This is seen in over 90% of infants with GER and is usually present by two months of age.[21, 62] This problem is much more common among infants than adults. Frequently, it may be quite forceful and may suggest pyloric stenosis; pylorospasm may be an associated problem that usually improves when reflux is controlled.[62, 68, 73, 88] In adults, reflux into the mouth or vomiting is less common, possibly because the esophagus is longer and has a greater capacity. The vomiting may be so voluminous that excessive calories are lost and there is a failure to thrive.[2, 40, 62] This is common in infants and is a major indication for surgery if medical therapy fails. It is a rare problem in adolescents or adults.

Once the refluxed material gets to the level of the pharynx, it may be aspirated and cause pulmonary problems. This is a major problem in children; pulmonary symptoms were present in 47% of patients from our center who had surgical repair.[65] These pulmonary problems my mimic those of recurrent obstructive bronchitis or recurrent aspiration pneumonia.[27, 29, 43, 91]

TABLE 2.—PROBLEMS RELATED TO GER

Direct
  Vomiting
  Failure to thrive
  Aspiration and pulmonary disease
Indirect
  Heartburn
  Esophagitis
  Waterbrash
  Stricture
  Short Esophagus
Unusual
  Apnea—blood pressure decreased
  Asthmatic bronchitis
  Syndromes
    Sandifer's syndrome
    Rumination
    Finger clubbing and protein-losing enteropathy
    Near-miss sudden infant death syndrome

In older patients and adults, usually the lower lobes are involved. Because infants spend a large portion of their time recumbent, there is a predilection for the upper lobes, especially the right. Choking and apnea may be a major problem, especially in the first year of life.[62] Usually it occurs during or just after feeding and may be associated with laryngospasm.

In some patients symptoms are most severe at night, with episodes of choking, coughing, asthma-like symptoms, and even cyanosis with laryngospasm.[22] Once pulmonary symptoms occur, rapid changes in abdominal pressure can augment reflux and make respiratory symptoms worse. Why some patients develop pulmonary symptoms is not fully understood. Patients with prolonged reflux are more likely to have respiratory symptoms perhaps related to the efficiency of the clearance mechanisms of the pharynx.[63] Patients with CNS disease may have severe reflux and are prone to respiratory symptoms.[65, 93] Many patients will aspirate or choke *only* toward the end of a feeding, when they are tired, or while asleep, when certain protective reflexes may not be as efficient.

Although patients with GER may have respiratory problems, it is also true that patients with primary respiratory disorders may have reflux. Coughing and sudden increases in abdominal pressure related to the respiratory disorder may make reflux worse, as may certain medications. Aminophyline relieves symptoms of asthma, but it also tends to decrease lower esophageal sphincter pressure and encourage reflux.[95] The physician is faced with the necessity of deciding if respiratory symptoms are related to GER. Even though there are no easily available tests that can prove the association, a careful history and observation of the child are useful. The authors, however, are very leery to ascribe asthma-like symptoms to reflux if there is a good history of allergies and if the patient responds well to bronchodilators. On the other hand, recurrent acute obstructive pulmonary symptoms (bronchiolitis) in patients who respond poorly to bronchodilators should arouse suspicions as to the presence of GER.[27, 29]

Symptoms secondary to reflux include waterbrash, heartburn, dysphagia, and neuropsychiatric complaints. Other secondary symptoms may be hematemesis or melena due to esophagitis and recurrent respiratory disease.[73]

Waterbrash is a common symptom in adults but occurs infrequently in children. Clear liquid suddenly appears in the mouth. The exact pathophysiology of this is unknown, and the chief difficulty is a social problem. Heartburn is the most common symptom of reflux in adults and is caused by esophageal irritation by acid gastric contents.[84] It is less common in young children, probably because they cannot voice the symptoms of substernal or high epigastric pain. In some infants the only symptoms of heartburn are irritability and crying episodes. Symptoms can often be elicited by certain foods, especially coffee, tomato juice, or citrus fruit.[85]

The most severe secondary effects of GER on the esophagus are shortening and stricture formation that can lead to dysphagia and even starvation.[2, 67, 73] It is now agreed that most cases of "congenital" short esophagus in children are caused by peptic esophagitis. With stricture formation there may be a decrease in vomiting or pulmonary symptoms, but signs of obstruction and dysphagia occur. If most reflux episodes occur at night, it is possible that signs of obstruction may develop without a long history of esophagitis or heartburn.[84] The patient with esophagitis may have either acute or chronic blood loss, which may cause iron deficiency anemia with occult blood in the stools, or in severe cases, hematemesis or melena.

At times some symptoms may not clearly suggest GER (see Table 2) and may seem neuropsychiatric in origin. Their importance lies not in their frequency, but rather in a recognition of these entities for rapid diagnosis of the problem and early effective treatment.

In 1964, Kinsborne[70] described a group of patients with what became known as Sandifer's syndrome. They had chronic iron deficiency anemia, emesis, and an intermittent head cocking trait. These patients had been referred for consideration of steriotactic surgery. Our experience is that these patients are frequently referred for psychiatric consultation. In one severe case it was noted that the head cocking always occurred after reflux to the superior esophageal sphincter.[55] The exact mechanism is not understood.

Bray and co-workers[17] have described another group of patients with neuropsychiatric problems. Episodes of unusual opisthotonic posturing usually occurred several times a day and often were associated with gurgling and cyanosis. Convulsions were a major consideration; several patients had been started on anticonvulsants without improvement. In others, unusual neurologic abnormalities or behavior ticks were postulated. All of their patients were shown to have GER, and effective treatment led to rapid resolution of the symptoms.

Rumination is an unusual syndrome wherein patients frequently will have opisthotonic posture and unusual sucking and tongue movements followed by regurgitation of parts of gastric contents into the mouth, where at least some are masticated and swallowed.[54] There has been a high mortality in the past related to inanition nd pneumonias.[67] Some maintain it is a psychotic condition.[77, 92] The authors agree with Botha that ruminant patients have some abnormality of esophageal function that allows bizarre psychiatric symptoms to develop. In our experience with 12 such patients, many had severe caloric loss and failure to thrive.[65] Surgical correction of GER terminated rumination and other problems related to GER.

Several patients with finger clubbing, protein-losing enteropathy, and iron deficiency anemia as the main presenting problems have been described. Upon investigation, all had GER, severe esophagitis, and decreased serum albumin.[55, 71] It is presumed that there was a severe seepage of protein from the grossly inflamed esophagus, and finger clubbing was related to a reactive mediastinitis noted at surgery. Surgical repair of GER resulted in a return of serum proteins to normal in several days and a regression of finger clubbing over a period of months. A strong case can be made for considering these problems as unusual manifestations of reflux rather than separate syndromes. Of three patients with GER, finger clubbing, and protein-losing enteropathy, one had rumination and another had Sandifer's syndrome.[55]

Two centers have reported a group of patients presenting with apnea and bradycardia who appeared to have aborted episodes of the sudden infant death syndrome (SIDS).[52, 72] How frequently reflux with choking and aspiration does lead to the SIDS is unknown. It is becoming obvious that these infants are not perfectly healthy prior to death, but have a number of problems, especially feeding problems.[80] At autopsy we have noted findings of GE reflux (increase in height of dermal papillae) in approximately 20% of patients with the SIDS.[50] Farrell[45] has noted that significant reflux is frequent in a group of infants presenting with apnea and bradycardia, but is only occasionally a major cause of symptoms.[45] Although the majority of such patients do not have GER as the initiating event, it is important to consider GER and identify the minority with reflux, institute effective therapy, and prevent morbidity and mortality.

Some patients, usually infants, may have recurrent episodes of obstructive bronchitis as their most obvious symptom.[29] The symptom may be incorrectly ascribed to asthma, other allergies, or repeated infections. GER should be considered and looked for, especially when such symptoms occur before the age of a year. In other patients respiratory symptoms may start at birth. In premature infants, especially, the symptoms of hyaline membrane disease and bronchopulmonary dysplasia may merge into symptoms of GER and aspiration. The radiologic and pathologic findings of chronic bronchopulmonary dysplasia and aspiration are very similar. A group of patients with GER and findings of typical sequelae of hyaline membrane disease were identified in Utah.[56] Many were having multiple apnea episodes per day or could not be weaned from a respirator. Once GER was controlled, there was dramatic improvement in the lung disease. Certainly not all chronic lung disease in premature infants is caused by GER, but our experience suggests that the situation is not rare. Even in the first weeks of life, prematures have intact sphincter mechanisms and do not normally reflux excessively.

Methods of Diagnosis

The patient's history is extremely important when one first considers the possibility of GER. Symptoms suggestive of reflux are often not volunteered. Many people expect some spitting in babies and do not consider that their child's spitting may be excessive or pathologic. This is especially true if other, more dramatic symptoms such as apnea, bradycardia, or cyanosis are present. Unless there is severe pulmonary disease or extreme failure to thrive, there are no specific physical findings.

A number of tests of esophageal function have been adapted for use in children. Unfortunately, none of them is infallible.[1, 6, 33, 87] As noted earlier, reflux is a normal physiologic phenomenon, especially after meals.[66] It is only when it is excessive that it may be pathologic. Thus, testing must distinguish degrees of reflux, not just its presence or absence. What follows is a discussion of the relative merits of different esophageal tests as they relate to reflux. Each measures a different parameter and should be used to answer specific questions. Only rarely does a patient need to have all of these tests performed, and many patients with mild symptoms require no specific tests at all.

BARIUM SWALLOW

The barium swallow is the most available and most commonly used test to demonstrate GER.[13, 31, 75] Usually a second review of the films will not add to the usefulness of the test, because multiple spot films are taken to demonstrate what the fluoroscopist has seen, and only he can tell if the barium-filled esophagus was filled from the mouth or stomach. Some indication of reflux can be deduced if overhead films of a small bowel series are taken. If several films show barium in the esophagus, reflux probably exists, since barium is usually not given throughout the exam. The accuracy of the procedure has varied from less than 40% to greater than 80% depending on the expertise and interest of the radiologist.[1, 6, 30, 62, 75, 87] It is not important to put pressure on the abdomen to induce reflux. If the patient is irritable and crying, he should be comforted and then rechecked for reflux. We have noted a number of patients who refluxed while quiet, but not when crying. A common error is to give insufficient barium; an amount approaching the volume of a normal feeding is a good guide. A major benefit of a barium study is that other disorders involving structural defects that might give similar symptoms, e.g., pyloric stenosis, partial small bowel obstruction, antral webs, etc., can be excluded. The barium swallow is also the simplest way to document the presence of a hiatal hernia. In adults there is no good correlation between the presence of a hiatal hernia and GER.[28] In children there is a strong correlation.[24] In children the presence of a hiatal hernia without reflux is unusual. Although there is debate in the pediatric radiologic literature on the criteria used to detect small herniae, 47 of 55 patients who underwent reflux surgery had an easily discernible hernia.[62] Unless the hernia is so huge as to fill a large portion of the thoracic cavity, surgical treatment is directed at the GER, not the hernia.

TUTTLE TEST

The acid reflux test (Tuttle) is an easily administered test for the presence of reflux.[26, 42, 62, 96] A pH probe is placed approximately 3 cm proximal to the lower esophageal sphincter and 300 ml/sq m of body surface of 0.1 N HCl is instilled into the stomach while the patient is supine. More than one episode of reflux (esophageal pH <4) in 30 minutes is indicative of pathologic reflux. So as not to exclude the patient with multiple episodes of reflux who does not clear the esophagus, we consider one episode involving greater than 30% of the first 30 minutes as indicating a positive test. Substituting apple juice (pH, about 4) does not change the results and this is easily fed by mouth, while 0.1 N HCl must usually be given by gavage.[50] As with all tests of reflux, there will be occasional patients with false positive or negative results, but the overall accuracy rate is about 85%.[1, 6, 42, 87]

EXTENDED pH MONITORING

In this test a pH probe is placed as in the acid reflux test, but pH is continuously monitored on a strip recorder over time, usually 18–24 hours.* Position as well as the sleep or waking state are recorded. The number of episodes of reflux (pH <4), number of prolonged episodes of reflux (<5 minutes), longest episode, and percent of time the patient experienced reflux can also be calculated. Since reflux normally occurs more frequently in the postprandial state, it is useful to separate the recording into periods less than and greater than 2 hours after feeding.[66] A numerical score can be assigned to the tracings. The mean in normal patients of each item is given two points, and each standard deviation above the mean is assigned an additional point. The test is quite sensitive, although some false positive and negative results do occur.[87] Evaluation of the re-

---

*References 3, 15, 32, 34, 59, 61, 64, 66.

sults can suggest the position most helpful in preventing reflux. The main disadvantage of the test is that it requires overnight hospitalization. The nasal probe is easily tolerated and hardly noticed after the first few minutes. Very young and older patients have no problem remaining within the three-foot radius of the recorder proscribed by the length of the pH cable. Only an occasional active toddler cannot understand the need for restraint.

GASTRIC SCINTISCAN

The gastric scintiscan, at first glance, has a number of theoretical advantages. A small amount of ^{99m}Tc is mixed with juice, milk, or other food and then ingested. Gastroscans are obtained by searching for reflux of the radioactive material into the esophagus.[1, 57, 76, 89]

The radiation dose is less than that for a single chest film, and multiple images may be obtained. For reasons not entirely clear, the accuracy of this test is less than that of others and there are a number of false positive and negative results.[87] The test has been adapted on an experimental basis to measure gastric emptying and clearance of impregnated food boluses from the esophagus. This is the most recently introduced test, and further refinement may improve its usefulness.

Tests of the Effect of Reflux

ESOPHAGOSCOPY

Since the introduction of fiberoptic endoscopy, esophagoscopy has been used much more frequently.[47] Flexible endoscopy with sedation and topical anesthesia to the pharynx has negated the need for general anesthesia or hospitalization. If one can exclude ingestion of a caustic chemical, visualization of a friable or erythematous mucosa is a sure sign of GER. A normal esophagoscopy, however, does not exclude the presence of reflux.[6, 33] The presence of a velvety patch of mucosa should tip one off to the possibility of columnar mucosa (Barrett's esophagus). With endoscopy, strictures can be visualized, and, if necessary, impacted foreign bodies can be removed. Large hiatal hernias can also be visualized, although they are more easily detected with barium contrast studies.

ESOPHAGEAL BIOPSY

This procedure is usually done in association with esophagoscopy, but it has major use as an independent procedure. A biopsy can be obtained through a flexible endoscope. Such biopsies can be useful if there is denudation of the epithelium or marked infiltration of inflammatory cells, but are of limited usefulness if one is searching for more subtle changes. Adequate biopsy samples are easily obtained with a Rubin multipurpose suction biopsy tube.[9] The procedure is safe and can be easily oriented so that sections perpendicular to the lumen can be obtained. Subtle hallmarks may be present in esophageal mucosa that appears normal at esophagoscopy, including an increased height of dermal papillae (exceeding more than 60% of the thickness of the mucosa) and a germinative layer greater than 10% of the thickness of the mucosa.[9] Both of these changes increase the percentage of proliferating cells in the epithelium and represent an adaptation to chronic irritation. Recently, the presence of even a rare eosinophil in the squamous epithelium has been reported as a regular finding in patients with reflux.[99] With severe disease there may be a breakdown of reparative mechanisms that leads to friability of the mucosa and ulcer formation. On biopsy there may be denudation of the epithelium and heavy infiltration of inflammatory cells. In some patients the ulcers may be lined with columnar epithelium that may resemble gastric or intestinal mucosa. It is not clear whether these columnar cells are an upgrowth of gastric tissue or a reversion of esophageal cells to a more primitive form.[11] In adults such tissue (Barrett's epithelium) is regarded as a metaplastic change and greatly increases the risk of adenocarcinoma.[51] The importance of such a finding in childhood is unknown, and it is uncertain if the columnar tissue will give way to squamous epithelium if GER is controlled.

Esophageal Motility

Esophageal manometry is often performed in conjunction with the Tuttle test. A catheter-like probe is inserted into the stomach and withdrawn into the esophagus. Usually there are at least three pressure-sensitive spots positioned 2.5 to 5.0 cm apart.[36, 41, 60, 62] Some workers use an external strain gauge and water-perfused catheters; others use a probe with the strain gauge built into the probe itself. No matter which technique is used, it must be realized that a foreign body is placed in the esophagus and that the size, rate of perfusion, and compliance of the catheters can affect the pressures recorded.[94] When comparing data from different centers it is important to know how pressure was recorded. In a rapid pull through, the catheter is withdrawn over a period of a few seconds, and the highest pressure recorded as the pressure-sensitive tip is withdrawn is considered the sphincter pressure.[41] In the slow pull-through method, the catheter is withdrawn a few millimeters at a time and pressures recorded for a period of time before further withdrawal.[62] The first method requires that the patient cooperate and not breathe during withdrawal. In the second method one must wait until the child is relaxed. It is important to know if the atmospheric or intragastric pressure is used as baseline pressure. Measuring pressure at inspiration, expiration, or mid-respiratory cycle can give different values.[36]

In spite of all these technical problems, some valuable information can be obtained. The presence of a lower esophageal sphincter can be identified, as can a decrease in pressure with deglutition. The presence of primary peristaltic waves initiated by a swallow, secondary peristaltic waves initiated by distention of the esophagus, or tertiary waves that are uncoordinated contractions of the esophagus, can be noted and related to a clinical disorder. Very high lower esophageal sphincter pressures that do not relax with deglutition and lack of primary waves in the distal esophagus are characteristic of achalasia.[60]

Patients with esophagitis may have mainly tertiary contractions of the esophagus. There is debate on the validity of esophageal sphincter pressure. Repeated studies in the same patients and studies with multilumen tube show wide changes in pressure.[25] It is now appreciated that there is not a good correlation between sphincter pressure and reflux, but patients with severe esophagitis tend to have very low pressures.[6, 53, 97] It is not clear whether esophagitis causes low pressures or vice versa. In adults the association between preoperative and postoperative sphincter pressure is not dramatic after antireflux surgery. Many patients with successful operations may have pressures lower than other preoperative patients.[39] In children, some authors note a consistent increase in sphincter pressure after successful surgery for reflux. We have not noted a good correlation between reflux and postoperative increase in sphincter pressure except in those with severe esophagitis.[53] The severity of esophagitis in patients may explain differences between the pediatric and adult experience. Adult patients usually come to surgery with a history of intractable heartburn that may have persisted for decades. In children the history is short, and chronic vomiting and failure to thrive is a common indication for surgery, and severe chronic esophagitis is usually absent.

The test takes effort to perform and expertise in interpretation and the equipment is quite expensive. It is not recommended as a primary test for the presence of reflux, but as an optional test when it is desirable to have further data on physiologic function of the esophagus.

BERNSTEIN TEST

This test is designed to determine whether perfusion of the esophagus with gastric acid (0.1 N HCl) can reproduce the patient's symptoms. It does not test for reflux. In practice, a catheter is placed into the proximal esophagus and connected to a slow drip of 0.1 N HCl. The patient does not know that the infusion is changed to 0.9% saline. If the patient's symptoms are brought on with HCl and relieved with saline, it is a positive test.[84] Some patients may have atypical pain, and in many it may be difficult to distinguish cardiac and esophageal pain. This test can be very helpful if there is a history of atypical pain and reflux, but has limited usefulness in pediatrics because the patients must cooperate and be able to describe symptoms during the infusions.

Diagnosis

The diagnosis of reflux is usually not difficult once one considers the possibility that the patient may have reflux. The amount of investigation performed should have a direct relationship to the seriousness of the problem and how typical the symptoms are. An infant who spits up frequently after feeding but has no respiratory symptoms and is growing well may need no testing. A patient with atypical symptoms who has respiratory symptoms and a failure to thrive or history of hematemesis would require a much more thorough evaluation.

Usually, the barium swallow or upper gastrointestinal series will be the first test ordered. Although there may be some differences from center to center, if the test is properly performed or interpreted, a correct answer should be obtained in approximately 80% of patients.[1, 87] More importantly, other disorders that might mimic symptoms of reflux can be detected or ruled out. These would include partial intestinal obstruction, pyloric stenosis, gastric webs, or malrotation. Vomiting is occasionally the main symptom in celiac disease, and a malabsorption pattern in the proximal small bowel can alert one to the possibility of a malabsorptive problem.

A barium swallow will be the only investigation most patients need. If results do not concur with the clinical picture or if further documentation of the problem is desired prior to more aggressive therapy or possible surgical intervention, it would be useful to choose another test.

In adults it has been shown that if two tests of esophageal function agree, they will accurately predict the presence or absence of GER.[6] In children two tests that agree will correctly predict the presence of GER approximately 95% of the time, while a single test may be correct only 80% of the time.[87] If the first two tests disagree, a third test will agree with one of them. In our experience, the use of a gastric scintiscan is not as effective in confirming the presence of GER as other tests, but if material can be identified in the lungs, it provides strong evidence that aspiration of refluxed gastric contents is occurring.[57]

Once GER is documented, the main value of esophagoscopy is in assessing the extent of esophageal damage. Esophagitis is an excellent indication of reflux but occurs in only a small minority of individuals.

As noted previously, the Bernstein test is useful in indicating that the patient's symptoms are related to reflux. It must be remembered that there is not a good correlation between severity of esophagitis and presence of heartburn. Esophageal manometry is most useful in detecting associated motor disorders of the esophagus. For patients with other problems (especially central nervous system disorders), one should proceed with great caution in surgical repair if there is an associated severe motor disorder of the esophagus, because any surgical repair may introduce some element of obstruction at the level of the lower esophageal sphincter. If surgery is performed, there is a great risk one may trade the problems of reflux for the problems of dysphagia.

Special Problems with Reflux

GER is not a single entity, but a problem that varies from patient to patient. Various groups of patients are now being recognized in whom different prognoses or responses to various medical or surgical interventions may be appreciated. In adults it is now appreciated that if patients have symptoms of gas or frequent burping in association with heartburn during the day but not at night, one should be very cautious in recommending surgical intervention.[38, 84] They may be classified as "upright refluxers," and once surgery is performed, there is a high incidence of bloating or the gas bloat syndrome, and the overall condition of the patient is likely to be unchanged. These patients rarely have pulmonary symptoms or develop esophageal stricture.

Certain pediatric patients are likely to have GER. Associated congenital problems were noted in 66 of 135 children who had surgical therapy for reflux, the majority of whom had disorders of the central nervous system.[65] Patients with reflux are common in institutionalized children, and gastroesophageal reflux is very common in retarded patients, especially those with Down's syndrome.[19, 93] One should be cautious in recommending surgery in these patients. Many will have poor esophageal motility, as mentioned above. In chronic care institutions, simple vomiting is often of much greater concern to caregivers than to the affected person. If major complications are lacking, e.g. bleeding or stricture, the quality of life of the individual should

be considered. Occasional or even daily vomiting may be of no
social significance compared to other common problems of
bowel or bladder function. On the other hand, if vomiting is so
frequent that attendants must spend all their contact time
cleaning and changing clothes rather than in individual training, surgical correction of GER can make a major improvement
in the quality of life of a handicapped person.

Two thirds of all patients with repair of esophageal atresia
and tracheoesophageal fistula in infancy will have dysmotility
of the distal esophagus and GER.[81, 82, 87] Recurrent respiratory
symptoms and anastomotic strictures are common postoperative problems frequently caused by GER.[38, 46, 83, 87, 98] Recent
studies have shown that recurrent esophageal anastomotic
strictures may be aggravated by esophagitis, and the poor motility of the distal esophagus interferes with mechanisms that
clear the esophagus of acid gastric contents. There may also be
subtle incoordination in pharyngeal or tracheal clearance
mechanisms that may occur in association with these major
malformations. Dysphagia is a common symptom in patients
with GER, but when it is the only symptom it is not associated
with GER. Awareness of these facts causes one to have a high
index of suspicion of GER in patients who have had repair of
esophageal atresia in infancy.

The natural history of GER in children was described by
Carre.[21] Most children will improve by 8–9 months, with complete resolution of symptoms in 60% by 18 months. Thus, one
can be quite optimistic in caring for these children. The situation is much different than that in adults, where reflux tends
to be a lifelong problem and therapy only helps to control
symptoms. Patients beyond the age of two tend to act much
more like adults. They are less likely to stop refluxing, and the
goals of treatment are more to control symptoms and prevent
esophagitis and strictures.

Because children and adults have had their esophageal pH
monitored over prolonged periods of time, it has become obvious that there is no constant pattern of reflux throughout the
day. Normally, reflux is more frequent while the patient is
awake than while he is asleep.[34] Reflux is more frequent during
the first two hours after feeding than it is afterward.[66] Because
of this, the period greater than two hours after eating, or use
of a single overnight sleeping recording, has been advocated for
some scoring systems. Although the exact mechanisms that

cause certain patients to develop respiratory symptoms are not understood, the mean duration of reflux episodes is a useful measurement to help predict which patients with reflux have respiratory symptoms induced by reflux and which have respiratory symptoms unrelated to it.

Patterns of reflux may bear some relationship to clinical symptoms. In one study, patients with reflux were grouped according to frequency of reflux episodes.[64] One group—continuous refluxers—had an abnormally high frequency of reflux for at least four hours after a meal. Another group—discontinuous refluxers—refluxed with a high frequency for only three hours and then rapidly decreased in frequency toward normal. A third group represented an intermediate minority. Statistically, class I continuous refluxers were older, much more likely to have large hiatal hernias, and more likely to require surgical repair of reflux. The class II discontinuous refluxers were younger, less likely to come to surgery, and were much more likely to have prolonged gastric emptying, higher lower esophageal sphincter pressures, respiratory symptoms, and nonspecific diarrhea. If it is assumed that respiratory symptoms develop more frequently in those with some subtle incoordination in airway protective measures, class II discontinuous refluxers represent more of a problem of coordination of motility along the intestine and are likely to improve with time, whereas class I continuous refluxers are more of a specific sphincter failure and are more likely to require surgical intervention.

Much has been made of the effect of lower esophageal sphincter pressure on sphincter competence, but this pressure is not constant. There are variations of pressure in the resting healthy patient.[12] Increases in abdominal pressure normally lead to slightly greater increases in sphincter pressure; such an increase is not noted in patients with chronic GER.[36]

Not all reflux occurs across a low pressure sphincter. Hauser et al.[49] have identified three types of reflux while constantly recording lower esophageal sphincter pressure in adults. There can be rapid transient decrease in sphincter pressure followed by reflux; reflux can occur across a sphincter with normal pressure, or across a sphincter with normal pressure associated with high abdominal pressure, e.g. such as would occur with a cough.

This variation in patterns and types of reflux helps to explain the inability of any single test to distinguish all patients with abnormal reflux. Barium esophagram and the acid reflux test sample only a short postprandial period when the distinction between normal and abnormal is not so obvious. The usual scoring of extended pH monitoring concentrates on the period greater than two hours after eating. A patient, then, may have just a few episodes of prolonged reflux leading to respiratory symptoms and have a false negative score.

As understanding of the various patterns and different mechanisms causing reflux are better understood, we will be better able to predict the outcome of therapy, tailor therapeutic efforts to the individual, and predict which patients will need surgical therapy.

Treatment

Once a tentative diagnosis of GER is made, whether based on history alone or confirmed by a series of esophageal function tests, the decision to treat and how vigorously to treat must be addressed. Most modes of medical therapy are based on physiologic reasoning, but not confirmed by clinical studies. The effects of surgical therapy are better documented, but there is great debate on the indications for surgery.

Not all patients with reflux need specific therapy, e.g., the infant with mild increased spitting after feeding or the older institutionalized child with cerebral palsy who may occasionally vomit shortly after eating. If there are no complications, vigorous 24-hour-a-day positional therapy is probably not worth the effort, and the effect of a short period of upright posturing is very debatable. Postural therapy with upright positioning is considered the mainstay of medical therapy.[23] Prolonged periods of esophageal pH monitoring would suggest that position has a physiologic role in the frequency of reflux. The effect of gravity may prevent regurgitation into the mouth and aid in clearing the esophagus.[78] Clinical experience in adults would indicate the effectiveness of position in preventing heartburn, and pediatric experience would indicate its usefulness in children. Infants spend most of their time prone, so special efforts are indicated to keep them upright throughout the day. Use of infant chairs can be a useful aid. Since most infants will slide to the bottom of a bed with the head elevated, we have found positioning of the child prone on a board elevated to 30 degrees useful. The child straddles a padded post to prevent sliding down the board. Rolled towels are placed on either side, and a loose strap keeps the child in the correction position. Infants tolerate this type of positioning very well.[17] It is reasonable to keep the child prone, for in this position the esophagus enters the most superior portion of the stomach. Unfortunately, as infants reach the age of one year, they demand more freedom to move about.

Extensive experience with prolonged esophageal pH monitoring indicates reflux is usually more frequent while the patient is awake than while he is asleep. We have noted clinically that some patients reflux much more frequently while they are asleep and upright. If lack of facilities or the seriousness of the situation do not indicate prolonged pH monitoring, one should heed parental statements that the child struggles whenever positioned upright or that vomiting is worse in such a position. Some patients with severe and recurrent aspiration may do better in the prone rather than the upright position. In the prone position, vomit is more easily expelled from the mouth, whereas gravity may predispose to aspiration in the upright position. Thickened feedings are usually advocated on the supposition that liquid gastric contents are more easily refluxed than semisolid ones. The authors are not impressed that the effect is a major one, although it is benign and worthy of a trial.[24] Although in adults the avoidance of corsets, girdles, or apparel that compress the abdomen and encourage reflux is stressed, the usual fashions of the pediatric patients makes this a minor therapeutic point.

Antacids and drugs that inhibit gastric acid secretion are frequently used in patients with reflux. Antacids are very effective in relieving heartburn and treating esophagitis. Cimetidine will also help relieve symptoms of heartburn and may help in healing of esophagitis, although the drug is not approved for this use.[7, 37]

Earlier papers indicated that alkalinizing the stomach contents would increase serum gastrin and thereby increase sphincter pressure and prevent reflux. It is now generally agreed that this is a pharmacologic effect of gastrin and not a physiologic effect.[58, 100]

Use of drugs to increase sphincter tone and prevent reflux

has limited appeal in adults, in whom the problem may have existed for decades, but it has great theoretical appeal in young children to tide them over until one can expect a spontaneous improvement of symptoms. Metoclopramide has been used successfully in adults, and a single report in pediatrics indicates that bethanechol chloride is helpful in treating reflux in children with vomiting and failure to thrive.[5, 37, 40] If these findings can be confirmed, it would be a major advance in treatment. These drugs do increase sphincter pressures, but recent studies indicate that prolongation of gastric emptying is a frequent occurrence in GER.[8] It is unknown whether their major therapeutic effect is related to raising the lower esophageal sphincter pressure or increasing the rate of gastric emptying.

If medical therapy is unsuccessful, one must balance the risks of surgical therapy with those of continuing reflux. A recent survey of several pediatric surgeons who frequently perform surgery for reflux would indicate that it is a relatively low-risk procedure. The mortality is approximately 0.5%, and many patients were premature and extremely ill, had associated heart disease, etc. In several large series there has been no operative mortality.[2, 65, 69, 86] Surgery will control reflux in approximately 95%, so it is quite effective. Choosing between the risks of continued medical therapy and surgical therapy often produces situations in which there is no clear consensus of opinion. A decision to operate on a patient with almost continuous vomiting in spite of vigorous medical treatment and who is failing to thrive and has iron deficiency anemia resulting from blood loss from a severely inflamed esophagus is not controversial. A decision to accept surgical risks in an infant with a poor home situation, protracted vomiting, a growth pattern approximating the third percentile for a period of six months, and two episodes of mild aspiration pneumonia instead of the subtle and unquantified risks of poor nutrition and pulmonary infections, can be defended or refuted with equal vigor.

Immediate recourse to surgical therapy is indicated in patients with severe life-threatening complications and in patients with strictures. We have had a number of infants with severe choking spells and recurrent apnea spells induced by reflux episodes who required multiple episodes of cardiopulmonary resuscitation.[52] To persist in medical therapy once the etiology was clear was to invite disaster. Patients with esophagitis and stricture will continue to reform the stricture so long as the reflux continues. Once reflux has been controlled, only a few dilatations will control the stricture. In very tight stricture formation it is often wise to do the first dilatation under direct visualization at the time of surgery.

At present, the Nissen fundoplication is the most widely used surgical procedure for reflux.[35, 90] In this procedure the fundus is wrapped about the distal esophagus. This procedure is effective if it must be performed within the thorax because of shortening of the esophagus. Surgical procedures tend to produce a supercompetent sphincter, and in postoperative studies very few if any reflux episodes are detected.[50] Occasionally these patients may be unable to vomit or burp when sick and develop acute gastric distention, a condition known as the gas bloat syndrome.[35] Fortunately, the symptoms of the gas bloat syndrome usually abate within a few months.

The Borema gastropexy is an anterior gastropexy that has been advocated for children.[14] Its concept is similar to a Hill posterior gastropexy, which is technically much more difficult. The sphincter is brought into the abdomen and anchored by suturing the lesser curvature to the diaphragm. Results are satisfactory, but we do not consider it a good procedure where there is severe esophagitis or shortening of the esophagus.

A Thal fundoplication is preferred by some, and a number of other operations have also been advocated.[2, 90] Properly performed, all of the procedures will give satisfactory results.

Summary

Information accumulated in recent years has provided answers to some, but not all, of the questions related to reflux. The various clinical presentations of GER are well described, and its natural history, especially in young childhood, is known. A number of tests to detect reflux have been adapted for children, and there has been good standardization in the performance of these tests. Criteria for diagnosis of GER are quite accurate, although consensus as to how extensive an evaluation is needed has not yet been reached. Medical therapy for reflux is reasonably effective. A number of surgical procedures have negligible morbidity and are very effective in controlling reflux. In spite of these advances, a number of areas require further study. Development of methods that clearly allow one to show a causal relation between GER and respiratory symptoms is an area of major importance. Development of criteria that would quickly identify those patients who would not benefit from a prolonged course of medical therapy would allow one to avoid the perpetuation of symptoms associated with ineffective medical therapy. Recent studies of the use of medication to prevent reflux open an exciting new vista. In view of recent studies demonstrating changes in gastric motility in adult patients with reflux, studies designed to further explore this area are indicated. If one could determine whether the therapeutic effect of bethanechol chloride and metocolpramide are related to esophageal or gastric effects, more effective drug therapy for GER might be devised.

BIBLIOGRAPHY

1. Arasu T.S., Wyllie R., Fitzgerald J.F., et al.: Gastroesophageal reflux in infants and children—comparative accuracy of diagnostic methods, *J. Pediatr.* 96:798, 1980.
2. Ashcraft K.W., Goodwin C.D., Amoury R.W., et al.: Thal fundoplication: A simple and safe operative treatment for gastroesophageal reflux. *J. Pediatr. Surg* 13:643, 1978.
3. Atkinson M., Van Gelder A.: Esophageal intraluminal pH recording in the assessment of gastroesophageal reflux and its consequences. *Am. J. Dig. Dis.* 22:365, 1977.
4. Batchelor M.D., Batchelor R.P.: Observations on a case of rumination with suggestions as to treatment. *Am. J. Dis. Child.* 17:43, 1919.
5. Behar J., Biancani P.: Effect of oral metaclopramide on gastroesophageal reflux in the post-cibal state. *Gastroenterology* 70:331, 1976.
6. Behar J., Biancani P., Sheahan D.G.: Evaluation of esophageal tests in the diagnosis of reflux esophagitis. *Gastroenterology* 71:9, 1976.
7. Behar J., Brand D.L., Brown F.C., et al.: Cimetidine in the treatment of symptomatic gastroesophageal reflux—a double blind controlled trial. *Gastroenterology* 74:441, 1978.
8. Behar J., Rambsy G.: Gastric emptying and antral motility in reflux esophagitis—effect or oral metaclopramide. *Gastroenterology* 74:253, 1978.
9. Behar J., Sheahan D.C.: Histologic abnormalities in reflux esophagitis. *Arch. Pathol.* 99:387, 1975.
10. Berenberg W., Neuhauser E.B.D.: Cardio-esophageal relaxation (chalasia) as a cause of vomiting in infants. *Pediatrics* 5:414, 1950.
11. Berenson M.M., Herbst J.J., Freston J.W.: Enzyme and ultrastructural characteristics of esophageal columnar epithelium. *Am. J. Dig. Dis.* 19:895, 1974.
12. Bloom A.A., Stekelman M., Varadee R., et al.: Resting pressures in the lower esophageal sphincter. *Am. J. Dig. Dis.* 19:1120, 1974.
13. Blumhagen J.D., Christie D.L.: Gastroesophageal reflux in children: evaluation of the water siphon. *Radiology* 131:345, 1979.
14. Boerema I.: Hiatus hernia: Repair by right-sided subhepatic, anterior gastropexy. *Surgery* 65:884, 1969.
15. Boix-Ochoa J., Lafuente J.M., Gil-Vernet J.M.: Twenty-four-hour pH monitoring in gastroesophageal reflux. *J. Pediatr. Surg.* 15:74, 1980.

GASTROESOPHAGEAL REFLUX
183

16. Botha G.S.: The Gastro-esophageal Junction. Boston: Little, Brown & Co., 1962, p 206.
17. Bray P.F., Herbst J.J., Johnson D.G., et al.: Childhood gastroesophageal reflux: Neurologic and psychiatric syndromes mimicked. J.A.M.A. 237:1342, 1977.
18. Brockbank E.M.: Merycism or rumination in man. Br. Med. J. 1:421, 1907.
19. Cadman D., Richards J., Feldman W.: Gastroesophageal reflux in severely retarded children. Dev. Med. Child. Neurol. 20:95, 1978.
20. Carre I.J., Astley R., Smellie J.M.: Minor degrees of partial thoracic stomach in childhood. Lancet 2:1150, 1952.
21. Carre I.J.: The natural history of the partial thoracic stomach ("hiatal hernia") in children. Arch. Dis. Child. 34:344, 1959.
22. Carre I.J.: Pulmonary infections in children with a partial thoracic stomach ("hiatus hernia"). Arch. Dis. Child. 35:481, 1960.
23. Carre I.J.: Postural treatment of children with a partial thoracic stomach ("hiatus hernia"). Arch. Dis. Child. 35:569, 1960.
24. Carre I.J.: Disorders of the oro-pharynx and esophagus, in Anderson C.M., et al. (eds): Pediatric Gastroenterology. Oxford: Blackwell Scientific Publications, 1975, pp 33–79.
25. Chattopadhyay D.K., Pope II C.E.: Lower esophageal sphincter pressure's variability destroys its usefulness. Gastroenterology 76:1111, 1979.
26. Christie D.L.: The acid reflux test for gastroesophageal reflux. J. Pediatr. 94:78, 1979.
27. Christie D.L., O'Grady L.R., Mack D.V.: Incompetent lower esophageal sphincter and gastroesophageal reflux in recurrent acute pulmonary disease of infancy and childhood, J. Pediatr. 93:23, 1978.
28. Cohen S., Harris L.D.: Does hiatus hernia affect competence of the gastroesophageal sphincter? N. Engl. J. Med. 284:1053, 1971.
29. Danus O., Casar C., Larrain A., et al.: Esophageal reflux—an unrecognized cause of recurrent obstructive bronchitis in children. J. Pediatr. 89:220, 1976.
30. Darling D.B., Fisher J.H., Gellis S.S.: Hiatal hernia and gastroesophageal reflux in infants and children: Analysis of the incidence in North American children. Pediatrics 54:450, 1974.
31. Darling D.B., McCouley R.G.K., Leonidas J.C., et al.: Gastroesophageal reflux in infants or children: Correlation of radiographical severity and pulmonary pathology. Radiology 127:735, 1978.
32. DeMeester T.R., Johnson L.F.: Evaluation of the Nissen antireflux procedure by esophageal manometry and twenty-four-hour pH monitoring. Am. J. Surg. 129:94, 1975.
33. DeMeester T.R., Johnson L.F.: The evaluation of objective measurements of gastroesophageal reflux and their contribution to patient management. Surg. Clin. North Am. 56:39, 1976.
34. DeMeester T.R., Johnson L.F., Joseph G.J., et al.: Patterns of gastroesophageal reflux in health and disease. Ann. Surg. 184:459, 1976.
35. DeMeester T.R., Johnson L.F., Kent A.H.: Evaluation of current operations for the prevention of gastroesophageal reflux. Ann. Surg. 180:511, 1974.
36. Dodds W.J.: Instrumentation and methods for intraluminal esophageal manometry. Arch. Intern. Med. 136:515, 1976.
37. Anonymous: Drugs for esophageal reflux. Med. Lett. Drugs Ther. 22:26, 1980.
38. Dudley N.E., Phelan P.D.: Respiratory complications in long-term survivors of esophageal atresia. Arch. Dis. Child. 51:279, 1976.
39. Ellis F.H., El-Kurd M.F.A., Gibb S.P.: The effect of fundoplication of the lower esophageal sphincter. Surg. Gynecol. Obstet. 143:1, 1976.
40. Euler A.R.: Use of bethanechol for the treatment of gastroesophageal reflux. J. Pediatr. 96:321, 1980.
41. Euler A.R., Ament M.E.: Value of esophageal manometric studies in gastroesophageal reflux in infancy. Pediatrics 59:58, 1977.

42. Euler A.R., Ament M.E.: Detection of gastroesophageal reflux in the pediatric age patient by esophageal intraluminal pH probe measurement (Tuttle test). *Pediatrics* 60:65, 1977.
43. Euler A.R., Byrne W.J., Ament M.E., et al.: Recurrent pulmonary disease in children: A complication of gastroesophageal reflux. *Pediatrics* 63:47, 1979.
44. Fabricius ab Aquapendente H.: *Tractus de Gula: Ventriculo et Intestinis.* Patav, 1618.
45. Farrell M.K., Keenan W.J., Wolske S., et al.: Gastroesophageal reflux (GER): Relation to apnea. *Pediatr. Res.* 14:498, 1980.
46. Fonkalsrud E.W.: Gastroesophageal fundoplication for reflux following repair of esophageal atresia: Experience with nine patients. *Arch. Surg.* 114:48, 1979.
47. Forget P.P., Meradji M.: Contribution of fiberoptic endoscopy to diagnosis and management of children with gastroesophageal reflux. *Arch. Dis. Child.* 51:60, 1976.
48. Guttman F.M.: On the incidence of hiatal hernia in infants. *Pediatrics* 50:325, 1972.
49. Hauser R., Dodds W.J., Patel G.K., et al.: Mechanisms of gastroesophageal reflux (GER) in patients with reflux esophagitis. *Gastroenterology* 76:1153, 1979.
50. Herbst J.J.: Unpublished data.
51. Herbst J.J., Berenson M.M., McCloskey D.W., et al.: Cell proliferation in esophageal columnar epithelium (Barrett's esophagus). *Gastroenterology* 75:683, 1978.
52. Herbst J.J., Book L.S., Bray P.F.: Gastroesophageal reflux in the "near miss" sudden infant death syndrome. *J. Pediatr.* 92:73, 1978.
53. Herbst J.J., Book L.S., Johnson D.G., et al.: The lower esophageal sphincter in gastroesophageal reflux in children. *J. Clin. Gastroenterol.* 1:119, 1979.
54. Herbst J.J., Friedland G.W., Zboralske F.F.: Hiatal hernia and "rumination" in infants and children. *J. Pediatr.* 78:261, 1971.
55. Herbst J.J., Johnson D.G., Oliveros M.A.: Gastroesophageal reflux with protein-losing enteropathy and finger clubbing. *Am. J. Dis. Child.* 130:1256, 1976.
56. Herbst J.J., Minton S.D., Book L.S.: Gastroesophageal reflux causing respiratory distress and apnea in newborn infants. *J. Pediatr.* 95:763, 1979.
57. Heyman S., Kirkpatrick J.A., Winter H.S., et al.: An improved radionuclide method for the diagnosis of gastroesophageal reflux and aspiration in children. *Radiology* 131:483, 1979.
58. Higgs R.H., Smyth R.D., Castell D.O.: Gastric alkalinization—effect on lower esophageal sphincter pressure and serum gastrin. *N. Engl. J. Med.* 291:486, 1974.
59. Hill J.L., Pelligrini C.A., Burrington J.D., et al.: Technique and experience with 24-hour esophageal pH monitoring in children. *J. Pediatr. Surg.* 12:877, 1977.
60. Ingelfinger F.J.: Esophageal motility. *Physiol. Rev.* 38:533, 1958.
61. Johnson L.F., DeMeester T.R.: Twenty-four-hour pH monitoring of the distal esophagus. *Am. J. Gastroenterol.* 60:325, 1973.
62. Johnson D.G., Herbst J.J., Oliveros M.A., et al.: Evaluation of gastroesophageal reflux surgery in children. *Pediatrics* 59:62, 1977.
63. Jolley S.G., Herbst J.J., Johnson D.J., et al.: Mean duration of gastroesophageal reflux identifies children with reflux-induced respiratory symptoms. *Gastroenterology* 78:1189, 1980.
64. Jolley S.G., Herbst J.J., Johnson D.G., et al.: Patterns of postcibal gastroesophageal reflux in symptomatic infants. *Am. J. Surg.* 138:946, 1979.
65. Jolley S.G., Herbst J.J., Johnson D.G., et al.: Surgery in children with gastroesophageal reflux and respiratory symptoms. *J. Pediatr.* 96:194, 1980.
66. Jolley S.G., Johnson D.G., Herbst J.J., et al.: An assessment of gastroesophageal reflux in children by extended pH monitoring of the distal esophagus. *Surgery* 84:16, 1978.
67. Kanner L.: *Child Psychiatry,* ed 3. Springfield, Ill.: Charles C Thomas, Publisher, 1957, p 484.

68. Keet A.D., Heydenrych J.J.: Hiatus hernia, pyloric muscle hypertrophy and contracted pyloric segment in adults. *Am. J. Roentgenol.* 113:217, 1971.
69. Kim S.H., Hendren W.H., Donahoe P.K.: Gastroesophageal reflux and hiatus hernia in children: Experience with 70 cases. *J. Pediatr. Surg.* 15:443, 1980.
70. Kinsborne M.: Hiatus hernia with contortions of the neck. *Lancet* 1:1058, 1964.
71. Krantman H.J., Rachelefsky G.S., Lipson M., et al.: Recurrent pulmonary infiltrates, digital clubbing and failure to thrive in a 4-year-old boy. *J. Allergy Clin. Immunol.* 61:403, 1978.
72. Leape L.L., Holder T.M., Franklin J.D., et al.: Respiratory arrest in infants secondary to gastroesophageal reflux. *Pediatrics* 60:924, 1977.
73. Lilly J.R., Randolph J.G.: Hiatal hernia and gastroesophageal reflux in infants and children. *J. Thorac. Cardiovasc. Surg.* 65:42, 1968.
74. Luschka H.: Das Antrum Cardiacum des menschlichen Magens, *Virchows Archiv (Pathol. Anat)* 11:427, 1857.
75. McCauley R.G., Darling D.B., Leonidas J.C., et al.: Gastroesophageal reflux in infants and children: A useful classification and reliable physiologic technique for its demonstration. *Am. J. Roentgenol.* 130:47, 1978.
76. Menin R.A., Malmud L.S., Petersen R.S., et al.: Gastroesophageal scintigraphy to assess the severity of gastroesophageal reflux disease. *Ann. Surg.* 191:66, 1980.
77. Menking M., Wagnitz J.G., Burton J.J., et al.: Rumination—a near fatal psychiatric disease of infancy. *N. Engl. J. Med.* 280:802, 1969.
78. Meyers W.F., Herbst J.J., Jolley S.G., et al.: Positioning a patient prone on a 30-degree inclined plane effectively decreases reflux. *Clin. Res.* 29:113A, 1981.
79. Morse J.L.: *Case Histories in Pediatrics*. Boston: William Leonard, Publisher, 1913, p 120.
80. Naeye R.L., Messmer J., Specht T., et al.: Sudden infant death syndrome temperament before death. *J. Pediatr.* 88:511, 1976.
81. Orringer M.B., Kirsh M.M., Sloan H.: Long-term esophageal function following repair of esophageal atresia. *Ann. Surg.* 186:436, 1977.
82. Parker A.F., Christie D.L., Cahill J.L.: Incidence and significance of gastroesophageal reflux following repair of esophageal atresia and tracheoesophageal fistula and the need for antireflux procedures. *J. Pediatr. Surg.* 14:5, 1979.
83. Pieretti R., Shandling B., Stephens C.A.: Resistant esophageal stenosis associated with reflux after repair of esophageal atresia: A therapeutic approach. *J. Pediatr. Surg.* 9:355, 1974.
84. Pope II C.E.: Gastroesophageal reflux disease, in Sleisinger M.H., et al. (eds): *Gastrointestinal Disease: Pathophysiology, Diagnosis, Management.* Philadelphia: W.B. Saunders Co., 1978, pp 541–565.
85. Price S.F., Smithson K.W., Castell D.O.: Food sensitivity in reflux esophagitis. *Gastroenterology* 75:240, 1978.
86. Randolph J.G., Lilly J.R., Anderson K.D.: Surgical treatment of gastroesophageal reflux in infants. *Ann. Surg.* 183:479, 1974.
87. Roberts C.C., Herbst J.J., Jolley S.G., et al.: Evaluation of tests for gastroesophageal reflux in patients operated on for tracheo-esophageal fistula. *J. Pediatr. Res.* 14:509, 1980.
88. Roviralta E.: Association de sténose hypertrophique du pylore et d'ectopie gastrique partielle (syndrome phrénopylorique), *Arch. Mal. App. Dig.* 39:1103, 1950.
89. Rudd T.G. Christie, D.L.: Demonstration of gastroesophageal reflux in children by radionuclide gastroesophagography. *Radiology* 131:483, 1979.
90. Shandling B.: Surgical techniques in the treatment of gastroesophageal reflux and hiatal hernia, in *Gastroesophageal Reflux Proceedings of the 76th Ross Conference on Pediatric Research.* Columbus, Ohio: Ross Laboratories, 1979, p 95.
91. Shapiro G.G., Christie D.L.: Gastroesophageal reflux in steroid-dependent asthmatic youth. *Pediatrics* 63:207, 1979.

92. Shegren T.G., Mangurten H.H., Brea F., et al.: Rumination—a new complication of neonatal intensive care. *Pediatrics* 66:551, 1980.
93. Sondheimer J.M., Morris B.A.: Gastroesophageal reflux among severely retarded children. *J. Pediatr.* 94:710, 1979.
94. Stef J., Dodds W.J., Hogan W.J., et al.: Intraluminal esophageal manometry: An analysis of variables affecting recording fidelity of peristaltic pressures. *Gastroenterology* 67:221, 1974.
95. Stein M.R., Weber R.W., Tower T.G.: The effect of theophylline on the lower esophageal sphincter pressure (LESP), abstracted. *J. Allergy Clin. Immunol.* 61:137, 1978.
96. Tuttle S.G., Grossman M.I.: Detection of gastroesophageal reflux by simultaneous measurement of intraluminal pressure and pH. *Proc. Soc. Exp. Biol. Med.* 98:225, 1958.
97. Welch R.W., Luckmann K., Ricks P., et al.: Lower esophageal sphincter pressure in histologic esophagitis. *Dig. Dis. Sci.* 25:420, 1980.
98. Whitington P.F., Shermeta D.W., Dexter S.Y.S., et al.: Role of lower esophageal sphincter incompetence in recurrent pneumonia after repair of esophageal atresia. *J. Pediatr.* 91:550, 1977.
99. Winter H., Madara J., Stafford R., et al.: Functional and morphological assessment of acid reflux in children. *Gastroenterology* 78:1293, 1980.
100. Wright L.F., Slaughter R.L., Gibson R.G., et al.: Correlation of lower esophageal sphincter pressure and serum gastrin concentration and lower esophageal sphincter pressure. *Am. J. Dig. Dis.* 20:261, 1975.

Some Health Care Needs of Young Athletes

NATHAN J. SMITH, M.D.

Professor of Pediatrics and Orthopedics,
University of Washington
Seattle, Washington

PARTICIPATION IN ORGANIZED SPORTS is an important part of the life of a majority of young people in the United States. The restricted environment in which most American children live allows little opportunity for spontaneous, self-generated play. Vitality and good health require regular energy-expending exercise. Without opportunities to create their own play, the play needs of children are more and more being offered as highly organized competitive sports programs patterned after the familiar model of varsity or professional sports. Such elaborate sports programs have become available because of economic affluence and abundant leisure time of parents. Both are essentials for highly organized youth sports programs. The extent of parental involvement is such that sports programs for youth are often accused of being designed more for the participation of the adults than they are for the young participants. That a great many children truly enjoy and gain much from participation both in youth sports and scholastic sports programs cannot be argued. There is no question that when there is informed and understanding involvement by adults, involvement free of the vicarious imposition of their own adult goals and aspirations, the programs can be appropriate, enjoyable, and maturing experiences.

Preadolescent and elementary-school-aged children have become regular participants in organized sports. At the same

0065-3101/81/0028-187-228-$03.75

time, junior and senior high school youths are participating in both community and scholastic sports programs in ever-increasing numbers. In many communities well over half of the boys and one third of the girls between 14 and 17 years of age are involved in organized, competitive scholastic sports. Thirty-nine sports for high school boys and 27 sports for girls are officially sanctioned as high school sports.[1] Little more than a generation ago, the typical American high school offered only three or four sports to boys (football, basketball, and baseball or track) and no interscholastic sports to girls. Nowadays it is proper to assume that healthy young people in middle-income and upper-income homes will be participants in some form of organized competitive sports.

Participation in competitive sports has a very significant meaning. It is more than just an opportunity for pleasant, healthful expenditure of energy. This can be deduced from a recent investigation by Coddington[2] of emotional stresses in youth. His study identified the relative degrees of anxiety perceived by junior and senior high school students that are generated by various life-stress situations. Failing in a competitive area with one's peers was perceived as being one of the most stressful events; it ranked with both divorce of parents and involvement in a teenaged pregnancy. Failure to succeed in an extracurricular event, such as not making an athletic team, was rated more stressful than failing a grade in school or even the death of a close friend. It is not unexpected that sports competition has the potential for producing severe stress and anxiety. Competition in sports serves as a testing ground of the competence of one's body, a focal point of great concern to all adolescents. Sports competition provides opportunities for comparison of one's physical prowess and skills with one's peers. Success and failure in sports can be a major determinant of acceptance by parents, teachers, and coaches and most particularly by peers.

The physician to the older child and adolescent deals with a patient population rarely threatened with life-endangering illnesses and thus there is little obligatory contact with any health professional. The adolescent is often reluctant to have health care contact. Encountering the doctor traditionally has meant finding or searching for something wrong with one's body, a concern with which the adolescent is innately insecure. As these youths experience few traditional reasons to have contact with the physician, those professionals with the interest and expertise to meet health concerns that now center on their sports activities may be perceived as an attractive and relevant health care resource.

Current experience in providing health care to young athletes documents that the management of major sports injuries is a minor part of their total health care. A variety of other health matters related to success and avoidance of failure in sports are more commonly encountered. Nutrition, stress management, fluid and electrolyte needs, specific energy needs for specific types of competitions, achieving optimal levels of body fatness, avoiding minor stress injuries, and the efficient and rapid rehabilitation of strains and sprains, are all questions that the junior or senior high school athlete will bring to an informed and concerned physician.

The Preparticipation Health Evaluation

The physician's entry into the athletic life of the young patient commonly occurs through the preparticipation health evaluation required for most scholastic sports programs. This provides an ideal opportunity to conduct a specifically sports-related history and physical examination and to demonstrate concern, expertise, and familiarity with the needs and anxieties of the athlete.

The required preparticipation health evaluation can be either an expensive, irritating, and perfunctory exercise, distasteful for both physician and athlete, or it can satisfy some very important and pertinent goals for both. In order to be meaningful, this medical contact of athlete and concerned physician should be designed to meet certain very definite objectives. The history and physical examination should be specifically directed to determining the suitability of the individual for sports participation. This examination is sports-directed and is *not* to be considered a comprehensive health appraisal. Detailed or comprehensive evaluation of an adolescent must be time-consuming and may often be needlessly repetitious and expensive for an individual who has been receiving previous comprehensive pediatric care. Equally important, a traditional health appraisal may not meet several of the needs that are pertinent to sports participation.

The   sports-directed   preparticipation   health   evaluation should be limited to accomplishing the following: It may discover acute medical conditions that are to be immediately treated. Conditions can also be found that will be worsened by athletic participation. These should be recognized as well as those conditions that may interfere with chances of success in a given sport. On occasion it might be possible to identify situations that place the individual at increased risk to injury, such as the grossly unconditioned aspirant, or the immature and small young person who is contemplating participation in a collision sport. Recognition of visual handicaps may prevent injury or failure. Legal needs are to be satisfied by the examination, as well as requirements for insurance coverage of the athlete.[3]

In addition to meeting these essential needs for the athlete and the sports program, the preparticipation physical evaluation provides the physician a valuable contact with the boy or girl about to become involved in sports. The physician can relate insight and interest in sports participation, an awareness of the needs of the athlete, and his or her availability in the future to offer guidance regarding health-related concerns that may arise.

A protocol for an efficient and effective group preparticipation examination has been described by Garrick.[4] The essentials of the medical history and physical examination are described for the examination to be efficiently conducted in the office or in a well-organized manner in a group setting of the school gymnasium or locker room. Although individual evaluation in the physician's office is traditionally looked on as the most desired setting in which to carry out any health evaluation, the very specialized needs to the preparticipation sports examination may be very effectively done as a team or group at the school. When done in this well-organized manner, the examination will better meet the specific needs of the athletes and the program than when it is performed in a busy office, clinic, or health center where the needs of an apparently healthy athlete must compete for attention with more urgent demands.

The athletic candidate should undergo a preparticipation health evaluation when he or she enters junior or senior high school athletic programs and need not have one for each sport, nor does the evaluation need to be redone every year. At the beginning of each academic year, or each sport season, an interval history review is needed to update the health and injury experience of the athlete. Whenever a transfer student enters a new school system the initial athletic preparticipation evaluation is carried out. The examinations should be scheduled several weeks prior to the beginning of practices for any given sport. This allows time to rehabilitate and strengthen the site of any previous injury and to implement any conditioning recommendations that are made.

The young people who seek sport-related health evaluations are the healthiest members of a very healthy segment of society. It becomes important to eliminate from the examination items unlikely to provide information pertinent to the specific needs and goals of suitability for safe sport participation. Time spent recording abundant negative data that are not pertinent is uneconomical and detracts from the effectiveness and validity of other data that is critical for the decisions that are to be made regarding sport participation. A history can be limited to four or five general screening questions concerning past health and injury experiences. The questions in the preparticipation history are the following:

1. Has any member of your family had a heart attack prior to age fifty?

2. Do you have to stop while running around a (quarter-mile) track twice?

3. Have you ever lost consciousness while participating in sports, either having fainted or been "knocked out?"

4. Are you taking any medication regularly?

5. Have you ever had an illness or injury that caused you to miss a game or a practice, caused you to go to the hospital overnight, or required an operation?

The first question deals with the identification of those families that may have hyperlipidemias or have experienced rare but important genetically transmitted heart disorders. The second question will identify limiting cardiopulmonary problems and the grossly underconditioned young boy or girl. The question regarding medication will identify the allergy patient requiring medication, the acne patient taking antibiotics, the seizure patient taking medication, and the insulin-dependent diabetic. The fourth question alerts one to the counseling needs of the individual in collision sports who has had a previous concussion and who will require decisions regarding continued participation, protective equipment, and the position to be played on the team. Fainting during exercise is not uncommon and may be an important indicator of the need for cardiology consultation to rule out congenital cardiac abnormalities that can be associated with sudden death during exercise. The implications of the questions regarding previous illness and injury are obvious.

When the preparticipation evaluations involve large numbers in the school setting, the athletes can complete their history forms in a group under the direction of a nurse or trainer in the presence of the coach. An affirmative answer to any of the questions will prompt a follow-up personal history by an examining physician. The athlete can complete the history form in the waiting room of the doctor's office.

The physical examination for the prospective athlete is limited to those things that will answer the needs and goals specifically related to sports participation. It does not follow the pattern or meet the needs of a detailed and complete physical evaluation. Usually, attention is directed only to the following items, specifically ignoring many aspects of a traditional physical examination. The skin is examined for the presence of pustular acne, impetigo, herpes, or fungal infections. Dental prosthesis and dental caries are looked for. Equality of the pupils is noted in inspection of the eyes. The heart is examined with care in a quiet area; specific note is made of irregularities in rhythm, altered sounds, or any evidence of enlargement. The lungs are not routinely auscultated, nor is it rewarding to routinely examine the ears, auditory canals, and tympanic membranes. Lymph nodes are palpated and enlargement of abdominal organs is identified in examination of the abdomen. The male genitalia are examined for the presence of both descended normal testes. An orthopedic examination is essential and may often be the most rewarding aspect of the examination. Evidence of inadequately rehabilitated previous sports injuries are the most commonly encountered abnormality in boys participating in high school sports.[3] The orthopedic exam can be done in a brief period of time; one looks for symmetric muscle development, full range of motion of all joints, and the presence of deformities, such as scoliosis or swollen, abnormal joints (Appendix).

Assessment of maturation of the young male athlete is a vital concern in the examination of the early high school and junior high school male athlete who may be contemplating participation in one of the collision sports, e.g., football, wrestling, and ice hockey.

Blood pressure and vision are tested. Vision testing may be limited to the use of Snellen's chart. The significance and management of abnormal or possibly abnormal blood pressure have been discussed recently.[5] After three or more repeated examinations document the presence of higher than normal blood pressure, a thorough diagnostic evaluation is indicated. Stress testing is mandatory before any restrictions of athletic participation are recommended.

Questions have been raised concerning the desirability of annual vision and blood pressure testing in those young people who may have no other health care contact during the year other than their preparticipation sports examination. If after their first evaluation only an interval history is demanded or required, blood pressure and vision abnormalities may develop and go undetected. These are appropriate concerns but only reinforce the concept that the preparticipation health evaluation for sports is not intended to be, and for reasons of economics and effectiveness cannot be, the mechanism through which complete health supervision is provided to the adolescent or preadolescent who happens to be participating in sports. The fact that there are more than six million high school athletes who need an annual health review dictates that there must be other more comprehensive, ongoing mechanisms to satisfy the multifaceted health care demands of the adolescent. Monitoring the vision and blood pressure of the young adolescent who happens to be an athlete is a high priority health care need that should not be monitored casually in relation to his or her athletic activity. If it is to be effective, the preparticipation sport health evaluation must be designed to meet the specific needs of the individual's participation in sports and not to satisfy the multifaceted goals of comprehensive health care.[3]

For the young male athlete, laboratory studies are not a necessary part of the sport-related preparticipation evaluation. Urinalysis in large populations of healthy young people are unrewarding and only serve to create undue anxiety.[6] The needs for assessing iron status are discussed below.

TABLE 1.—Disqualifying Conditions for Sports Participation*

CONDITIONS	COLLISION	CONTACT	NONCONTACT	OTHER
General				
Acute infections:				
Respiratory, genitourinary, infectious mononucleosis, hepatitis, active rheumatic fever, active tuberculosis	X	X	X	X
Obvious physical immaturity in comparison with other competitors	X	X		
Hemorrhagic disease:				
Hemophilia, purpura, and other serious bleeding tendencies	X	X	X	
Diabetes, inadequately controlled	X	X	X	X
Diabetes, controlled				
Jaundice	X	X	X	X
Eyes				
Absence or loss of function of one eye	X	X		
Respiratory				
Tuberculosis (active or symptomatic)	X	X	X	X
Severe pulmonary insufficiency	X	X	X	X
Cardiovascular				
Mitral stenosis, aortic stenosis, aortic insufficiency, coarctation of aorta, cyanotic heart disease, recent carditis of any etiology	X	X	X	X
Hypertension on organic basis	X	X	X	X
Previous heart surgery for congenital or acquired heart disease†				
Liver				
Enlarged liver	X	X		
Skin				
Boils, impetigo, and herpes simplex gladiatorum	X	X		
Spleen				
Enlarged spleen	X	X		
Hernia				
Inguinal or femoral hernia	X	X	X	
Musculoskeletal				
Symptomatic abnormalities or inflammations	X	X	X	X
Functional inadequacy of the musculoskeletal system, congenital or acquired, incompatible with the contact or skill demands of the sport	X	X	X	
Neurologic				
History or symptoms of previous serious head trauma, or repeated concussions	X			
Controlled convulsive disorder‡				
Convulsive disorder not moderately well controlled by medication	X			

TABLE 1.— *Continued*

Previous surgery on head	X	X		
Renal				
Absence of one kidney	X	X		
Renal disease	X	X	X	X
Genitalia§				
Absence of one testicle				
Undescended testicle				

*"This list of recommendations was created by members of the Committee and reflects only their opinion in 1966. The recommendations are not based on the analysis of any epidemiologic data defining true injury experience or the risk of injury of present-day sports participation. These recommendations are, however, the only recognized recommendations for disqualification for sports that are in print and may be used as a general guideline in counseling athletes and parents." Courtesy of the American Medical Association Committee on the Medical Aspects of Sports: *A Guide for Medical Evaluation of Candidates for School Sports.* Chicago: American Medical Association, 1966. Copyright 1966, American Medical Association.

Sports categories are: collision—football, rugby, hockey, lacrosse, etc.; contact—baseball, soccer, basketball, wrestling, etc.; noncontact—cross country, track, tennis, crew, swimming, etc.; other—bowling, golf, archery, field events, etc.

†Each patient should be judged on an individual basis in conjunction with his cardiologist and operating surgeon.

‡Each patient should be judged on an individual basis. It is probably better to encourage a young boy or girl to participate in a noncontact sport rather than a contact sport. However, if a particular patient has a great desire to play a contact sport, and this is deemed a major ameliorating factor in his/her adjustment to school, associates, and the seizure disorder, serious consideration should be given to letting him/her participate if the seizures are moderately well controlled or the athlete is under good medical management.

§The Committee approves the concept of contact sports participation for youths with only one testicle or with an undescended testicle(s), except in specific cases such as an inguinal canal undescended testicle(s), following appropriate medical evaluation to rule out unusual injury risk. However, the athlete, parents, and school authorities should be fully informed that participation in contact sports for such youths with only one testicle does carry a slight injury risk to the remaining healthy testicle. Following such an injury, fertility may be adversely affected. But the chances of an injury to a descended testicle are rare, and the injury risk can be further substantially minimized with an athletic supporter and protective device.

The preparticipation health evaluation should be conducted in an adequate period of time before the beginning of the practice season to allow for implementation of those recommendations that are to be made regarding specific rehabilitative needs and needs of conditioning. The recorded findings from group examinations are reviewed soon after the examination session is over and only then are decisions made as to any limitation as to participation or further examinations that are needed.

Guidelines have been published regarding disqualifying medical conditions for various types of sport participation (Table 1). It is recommended that those who lack any of the paired organs, e.g., a lung, an eye, a kidney or testes, not be permitted to participate in collision sports such as football, wrestling, ice hockey, or lacrosse. In recent years, when such recommendations have been challenged, the courts have ordered schools to allow participation in collision sports of young boys with such health handicaps. In most instances it is recommended that patients with poorly controlled seizure disorders do not participate in water sports, such as swimming, rowing, or water polo. Those with hepatosplenomegaly should avoid participation in collision sports, as should those with hemorrhagic disorders. Valid reasons for exclusion from participation are quite limited, and the increasing number of sports in both community and school-based programs makes some form of participation available to essentially every child. The physician will best serve the needs of aspiring young athletes with chronic health problems by identifying a specific sports activity in which the individual can be competitive rather than placing undue emphasis on exclusions. A boy with cystic fibrosis, for example, has been a coxswain in a rowing program. A young man with osteogenesis imperfecta tarda is very competitive on a swimming team, and another boy with a word-processing learning disorder participates in a karate program where the coach gives minimal instruction by written or spoken word.

The information from the preparticipation evaluation is made available to the school sports program, parents, the team physician, and the school's athletic trainer.

Maturation Assessment and Sports Participation

The impact of both physical and behavioral maturation on the success and enjoyment of sports participation makes assessment of maturational status an important factor in counseling the child and parents about participation in organized sports. It is obvious that certain types of athletic activities, even though available, are inappropriate for the child of early elementary school age. Preadolescents and early adolescents experience great variation in both physical and behavioral maturation rates and are at particular risk of finding themselves mismatched in athletic contests. Regardless of their size, these late maturers are noncompetitive and often unable to satisfy the expectations of parents and coaches. One of the few positive things that the physician is able to do in injury prevention is identify the late-maturing individual and advise against participation in the collision sports of football, wrestling, or ice hockey until an appropriate level of physical maturation is reached.

Proficiency and success in youth sports is greatly influenced by maturational status. When sexual maturation was assessed according to either pubic hair distribution or skeletal age, over half of the highly proficient baseball players in the Little League World Series were found to be maturationally advanced for their chronological age. Pitchers, catchers, and cleanup batters are the most advanced. The close correlation with sexual maturation and athletic performance in many of the popular sports should prompt the physician to carefully consider maturation status in counseling boys or girls who contemplate participation in competitive sports. Assessment of sexual maturation is effectively done using Tanner staging techniques, which correlate with tests of muscle strength in both boys and girls. Some strength tests, such as grip strength testing, along with Tanner staging of sexual maturity, may be helpful in impressing an eager young aspirant of the significance of his or her maturation level in relation to his or her potential in sports.

There are obvious risks for the slow, late-maturing individual. These individuals are handicapped in two very significant ways when they are obliged to participate and compete with individuals of the same chronologic age but who are sexually and physically more advanced than they. The late maturer will compete at a decided disadvantage for a position on the team and, at best, will probably become a noncontributing bench warmer. If the team is such that he is to become a regular player, they are probably so devoid of talent that the outcome of most contests will be defeat for his team for which he will soon believe he is, in part, responsible. One way or the other, he is destined to be a loser and suffer considerable loss of self-esteem and the desire to pursue rewarding athletic endeavors later. The late maturer is also at increased risk to injury in collision sports. Although serious injury is not common among small preadolescent players in the peewee league of collision sports, one can hardly expect the smaller, late maturer to look with favor on a play experience in which he must suffer an inordinate number of bumps and bruises at the hands of stronger and more mature adversaries and teammates.

Parents of the late-maturing young boy and girl should be advised to discourage participation in collision sports during preadolescence and the early years of adolescence, i.e., while the child is in grade school and junior high school. Until children of this age can be matched on the basis of their physical maturation status, collision sports are inappropriate for early and preadolescents in junior high schools where maturation varies so greatly. Football and wrestling are inappropriate sports for junior-high-school-aged children. There are other team and individual sports that can be made available and that are appropriate for children of this age, sports in which size and strength are not major determinants of proficiency.

Increasing concern is being expressed for the young athlete who experiences high levels of success in youth sports because of advanced physical maturity with advanced size and strength for his chronological age. This is the highly successful pitcher on the Little League baseball team, the star quarterback on the juvenile football team, the player every coach wants to have on his community-based sports team every season. This young all-star is outstanding, not because of exceptional skill or remarkable talent but because of his or her advanced biologic age. Such athletes are bigger, stronger, have better muscle control and endurance because of advanced physical development. The skills these early maturers learn in their sport experience are usually learned at the hands of the nonprofessional volunteer coach; they are poorly taught and difficult or impossible to improve later under more sophisticated coaching. The expectations of continued outstanding performance may become a significant burden and an increasing problem as the athlete gets older and his peers begin to achieve a comparable degree of physical maturity. Maintaining all-star status becomes increasingly difficult and sooner or later it becomes essentially impossible. Parents and coaches alike can become disenchanted with the fading stardom of the early maturer who is often assumed by all of the admiring adults not to be "putting out." Loss of adult acceptance, loss of the admiration and attention of teammates and peers, and the eventual loss of self-worth and esteem are all significant hazards for the early maturer who experiences excessive adoration in the highly organized sports programs. The pediatrician will recognize the early maturer. The child and parents should be advised to take whatever steps may be necessary to participate with individuals of comparable maturational age where skills can be learned from appropriate coaches and where the child can be properly compared and his or her potential can be tested against proper opponents. The early maturer will thus grow up with an athletic performance in proper perspective.

There are two situations in high school sports programs where maturation assessment is particularly important. Late-maturing boys of small size are often tempted to participate in the high school wrestling programs in the lower weight classes. Small size per se is not a disadvantage in wrestling, as competitors are matched on the basis of weight. However, the small boy who is a late maturer is an inappropriate opponent for the small boy of similar weight who is genetically destined to be small and has reached a more advanced stage of physical maturity. Wrestling is a high-injury sport. Competition between individuals of the same size but of widely varied stages of maturation increases the risk of injury. Boys less than a Tanner stage four in sexual maturation are not suitable candidates for high school wrestling programs.

A second area of concern for maturational status is in the assessment of the tall, linear, late-maturing young boy who is a sought-after candidate for the basketball team. Many very tall boys are attracted to this sport but often lag far behind the average in physical maturation. Such a boy may experience his peak velocity in height attainment as late as the sophomore or junior year in high school. It is well established that significant increases in both strength and endurance are not acquired until at least twelve to twenty-four months after the peak velocity in height attainment has been experienced. Thus, the parent and coach soon may experience considerable disappointment and frustration at the lack of endurance and performance of the very tall and unusually well-endowed physical specimen on the basketball court. They will profit from counseling to allow time for development of the strength and endurance that are essential to be competitive in this sport, even though an enviable height has been achieved. Many of the truly outstanding, very tall basketball players active in professional basketball today were not outstanding players until late in their high school careers, when they became physically capable of exploiting their unusual height advantage in playing the game. It is unfortunate indeed that there is a commonly accepted precept in American coaching that, for the physically advantaged, lack of competitive success is always due to simple lack of effort—a fallacy that can negate a positive sport experience for the tall, linear, late maturing boy who has not as yet developed the muscle strength and endurance necessary for an acceptable performance. The frustrations of the coach and parent are painful indeed as they contemplate a winning season or a college scholarship with a six-foot-eight-inch high school junior who is still growing but who lacks the stamina to run up and down the basketball court twice.

Counseling Parents about Youth Sport Participation

Because nearly 90% of American children live in so-called urban communities, communities that provide little place for safe, self-generated, and unsupervised play, the active exercise desired and needed by young people may be limited to play experiences organized by adults in today's youth sport programs. The youth sport phenomenon has proliferated at a tremendously rapid rate in the past two decades, so that in some communities there is hardly a sport that is not available as a highly organized activity for children as young as four or five. The majority of American children between the ages of eight and 15 years in a physician's practice today are involved in one or more sports organized on a local, regional, and national level. Most programs have been patterned after the varsity or professional sports model made familiar and attractive by the mass media, a model to which the child and parent can readily relate. With excessively long seasons and practice schedules, inappropriate matching of competitors, untrained volunteer coaching, little concern for health and safety, and a variety of parental excesses, it is often difficult to accept many youth sport programs as a desired answer to the play and recreational needs of the preadolescent and elementary-school-aged child. As the pediatrician's patient reaches the age where decisions regarding youth sport participation must be made, thoughtful counseling is now becoming an important part of health guidance. Knowledge of the youth sport programs in the community, the goals and priorities of the family, the social and physical maturity of the child, are all factors to be considered in avoiding family conflicts and contributing to a healthy sports experience for the child patient.

It is lamentable that, considering the dimensions of the youth sport participation in this country, there is little sound data on the physical or emotional impact of youth sport participation on the child. There is some documentation that generally the risk of injury in most youth sport programs is not great, considerably less than for participants at older age levels.[8] Even in the collision sports, the size, speed, and power of the small preadolescent athlete fails to generate forces that will cause many injuries. Behavioral impacts are less well documented. Stress has been evaluated in Little League baseball players through monitoring pulse rates in a study conducted by Hanson.[9] When they sat on the bench their average pulse rates were 95 per minute. When they played in the field the pulse rates rose to an average of 127, and as the Little Leaguer stood in the batter's box the pulse rate rose to 167 per minute. How much emotional stress is reflected in a pulse rate of 167? This is obviously a question to which only a subjective answer may be given.

More recently, Simon[10] has used a psychological scale designed to measure emotional states in children and compared the anxiety experienced in seven different sports, in physical education class activities, in taking academic tests, and in performing in musical competitions either as soloists or as a member of the school band. The children could score from as low as 10 (low anxiety) to as high as 30 (high anxiety) on the particular scale that was used. Academic tests and physical education classes created little anxiety. Individual sports such as wrestling and gymnastics are the most emotionally demanding experiences, but performing the musical solo was by far the most anxiety-generating activity. It is pointed out that the average anxiety score for each of the sports did not reach even the midpoint in the anxiety scale used by Simon.

Smoll and Smith[11] have documented the responses of Little League baseball players to encouraging-reinforcing coaching techniques compared to the responses of the preadolescent players to the threatening and punitive coaching behavior of other coaches. Their data indicates that children are more responsive to the former than the latter and that the win-loss records of the teams were no different regardless of the coaching philosophy and techniques that were used.

The most threatening emotional consequences of participation in highly structured sports programs now available to very young children will come from parental, and to a lesser extent, sibling reactions to a child's athletic activities. The perplexity of competitive stress from sports is focused in the home, where parental and family reactions determine whether the uncertainty of outcome, which is the nature of the sport participation, will be a healthful, maturing challenge or whether it will be overly stressful and destructive. Where this fine line is to be drawn varies with each child and each family. One child's challenge is another child's stress. A major determinant will be how confident and secure the child finds himself in relation to the important adults in his life. Children will grow from the challenges of sport if they know that their parents and family, their peer group, and their coaches will consider them worthy persons regardless of the outcome of their performance in any game or athletic contest. Knowing that their worth does not depend on the outcome of some game or contest will give the young athlete the confidence to risk and cope with losing and thus confidently enjoy the benefits of sport participation.

How can the all too frequent pitfalls of youth sport participation be avoided? With guidance from the child's physician regarding maturational status, involvement in an inappropriate sport should be avoided. Some familiarity with community youth sport programs will allow the physician to advise against participation in those that involve inappropriate goals, scheduling, commitments, etc. Most important, parents can be prompted to ask themselves certain pertinent questions regarding youth sport involvement. Answers to such questions will form the basis of thoughtful and appropriate decisions helpful in avoiding trouble when such questions are considered prospectively rather than after a sports participation problem has developed. Some such questions are the following:

Who really wants to get involved in the sports program?— the child, the parent, the coach, or the program organizers? Is this a proper sport for a child of this maturation age? What advantage will this sport program provide for my child—fun?

exercise and fitness? learning skills? teamwork? Does our child appreciate the time commitment that signing up for the program represents, time that will be taken away from other forms of play? What will participation in the program mean to family life and scheduling of family activities such as meal times, vacations, weekends, etc.? What will it do to the relationships with the other children in the family? What do we know about the program's goals? About the objectives and qualifications of those who run the program? Are the practices and competitions conducted in a safe and well-supervised manner? How are the competitors matched and assigned to teams? Do all children get to play? What is the degree of parental involvement expected to be? What are the expected financial obligations for uniforms, equipment, travel, etc.? Are parents expected to be at practices, games, provide chauffeuring services, laundry service, etc.? Is our child prepared emotionally to handle winning and losing? Can he or she accept instruction and criticism from a coach? Are we ready to be the parents of a bench warmer or a loser and accept the decisions of the coach about our child? How will we get out of the program if we want to? What will we do if our child wants to quit?

Youth sport programs can be organized on a very low-key recreational basis so that all children may participate. Parental involvement can be kept to an absolute minimum and the goals of the programs concentrated on learning skills, social growth, and healthy energy-expending exercise. All too many programs, however, in the hands of the untrained volunteer staffs, are directed at producing league champions with winning an overstressed goal for the age of the competitors. These youth sport programs then become more a program for entertainment and gratification of the adults than a healthy play experience for children.

American public schools have not accepted the responsibility for appropriate instruction in physical education for children, and by default the youth sport program has exploited the need for exercise and play experiences of our young people. As a result, the American child has the least desirable opportunity for physical fitness of any childhood population in the industrialized nations of the world. The child's physician has the responsibility of alerting parents to the pitfalls as well as the advantages of youth sport participation and, hopefully, will assume a leadership role in the community to minimize the negative aspects of youth sports programs active there. Who else will speak up for children in this critical area?

Nutritional Concerns of Young Athletes

It has been well established in a series of nutrition and health surveys that American adolescents and preadolescents are the segments of the population at greatest risk of inadequate and undesirable dietary practices.[12] It is likewise becoming recognized that participation in sports can be a highly effective motivating force to improve dietary intakes. Young people often desire to upgrade their nutrition practices to improve their athletic performance and thus the athletic coach or trainer has become a more effective nutritional educator, even though he or she all too often teaches from an inadequate and misinformed base of information about nutrition.

Athletes recognize that food intake is an important determinant of two major factors affecting their athletic performance. The first is body composition—i.e., how fat or thin they are, their weight, their state of hydration, etc.—and the second, food as a source of energy. The serious young competitor often approaches a training diet plan with the same intense commitment of his or her training program and goes to extremes in an effort to find a diet thought to improve performance. Thus, the serious athlete is particularly vulnerable to any of a host of fads and food fallacies that are often vigorously promoted to a very vulnerable population of athletes. Energy supplements, so-called muscle-building supplements, and, most particularly, high-potency vitamin supplements are all used by the athlete to such an extent that there is a widely quoted adage that one can always tell the American athlete in international competition because he or she has the most expensive urine in the world.

The first information the young athlete should receive regarding his or her nutritional needs is the fact that intense training and energy-expending competition doesn't increase the body's need for any specific nutrient. These will be only increasing the needs for energy and water. Well-controlled studies of the impact of dietary supplementation with most of the vitamins have been carefully carried out with populations of athletes and military personnel. This research has demonstrated an absence of any effect on physical work performance and endurance of a variety of vitamin and mineral supplements when added to a mixed American diet adequate in amount to meet the athlete's energy needs. Of particular interest are those studies involved with evaluating vitamin E supplementation. A well-controlled study of competitive swimmers demonstrated no effect in performance or in endurance. Years before the current enthusiasm for intakes of massive doses of vitamin C, the nutritional performance laboratory of the United States Army had investigated the impact of large doses of vitamin C on work performance and found such intakes to be without effect in increasing either performance or endurance.

The enthusiastic and uninformed athlete is at risk to the hazards of uncontrolled intakes of vitamin or protein supplements. Vitamin A intoxication should be suspected in the young athlete who presents with consistent headache, malaise, and bone pain. No more than 50 to 100,000 units of vitamin A daily may induce toxicity. Likewise, vitamin E intoxication can occur with muscle pains, weakness, and gastrointestinal symptoms. A syndrome of pseudogout is recognized and is caused by ingestion of large quantities of protein supplements. Joint pains and hyperuricacidemia are seen with certain young men who attempt to gain body weight and increase muscle mass with the injudicious use of supplements and extreme intakes of protein-rich foods.

If young athletes are to avoid needlessly expensive and potentially dangerous vitamin, mineral, and protein supplementation, they need guidelines that they can use confidently in evaluating their nutrient intakes. Some practical assessment scheme will permit the athlete to be confident that an adequate amount of all essential nutrients is being provided by the daily diet. The interested or insecure individual may record his food intake for a few representative days and with one of the currently taught food group systems, determine whether or not the diet is suitably varied. The widely taught four food group system is adequate for these evaluations and is a system most young people have been exposed to in school. Knowing that they have received two servings of both high-protein foods and foods from the dairy group and four servings each from the groups of grain foods and from the fruit-vegetable group, the boy or girl athlete can be assured that he or she gets adequate amounts of all of the 60 or more essential nutrients. Supplementation of such a varied diet is only potentially dangerous and needlessly expensive.

The generous and varied American diet eaten by the active youngster will meet the needs of essential nutrients for the young athlete. The most frequently encountered problem area concerns the adequacy of energy intake provided by the diet. Achieving and maintaining a desirable competing weight for a given sport depends on controlling the total energy content of the diet. Once a desired weight and level of body fatness has been achieved, regular periodic weighings once or twice a week will detect any unintentional weight losses. Unintended weight loss results only from energy intakes inadequate to meet the demands of training and other energy expenditures in the daily life style of the athlete. The loss of only a few pounds may be very significant, for this negative energy balance will be accompanied, sooner or later, by a deterioration of performance.

Where emotional commitment to training and weight control is unusually intense, weight loss can occur rapidly and become extreme and simulate the true anorexia nervosa commonly encountered in teenaged girls and young women. Both male and female participants in a variety of sports may be seen with so-called anorexia nervosa of the athlete. These athletes may continue high energy-expending athletic performance yet rapidly lose weight. Weekly or twice-weekly weighings should identify early the individual developing anorexia, food aversion, and extreme weight loss. Reassurance and counseling designed to modulate the emotional stresses of training and competition, school achievement, peer relationships, etc., are usually helpful with the prognosis of this food aversion syndrome of the athlete, about which the physician may be more optimistic than he can with the guarded prognosis of classical anorexia nervosa in the young female population.

Food energy intake inadequate to meet the needs of training and competition can be a significant contributor to underperformance and so-called staleness. Workers in the Exercise Physiology Laboratory at Ball State University have measured muscle glycogen concentrations in muscle biopsy samples taken periodically during intense training.[13] Subjects in these studies were training with daily ten-mile runs. The muscle glycogen content of quadriceps muscle fibers became progressively less with each day's vigorous training, even though the athletes were taking unrestricted high carbohydrate diets (60% of total calories). While they continued on the high carbohydrate diet, it took three days of markedly reduced training activity before the muscle glycogen concentration returned to a pretraining level. Decreasing energy expenditure and maintaining of a good caloric intake is essential in preparing for important competitions. Much of the adverse consequence of so-called overtraining can be energy depletion of specific muscle fibers.

The athlete's most common concern regarding energy balance is directed to achieving an optimal competitive weight. This problem occupies a prominent place in the training of all individuals in weight-matched sports such as wrestling, lightweight rowing, boxing, and weightlifting. Most athletes and coaches identify a level of fatness and body weight at which athletes are most competitive. This may be a very minimal level of fatness in such sports as gymnastics and figure skating, competitive diving, etc. In sports such as football and ice hockey, minimal fatness may not be so essential. However, it is recognized that well-controlled, moderate levels of fatness are associated with optimum endurance and quickness. What most athletes are trying to achieve is the greatest level of strength, endurance, and quickness for each unit of body weight. This body composition is associated with a given degree of fatness and identified as a desired competing weight. Fatness in excess of a desired minimum that contributes nothing but excess weight will reduce speed and quickness as well as compromise endurance.

The most convenient and practical method of estimating body fatness is by measuring skin-fat fold with an appropriate caliper. By applying a formula such as the one developed by Wilmore,[14] it is possible to translate one or more skin-fat fold measures into a calculated percentage of body weight that is made up by body fat. Many coaches and physical education specialists are skilled in estimating body fat by using underwater weighing. Body density is calculated from this measure with that percentage of the body weight that is made up of body fat readily determined. Other methods such as counting the body's

TABLE 2.—RELATIVE BODY FAT VALUES
FOR MALE AND FEMALE ATHLETES IN
VARIOUS SPORTS.*

SPORT	MALES FAT(%)	FEMALES FAT (%)
Baseball/softball	12–14	16–26
Basketball	7–10	16–27
Football	8–18	—
Gymnastics	4–6	9–15
Ice hockey	13–15	—
Jockeys	12–15	—
Skiing	7–14	18–20
Soccer	9–12	—
Speed skating	10–12	—
Swimming	5–10	14–26
Track and field		
Sprinters	6–9	8–20
Middle distance runners	6–12	8–16
Distance runners	4–8	6–12
Discus	14–18	16–24
Shot put	14–18	20–30
Jumpers and hurdlers	6–9	8–16
Tennis	14–16	18–22
Volleyball	8–14	16–26
Weightlifting	8–16	—
Wrestling	4–12	—

The values represent the range of means reported in various published and unpublished studies.
From Wilmore J.H., in Smith N.J. (ed): *Sports Medicine for Children and Youth: Report of Tenth Ross Roundtable on Approaches to Common Pediatric Problems.* Columbus, Ohio: Ross Laboratories, 1979. Used by permission.

content of 40 K in a total body counter or measuring body fat by calculating the amount of fat-soluble gases retained in breathing tests are less commonly employed procedures and are obviously more complex and require extensive equipment. Table 2 shows the percentage of body fat found in high-performing athletes in various sports. These values can serve as a general guideline in counseling the serious athlete as to degree of fatness and desired competitive weight associated with high performance in a given sport.

Once a present level of fatness has been estimated and the desired level of fatness identified, the athlete can proceed with a fat and weight reduction program. Usually fat should not be lost at a rate that exceeds two or three pounds each week. It is necessary to initiate any conditioning and fat reduction program well in advance of the schedule of competitions. Secondly, during the period of fat reduction the athlete should ingest adequate calories to protect the lean body tissues. This will be approximately 2,000 calories a day for an active young male athlete and no less than 1,600 calories for an average high school female athlete. Lesser caloric intakes than these can result in use of lean body tissues, i.e., muscle, as a source of energy.

If the average young high school boy eats three meals a day with single servings of modest size, avoids desserts and excessive milk intake, and most importantly, avoids all between-meal eating, he will probably be reducing his caloric intake by 500 to 1,000 calories below that needed to maintain his weight with normal school activity. If he increases energy expenditure with an hour to an hour and a half conditioning workout, he will increase his daily energy expenditure by 500 to 750 calories. In general, we would hope the young athlete trying to reduce his or her body fat would create a negative energy balance of approximately 1,000 calories each day, totalling 7,000 calories a week. This is the energy equivalent of two pounds of body fat. (The energy of one pound of body fat is the equivalent of 3,500 calories.)

Few things will be appreciated more by the serious young competitor than having guidance as to a desired level of body fatness for his or her sport and how to achieve that level of fatness while maintaining an adequate energy intake to meet the training demands and function in school while feeling like a reasonable human being. No change in body weight, whether by gaining muscle mass through muscle training and increases in energy intake or by reducing body fat through training and modest diet restriction, can be accomplished rapidly. Starting early and proceeding with a deliberate gradual rate of change is an absolute essential.

Especial Concerns of the Female Athlete

During the past decade, large numbers of girls began participating in organized competitive sports for the first time. Nowadays the typical girl in the middle-income or upper-income American family is as likely to be involved in organized sports as is her brother, first at the community level of youth sports and later in the rapidly expanding sports programs in junior and senior high schools. Neither the new female athlete nor her mother has little, if any, previous experience or tradition to call on in guiding her in her new adventures in training, conditioning, and competition. One obvious answer to questions concerning sports is to adopt many of the procedures and mannerisms of their male counterparts and to try harder. The results may often be undesirable and at times awesome. In the latter category is the "new" girl, the third basewoman who comes to bat with a large wad of chewing tobacco in her cheek.

The more serious consequence of the inexperience of many young female athletes is their lack of experience in modifying and regulating their training and conditioning programs. As a result, many injuries from overuse and stress may be encountered in many of the girls' sports programs. Muscle strains, shin splints, stress fractures, and particularly retropatellar pain syndromes are not uncommon. Osgood-Schlatter disease, previously thought to be an affliction of active boys, is not uncommon among junior high and high school female athletes. Girls often need guidance in the intensity of early training efforts and their need to rest and reduce their training schedules when symptoms of overuse begin to appear.

Girls are not commonly involved in the collision sports of football, wrestling, ice hockey, etc., and thus avoid the high risk of injury in these activities. However, in other sports the injury experience is essentially the same as with male participants in the same sport. Early concern that the female breast might suffer serious injury in sport participation has not been borne out. In a few situations in such sports as basketball or soccer, where the breasts have been bandaged and immobilized against the chest wall, severe hematomata has developed as a result of a significant blow. Unless bound down firmly to the thoracic cage wall, the mobile breast tissues are not particularly vulnerable to trauma.

Proper breast support for the female athlete is an important concern and only recently have suitable brassieres for the female athlete become available. Protection from trauma is not an important consideration except in a sport such as fencing and for baseball catchers, where traditionally suitable chest protection has been provided for both male and female. Effective support for the female breast is essential for comfortable and acceptable active sport participation. In those running and jumping sports where there is vertical body motion, the breasts will move uncomfortably and if such activity is pursued for a significant period there will inevitably be stretching of integument and other supports, leading to permanent, undesirable sagging of the breasts. Without some supporting control of breasts in the high-school-aged female athlete, discomfort and aversion to excessive breast movement will prompt a large number of girls to forgo the many advantages of sport participation. It is fortunate that the recent research efforts of Haycock[15] have designed a highly effective breast support for the active girl athlete. Girls should be counseled in regard to use of such well-designed bras. Though there are many so-called athletic bras on the market, only two or three can be recommended. These include the Lady Duke and Lilly of France.

Menstrual irregularity is often associated with intense sport participation, and girls seriously committed to training and competition may have prolonged periods of amenorrhea. The emotional stress alone of competing for a position on the team can be a causative factor. Where intense training is associated with marked reduction in body fat, as in figure skating, gymnastics, distance running, etc., amenorrhea will usually occur when body fat is reduced to an estimated level of less than 10% to 12% of total body weight. These lean young women should know that even without experiencing their normal menses they may continue to be ovulating and can become pregnant. The amenorrhea associated with training and fatness reduction is temporary and to date no adverse consequences have been documented as resulting from the prolonged periods of amenorrhea associated with dedicated athletic training. The regular menstrual cycle should be expected quite promptly after decreasing the intensity of training and acquiring increased levels of body fat.

Iron Deficiency, Depletion, and Deficiency Anemia in the Female Athlete

The health and nutrition surveys of the past decade have documented that varying degrees of iron lack are common among women of childbearing age in the United States. Best estimates suggest that nearly 15% of females from 14 to 45 years of age will be found to have less than desired iron nutrition when assessed with one or more biochemical methods of assessing iron status. In the population of teenaged girls, there is little difference in the frequency of iron lack in relation to family income; girls from middle-income and upper-income families have essentially the same incidence of iron depletion as those from poverty-stricken families. Several hundred women varsity athletes at the University of Washington have been surveyed with erythrocyte protoporphyrin levels used as the screening method. Approximately 8% of these women were found to be iron-depleted. Recently, Finch et al. have documented the consequences of iron depletion unrelated to any reduction in hemoglobin concentration in animals in the laboratory. These studies strongly suggested that iron-depleted athletes may be significantly limited in their endurance because of their limited iron status. Iron-depleted rats with normal hemoglobin concentrations had limited exercise tolerance, which was associated with exaggerated exercise-induced lactic acidosis. The altered energy metabolism was related to compromised function of the iron-dependent α-glycerophosphate dehydrogenase system. Studies in women athletes with normal hemoglobin levels but elevated protoporphyrin concentrations in their erythrocytes and reduced plasma ferritin concentrations suggest that similar increases in postexercise lactic acidosis are experienced by the iron-depleted woman athlete. Until definitive human studies are completed, it is probably important to provide some biochemical assessment of iron status for every young woman seriously committed to a sports program. Either erythrocyte protoporphyrin determination, transferrin saturation, or a serum ferritin determination can be used to identify the young woman who will benefit from an increase in iron intake. The individuals found to be iron-depleted should have the causative factor identified and receive a full therapeutic course of iron. Most commonly, normal but greater than average menstrual iron losses will be the cause of iron deficiency, and long-term medicinal iron supplementation will be needed.

Sports Injuries

Orthopedic and surgical management of sports injuries is not a common concern of the physician who treats young athletes. In a sports medicine clinic serving the medical needs of a population of university level varsity athletes, a trauma-related surgical decision was required eight times in each 100 typical visits and a surgical procedure was performed no more than once. Minor infectious illnesses, skin care, conditioning concerns, stress management, nutrition, and weight control problems prompt the majority of visits to the clinic.

The injury experience to be expected in a present-day high school sports program has been documented in a detailed study by Garrick.[16] Using highly skilled certified athletic trainers stationed full time in four Seattle high schools, they observed and recorded the injury experience in 19 sports over a two-year study period. Most of the sports-related injuries were of a minor nature; 70% of the athletes missed less than a week of sport participation and 29% missed only one day. The trainers referred 42% of those injured to a physician for care. Of those seen by a physician, 71% had an x-ray examination and 2% were hospitalized, including 1.7% of those injured who required a surgical procedure.

In essentially all sports most of the injuries occur during practice sessions when the only responsible adult present is the coach. Thus, upgrading the competence of the coach in the prevention, early management, and recognition of injuries is the most effective action that can be taken in improving the medical handling of common sports injuries.

The majority of sports injuries are first seen by the coach and because of their minor nature are treated by the athlete and/or the parent. All of these individuals should be instructed as to the application of proper first aid based on the well-accepted concept of ICE: *i*ce, *c*ompression, and *e*valuation. When first aid and home management of injuries are limited to these modalities, and when the latter are properly and effectively applied, it is essentially impossible to compound or further damage a sports injury. The strict avoidance of all drugs as well as prohibiting taping or strapping of a sports injury without a physician's supervision are important guidelines for the parent, young athlete, and coach. The persistence of symptoms that do not respond promptly to simple ICE first aid requires prompt evaluation by a physician. Any therapy beyond the short-term use of ICE demands a specific diagnosis by a physician. Not only does this apply to the use of any drugs, supports, and manipulations, but most particularly to the initiation of any rehabilitation program.

Injured athletes experience reinjury with disturbing frequency when they return to training and competition. They are not only at risk to reinjury of the previously injured part, but new and unrelated injuries are common. This very disturbing experience relates in large part to the usual lack of an adequate rehabilitation program. The athlete adequately rehabilitated after an injury should have adequate strength, agility, and complete ability to normally protect himself or herself from recurrent injury. As little as 48 hours of immobilization of the knee will cause a measurable loss of strength in the quadriceps muscles. As little as a 10% loss of quadriceps strength increases the risk of reinjury of the knee. A sprained ankle, when immobilized in a cast for one month, requires two months of active rehabilitation in order to regain normal, safe function. Rehabilitation of the sports injury is the critical factor that determines whether or not a sports injury has been successfully managed. The required modalities and rehabilitative techniques are not complicated and could be provided by interested primary care physicians and their office personnel. As mentioned earlier, evidence of an inadequately rehabilitated previous sport injury is the most common finding in the preparticipation evaluation of the older high school athlete.

Life-Threatening Sports Injuries

Serious life-threatening sports injuries occur rarely but they are an ever-present potential danger whenever young athletes are actively training and competing. Life-threatening injuries include severe head or neck injury, cardiac or respiratory arrest, severe hemorrhage, and shock, particularly in relation to heat exposure. Any young athlete experiencing these calamaties can die before professional health assistance can be obtained. As with less serious injuries, life threatening injuries are most apt to occur during practice when the coach is the only responsible adult present. Every coach, therefore, should be certified in cardiopulmonary resuscitation. In addition, the coach should be prepared at all times to call for emergency assistance; this means immediate and constant access to a functioning telephone, knowing whom to call, and being assured at all times that there is unlocked access to the practice area for an emergency vehicle and crew. Active young people should have an opportunity for cardiopulmonary resuscitation training and certification by the time they enter high school, with plans for suitable refresher experiences during their high school careers. At every practice and at every game the coach should be certain that emergency medical assistance is effectively and immediately available and that he or she, as the coach, is trained in the techniques that will keep an injured athlete alive until medical help arrives.

Appendix

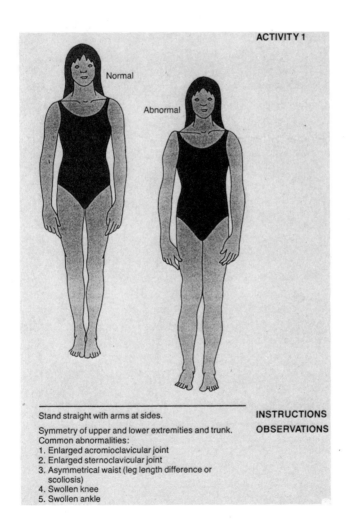

ACTIVITY 1

Normal

Abnormal

Stand straight with arms at sides.   **INSTRUCTIONS**

Symmetry of upper and lower extremities and trunk.   **OBSERVATIONS**
Common abnormalities:
1. Enlarged acromioclavicular joint
2. Enlarged sternoclavicular joint
3. Asymmetrical waist (leg length difference or
   scoliosis)
4. Swollen knee
5. Swollen ankle

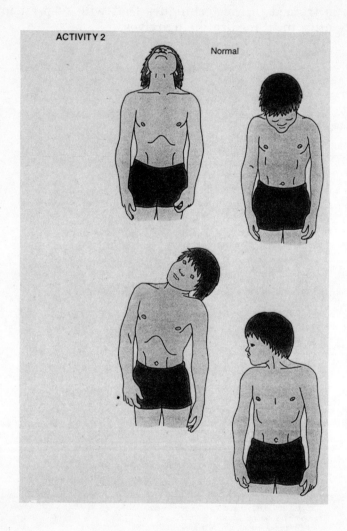

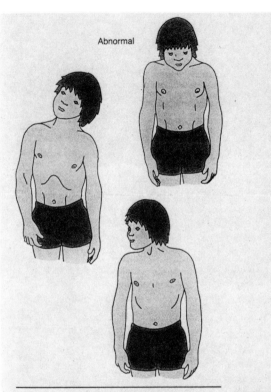

Abnormal

Look at ceiling; look at floor; touch right (left) ear to shoulder; look over right (left) shoulder.	**INSTRUCTIONS**
Should be able to touch chin to chest, ears to shoulders and look equally over shoulders. Common abnormalities (may indicate previous neck injury): 1. Loss of flexion 2. Loss of lateral bending 3. Loss of rotation	**OBSERVATIONS**

ACTIVITY 3

Normal

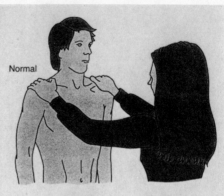

Abnormal

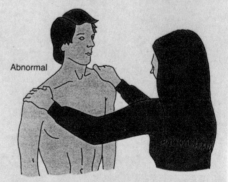

INSTRUCTIONS   Shrug shoulders while examiner holds them down.

OBSERVATIONS   Trapezius muscles appear equal; left and right sides equal strength.
Common abnormalities (may indicate neck or shoulder problem):
1. Loss of strength
2. Loss of muscle bulk

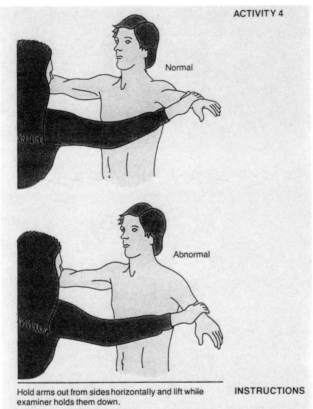

ACTIVITY 4

Normal

Abnormal

Hold arms out from sides horizontally and lift while   **INSTRUCTIONS**
examiner holds them down.

Strength should be equal and deltoid muscles should   **OBSERVATIONS**
be equal in size.
Common abnormalities:
1. Loss of strength
2. Wasting of deltoid muscle

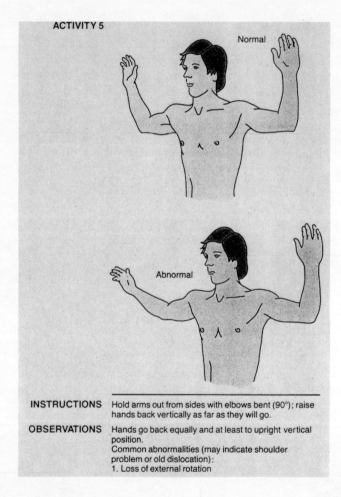

ACTIVITY 5

Normal

Abnormal

| INSTRUCTIONS | Hold arms out from sides with elbows bent (90°); raise hands back vertically as far as they will go. |
| OBSERVATIONS | Hands go back equally and at least to upright vertical position.
Common abnormalities (may indicate shoulder problem or old dislocation):
1. Loss of external rotation |

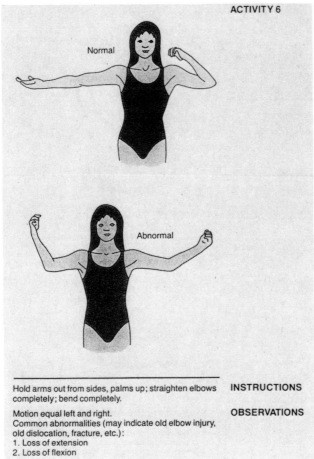

ACTIVITY 6

Normal

Abnormal

INSTRUCTIONS

Hold arms out from sides, palms up; straighten elbows completely; bend completely.

OBSERVATIONS

Motion equal left and right.
Common abnormalities (may indicate old elbow injury, old dislocation, fracture, etc.):
1. Loss of extension
2. Loss of flexion

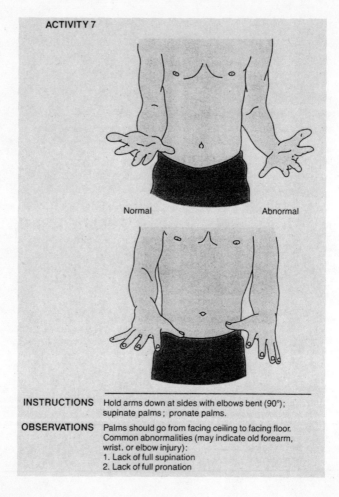

ACTIVITY 7

Normal   Abnormal

INSTRUCTIONS   Hold arms down at sides with elbows bent (90°);
                supinate palms ; pronate palms.

OBSERVATIONS   Palms should go from facing ceiling to facing floor.
                Common abnormalities (may indicate old forearm,
                wrist, or elbow injury):
                1. Lack of full supination
                2. Lack of full pronation

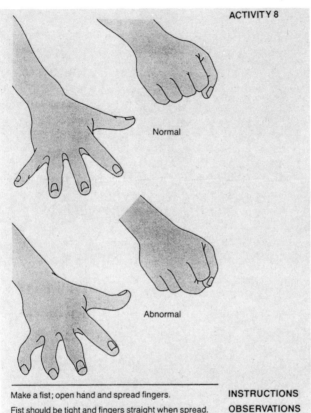

ACTIVITY 8

Normal

Abnormal

Make a fist; open hand and spread fingers.	**INSTRUCTIONS**
Fist should be tight and fingers straight when spread.	**OBSERVATIONS**

Fist should be tight and fingers straight when spread.
Common abnormalities (may indicate old finger
fractures or sprains):
1. Protruding knuckle from fist
2. Swollen and/or crooked finger

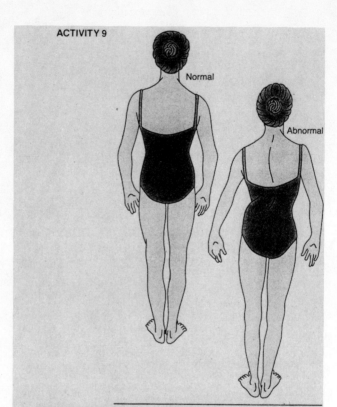

ACTIVITY 9

Normal

Abnormal

INSTRUCTIONS   With back to examiner stand up straight.

OBSERVATIONS   Symmetry of shoulders, waist, thighs, and calves.
Common abnormalities:
1. High shoulder (scoliosis) or low shoulder (muscle loss)
2. Prominent rib cage (scoliosis)
3. High hip or asymmetrical waist (leg length difference or scoliosis)
4. Small calf or thigh (weakness from old injury)

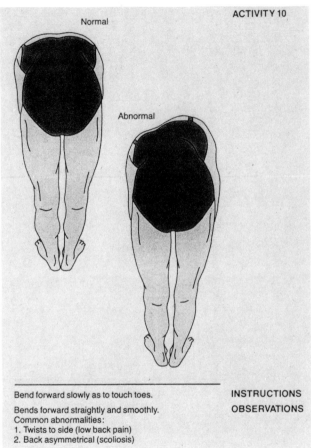

ACTIVITY 10

Normal

Abnormal

Bend forward slowly as to touch toes.   INSTRUCTIONS

Bends forward straightly and smoothly.   OBSERVATIONS
Common abnormalities:
1. Twists to side (low back pain)
2. Back asymmetrical (scoliosis)

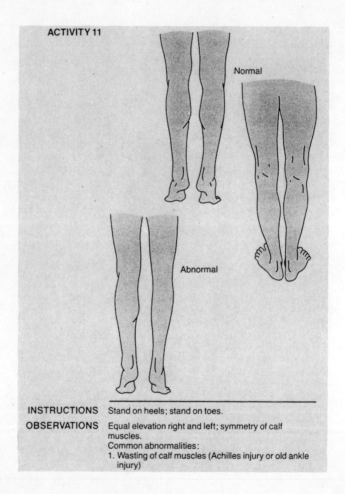

ACTIVITY 11

Normal

Abnormal

INSTRUCTIONS   Stand on heels; stand on toes.

OBSERVATIONS   Equal elevation right and left; symmetry of calf
muscles.
Common abnormalities:
1. Wasting of calf muscles (Achilles injury or old ankle
   injury)

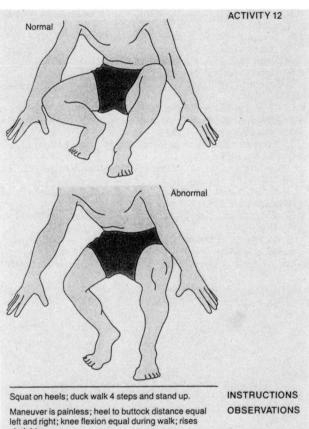

ACTIVITY 12

Normal

Abnormal

Squat on heels; duck walk 4 steps and stand up.   **INSTRUCTIONS**

Maneuver is painless; heel to buttock distance equal   **OBSERVATIONS**
left and right; knee flexion equal during walk; rises
straight up.
Common abnormalities:
1. Inability to full flex one knee
2. Inability to stand up without twisting or bending to
   one side

REFERENCES

1. Shaffer T.E., in Smith N.J. (ed): *Sports Medicine for Children and Youth: Report of the Tenth Ross Roundtable on Approaches to Common Pediatric Problems.* Columbus, Ohio: Ross Laboratories, 1979.
2. Coddington R.D.: The significance of life events as etiologic factors in the diseases of children. *J. Psychosom. Med.* 16:205, 1972.
3. Garrick J.G., Smith N.J.: Preparticipation sports assessment. *Pediatrics* 66:803, 1980.
4. Garrick J.G.: Sports medicine. *Pediatr. Clin. North Am.* 24:737, 1977.
5. Mitchell S.C., Blount S.G. Jr., Blumenthal S., et al.: The pediatrician and hypertension. *Pediatrics* 56:3, 1975.
6. Strong W.B.: Hypertension in sports. *Pediatrics* 64:693, 1979.
7. Goldberg B., Saranti A., Witman P., et al.: Preparticipation sports assessment. *Pediatrics* 66:736, 1980.
8. Garrick J.G., in Smith N.J. (ed): *Sports Medicine for Children and Youth: Report of the Tenth Ross Roundtable on Approaches to Common Pediatric Problems.* Columbus, Ohio: Ross Laboratories, 1979.
9. Hanson D.L.: Cardiac response to participation in Little League baseball competition. *Res. Q.* 38:384, 1967.
10. Simon J.A.: *Children's Anxiety in Sport.* Champaign-Urbana, Ill.: University of Illinois, 1977.
11. Smoll F., Smith R.E. (eds): *Psychological Perspectives in Youth Sports.* Washington, D.C.: Hemisphere Press, 1978.
12. Hodges R.E., Krehl W.A.: Nutritional status of teenagers in Iowa. *Am. J. Clin. Nutr.* 17:200, 1965.
13. Costill D.L., Bennett A., Branam G., et al.: Glucose ingestion at rest and during prolonged exercise. *J. Appl. Physiol.* 34:764, 1973.
14. Wilmore J.H.: *Athletic Training and Physical Fitness.* Boston: Allyn & Bacon, 1977.
15. Haycock C.: Personal communication.

Thymic Hormones and the Immune System

DIANE W. WARA, M.D.

Associate Professor of Pediatrics
University of California, San Francisco
School of Medicine
San Francisco, California

Introduction

FROM THE TIME a newborn infant leaves the sterile environment of the uterus, it is continually assaulted by foreign antigens in the form of microbial agents (bacteria, viruses, fungi, and protozoa) and inert agents inhaled from the atmosphere or ingested during feeding. The function of the immune system is to prevent or retard the local establishment and systemic spread of these agents; the immune system also acts to prevent the development of autoimmune disease and malignancy. The development of competent immunity in man follows the division of stem cells (precursor bone marrow cells) into at least two populations. B-lymphocytes or bone-marrow-derived lymphocytes are influenced by the human bursa equivalent and are capable of differentiating into plasma cells, which then can synthesize and secrete specific antibodies. Alternatively, stem cells may pass through the thymus gland,[1, 2] where they presumably are matured by direct contact with the epithelial portion of the thymus or by means of a hormonal "induction." They are then exported into the peripheral lymphoid compartment, where they function as competent T-lymphocytes.

NOTE: The author of this chapter is a recipient of Research Career Development Award HD 00170-01.

0065-3101/81/0028-229-270-$03.75

TABLE 1.—MURINE THYMOCYTE DIFFERENTIATION: CELL SURFACE
ANTIGENS AND CELL FUNCTION

CELL	TL	THY-1 (θ)	CON A*	TDT†	LYT	PHA‡	MLC§
Prothymocyte (precursor bone marrow cell)	−	+/−	−	+/−	−	−	−
Cortical thymocyte (T₁)	+	+	+	+	+	−	−
Medullary thymocyte (T₂)	−	+	+	−	+ +	+	+
Circulating T-lymphocyte	−	+	+	−	+ +	+	+

*Cell division in response to concanavalin A.
†Terminal deoxynucleotide transferase activity.
‡Cell division in response to phytohemagglutinin.
§Cell division in response to foreign (allogeneic) cells.

There is evidence in animals and in man that subpopulations of lymphocytes exist which are defined both by functional activity and by selective surface markers. As precursor bone marrow cells differentiate to competent T-lymphocytes, their cell surface antigens change, and they acquire new functional capacities[3-8] (Tables 1 and 2). Although the murine system in animals has been more carefully defined than the one in man, both are characterized by prothymocytes with surface antigens that are maintained throughout differentiation. In the mouse, the theta (thy-1) antigen is present on both prothymocyte and circulating T-lymphocyte; in man, human T-lymphocyte differentiation antigen (HTLA) persists. The enzyme terminal deoxynucleotide transferase is present during early differentiation in both murine and human systems but is lost with maturation. During differentiation within the thymus gland, diversi-

TABLE 2.—HUMAN THYMOCYTE DIFFERENTIATION: CELL SURFACE
ANTIGENS AND CELL FUNCTION

CELL	HTLA*	T CELL ROSETTE	TDT†	OKT/LEU‡	CON A§	PHA‖
Prothymocyte	+ +	−	+	−	−	+/
Cortical thymocyte	+ +	+	+	+/−	+	−
Medullary thymocyte	+	+	−	+	+	+
Circulating T-lymphocyte	+	+	−	+	+	+

*Human T-lymphocyte differentiation antigen.
†Terminal deoxynucleotidyl transferase.
‡T-lymphocyte differentiation antigens.
§Lymphocyte responsiveness to concanavalin A (Con A).
‖Lymphocyte responsiveness to phytohemagglutinin (PHA).

fication of cell surface antigenicity and cell function occurs. The LyT antigens in mice and the OKT or Leu antigens in man are expressed differentially on subpopulations of T-lymphocytes destined to function in a "helper" or "suppressor" capacity.[9] In man, T-lymphocytes function as cytotoxic cells, producers of various lymphokines, participants in delayed hypersensitivity reaction, and as helper and suppressor cells for the production of specific antibody by B-lymphocytes. The control of antibody production by B cells is modulated by T cell help and T cell suppression. Peripheral blood T-lymphocytes adhere to sheep red blood cells and form T cell rosettes; they respond to phytohemagglutinin and other lectins by dividing.

The central role of the thymus gland in the ontogeny and function of lymphoid tissue and in the maintenance of immune balance is fully recognized. Thymus-deprived animals and children born with primary cellular immunodeficiency disease secondary to thymic hypoplasia have characteristic T-lymphocyte abnormalities with associated B-lymphocyte abnormalities. Implantation of a syngeneic neonatal thymus graft into thymus-deprived mice is effective in abolishing immunologic unresponsiveness.[10] Fetal thymus transplantation in children with primary cellular immunodeficiency disease may result in partial reconstitution of their immune systems.[11] Transplantation of thymus in cell impermeable chambers, through which only soluble factors may pass, results in partial restitution of immunity to thymus-deprived animals and man.[12, 13] Assessment of the effect or effects of thymus transplantation in cell impermeable chambers resulted in the concept that the thymus gland produces a factor or factors capable of interacting with immature stem cells in the thymus-deprived animal and of partially replacing the function of the normal thymus gland.

As early as 1940 extracts of normal thymus were reported to produce a lymphocytosis when injected into rats, guinea pigs, and pigeons.[14] Subsequently, a series of thymus extracts were produced that had various effects on the immune system. Thymosin fraction V, thymic humoral factor, serum thymic factor, and thymopoietin are four thymic hormones that have been characterized biochemically and biologically during the past decade. In this chapter we emphasize these hormones and their components, recognizing that other factors have been isolated and partially characterized. At the present time, it is not

known whether a single or multiple thymic factors are important in the maturation and regulation of the cellular immune
system. Available evidence suggests that a series of hormones
acts sequentially on stem cells to mature them to competent T-
lymphocytes and to maintain a population of circulating T
cells.

The Thymus Gland and Thymic Hormones

THE IMMUNE SYSTEM IN THYMUS-DEPRIVED ANIMALS AND MAN

The essential role of the thymus in the differentiation and
functional maturation of bone-marrow-derived precursors into
circulating immunocompetent T-lymphocytes is well established.[15, 16] It is clear that most of the cell maturation occurs
within the thymus itself; there is some evidence that not all
peripheral blood T-lymphocytes are completely mature, and
that a subpopulation may require the presence of the thymus
or thymic hormones for full development.[15] The impact of the
thymus gland on the development of competent cellular immunity is best understood in the murine system. The importance of the thymus gland was suggested as early as 1909,
when Maximow, in his studies on thymus histogenesis, observed a close interaction between thymic cells and the epithelial anlage of the thymus gland. He concluded that the thymic
epithelial cells attracted "wandering lymphoid cells" migrating
from elsewhere. Further, as summarized by Trainin,[17] Maximow suggested that the epithelial cells of the thymus had a
stimulating influence on these lymphoid elements. In a series
of studies begun during the 1930s and spanning more than 25
years, Comsa[18] defined the interaction between lymphoid elements and epithelial elements in the thymus and began to determine the significance of the various components involved.
Comsa and his colleagues assessed the effect of thymectomy on
one-month-old guinea pigs and described a subsequent syndrome characterized by weight loss, retarded growth, weakness, and death in up to 70% of the animals operated on. Thus,
the "wasting syndrome" following thymectomy was defined.

Early studies on the effect or effects of thymectomy on the

immune system in mice were performed in animals older than age one month. Subsequently, the experiments of Good and associates[19] and of Miller[20] in 1962 established the thymus as an organ essential for the development of cellular immunity. They documented that the results of thymectomy in animals after the first few days of life, especially in adult animals, are not as dramatic as the results of thymectomy in neonatal animals. Total white blood cell counts of neonatally thymectomized mice are approximately one half of those of normal mice; this decrease is due primarily to a decrease in the small lymphocyte population.[20] Following neonatal thymectomy, the lymphocyte count continues to decrease with age. Neonatal thymectomy performed in animals in which lymphatic tissue is not yet complete results in the depletion of small lymphocytes in thymus-dependent tissues; further development of these tissues stops with thymectomy. In animals thymectomized at birth, there is an impaired primary antibody response to a variety of antigens, including sheep erythrocytes and bovine serum albumin. Antibody responses to other antigens in other animal species may be normal.[21]

In addition to producing lymphopenia, neonatal thymectomy impairs an animal's capacity to reject skin homografts.[19] Neonatal animals undergoing thymectomy are more susceptible to graft versus host reactions (GVHR). Animals thymectomized during the neonatal period die following progressive weight loss, diarrhea, ruffling of the fur, hunching, and lethargy, which are characteristic of the "wasting syndrome."[20]

Children born with absent, small, or abnormally functioning thymus glands were reported as early as 1964[21] to have a morphologically abnormal thymus gland and abnormal cell-mediated immunity, as manifested by impaired skin homograft rejection, and abnormal peripheral blood lymphocyte responsiveness to phytohemagglutinin. A developmental failure of the third through sixth pharyngeal pouches results in diminished or absent thymus and parathyroid tissue. The immunologic deficits consequent to this developmental defect were first recognized in a patient and reported by DiGeorge.[22] Although cell-mediated immunity was abnormal in the first reported child, antibody-mediated immunity was relatively intact.

Thus, in mice undergoing thymectomy shortly after birth, development of the thymic-derived lymphocyte system is arrested at the time of thymectomy. There is some evidence of residual antibody-mediated immunity. In infants born with the DiGeorge syndrome, abnormal cell-mediated immunity can be correlated with histologic absence of T cell-dependent areas in the thymus gland, lymph nodes, and spleen.

RECONSTITUTION OF THE IMMUNE SYSTEM IN THYMUS-DEPRIVED ANIMALS AND MAN BY THYMUS TRANSPLANTATION IN CELL-IMPERMEABLE CHAMBERS

Complete removal of the thymus in neonatal mice usually leads to several syndromes that are felt to be interdependent. These include failure to gain weight normally, subsequent deterioration in overall physical condition, lymphopenia expressed by a reduction in the lymphocyte cell populations of lymphoid organs and peripheral blood, impairment of some immunologic capacities, and subsequent death.[20] Animals thymectomized as adults and subsequently irradiated develop most of these same symptoms. In 1961, Miller[23] observed that after neonatal thymectomy the subcutaneous implantation of a syngeneic neonatal thymus graft abolished immunologic unresponsiveness, prevented or reversed the changes in lymphoid tissue, and prevented the development of "wasting disease." Subsequently, experiments were performed to evaluate the possible role of hormone-like thymic factors. The first such experiments were designed to assess the reconstitution obtained by implanting thymus-deprived animals with thymus grafts enclosed in cell-impermeable chambers; only soluble factors passed through the chambers into the mice. Following implantation of neonatal thymus glands in cell-impermeable chambers, it was observed that the "wasting syndrome" did not occur with the intensity usually manifest in thymectomized control mice.[24-26] Body weights of the animals in these experiments increased steadily though they often remained below normal values.[24, 26] The decline in peripheral blood lymphocytes was usually arrested.[24] The growth and microscopic appearance of lymphoid organs was similar to normal.[24] Reconstituted neonatally thymectomized mice did not demonstrate as significant an impairment in their antibody response to sheep red blood cells as did nontransplanted mice. However, the average antibody titer remained lower than those in intact normal control animals.[26]

The results in these early studies suggested that thymus tissue enclosed in cell-impermeable millipore chambers was capable of preventing most of the deficit that followed neonatal thymectomy in mice. Endotoxin-contaminated chambers, empty chambers, and chambers containing a variety of normal and neoplastic tissues were ineffective in restoring the impaired functions of the thymectomized hosts. Therefore, the reconstitution was felt to be specific to the thymus gland. When the repopulated lymphoid organs of the reconstituted animals were examined, the chromosomal markers in the mitotic cells were of the host type,[25, 26] indicating that the donor thymus did not provide a cell population for the repair process. The investigators concluded that the inductive activity of the thymus in these early experiments could be attributed to a noncellular diffusible factor that passed out from the chambers into the systemic circulation of the animals.

Fetal thymus transplantation has restored cellular immunity in several patients with the DiGeorge syndrome (thymic hypoplasia with hypoparathyroidism).[27, 28] Reconstitution of cellular immunity occurs rapidly and appears to be permanent; lymphoid cell chimerism is absent. A single patient with this syndrome had partial reconstitution following fetal thymus transplantation in a millipore chamber; this was presumably mediated by a cell-free product[13] and suggests that, at least in the DiGeorge syndrome, reconstitution of cell-mediated immunity by fetal thymus transplantation results from release of an inducing substance by the transplanted thymus, a substance that stimulates the patient's own thymic precursor cells.

Purification and Chemical Characterization of Thymic Humoral Factors

HISTORY OF THYMIC EXTRACTS

The reconstitution of immune functions with thymic extracts was assessed experimentally as early as 1896, when Abelous and Billard[29] described restoration of muscle tone in thymectomized frogs given crude thymic extracts. During the next six decades, numerous investigators attempted to isolate thymus gland extracts that could replace the function of an intact thymus gland and reconstitute thymectomized animals or enhance immunologic competence in intact normal animals. The earliest thymic extracts with presumed specific effects on the immune system induced lymphopoietic hyperplastic changes in lymph nodes or a peripheral blood lymphocytosis in normal animals. Gregoire and Duchateau[30] used pig and rabbit thymus tissue to produce a saline extract, injected the extract into rats, and produced lymphopoietic changes in regional groups· of lymph nodes. They concluded that the extract was obtained primarily from the epithelium, for the animal thymic tissue had been irradiated and depleted of cortical thymocytes prior to preparation of the extract. Metcalf[31] injected newborn or baby mice intracerebrally with a factor collected from the plasma of patients with chronic lymphatic leukemia and observed increased numbers of peripheral blood lymphocytes. Subsequently, this lymphocytosis-stimulating factor (LSF) was found in higher concentrations in the thymus than in the plasma of mice and human beings with leukemia.

These data, accumulated primarily between 1940 and 1965, established the thymus as an endocrine gland capable of producing cell-free products that could modulate the immune system. However, prior to 1972, most of the experiments were carried out with crude thymic extracts that were poorly characterized biochemically. The effects of these extracts on the immune system in animals were diverse and included the induction of lymphocytosis in rats, guinea pigs, and pigeons; prevention of the "wasting syndrome" in newborn thymectomized mice; induction of thymocyte division; and variable lymphopoietic effects.[17] Since 1970, factors with thymic hormone activity have been isolated from thymus tissue,[32-34] peripheral blood,[35] and culture fluid from thymic epithelial cell lines.[36] The thymic humoral factors have been well characterized biochemically, and in some instances amino acid-sequenced and -synthesized.[35, 37-39] One humoral factor, thymosin α-1, has been synthesized in *Escherichia coli* using recombinant DNA cloning techniques.[40] The biologic activity of these hormones has been assessed in three primary systems. The ability of a biochemically characterized compound to reconstitute cellular immunity in thymus-deprived animals has been evaluated for most products. The effect or effects of a product on the maturation of an immature precursor cell to a functioning thymic-derived lymphocyte has been investigated in mice and human beings in laboratory culture systems. Finally, the ability of thymic hormones to enhance T-lymphocyte function and/or to alter the course of disease has been assessed in man. Children with primary immunodeficiency disease and adults with various malignancies have received regular injections of thymosin fraction V.

In this chapter we will restrict our review of thymic hormones to thymosin fraction V and polypeptides contained within it, thymic humoral factor, thymopoietin and its chemically characterized active component, and serum thymic factor (Table 3). During the 1970s, many additional products have been isolated from animal thymus, cell cultures, or blood and demonstrated to have biologic activity. During the 1980s those products with specific hormonal activity and necessary for the induction and maintenance of cellular immunity in man hopefully will be identified.

THYMOSIN FRACTION V, THYMOSIN α-1

Studies by A. L. Goldstein and associates have demonstrated that a partially purified thymus extract, termed thymosin fraction V, can correct some of the immunologic abnormalities resulting from the lack of thymic function in thymus-deprived

TABLE 3.—PHYSICAL AND CHEMICAL PROPERTIES OF THYMIC FACTORS

COMPOUND	MOL WT	CHEMICAL PROPERTIES	ORIGIN
Thymosin fraction 5	1,000 to 15,000	Family of heat-stable, acidic polypeptides	Bovine thymus
Thymosin α-1	3,108	28 amino acid residues, pI 4.2	Bovine thymus + synthetic
Thymopoietin	5,562	49 amino acid residues, heat stable, pI 5.2	Bovine thymus + synthetic
Thymopoietin pentapeptide		Amino acid residues, 32−36 in thymopoietin	Synthetic
Thymic humoral factor	3,200	31 amino acid residues, heat labile, pI 5.7−5.9	Bovine thymus
Serum thymic factor	857	9 amino acid residues, heat labile, pI 7.3	Mouse, pig serum

animals as well as in some children with primary cellular immunodeficiency disease. Thymosin fraction V is composed of a group of polypeptides with molecular weights ranging from 1,000 to 15,000. Several of these polypeptides have been purified and their biologic activity has been studied. It appears that the polypeptides contained within thymosin fraction V act individually, sequentially, or in concert to influence the development and maintenance of T cell immunity.

In 1966, Klein et al.[41] isolated a lymphopoietic factor in rat and mouse thymus extracts. Subsequently, a biologically active fraction was isolated from calf thymus and was termed thymosin.[32] In 1975, thymosin fraction V was prepared in large quantities for clinical trials.[42]

Thymosin fraction V is obtained from bovine calf thymus. The tissue is homogenized and centrifuged. The supernatant is filtered through glass wool and processed through an 80-C heat-step, acetone precipitation, and ammonium sulfate precipitation. The 25% to 50% ammonium sulfate precipitate is further subjected to ultrafiltration in an Amicon DC-2 hollow fiber system and then desalted on a Sephadex G-25 column to yield fraction V. Analytic isoelectric focusing of thymosin fraction V reveals multiple components in the preparation. The polypeptides are a family of heat-stable, acidic polypeptides and contain less than 10% lipid, carbohydrate, and polynucleotide.

The first thymosin polypeptide isolated from the acidic region of fraction V was termed thymosin α-1.[38, 39] Thymosin α-1 is isolated from fraction V by ion-exchange chromatography and gel filtration. The yield of thymosin α-1 from fraction V is about 0.6%. Amino acid sequencing of thymosin α-1 revealed a polypeptide consisting of 28 amino acid residues and a molecular weight of 3,108. The amino acid sequence of thymosin α-1 shows no homology with the published sequence of other thymic factors. Recently, Wetzel and associates[40] have succeeded in synthesizing thymosin α-1 in *E. coli* using recombinant DNA cloning techniques.

THYMIC HUMORAL FACTOR (THF)

Trainin and associates first prepared cell-free extracts of thymus from sheep, calf, and rabbit by crude homogenization of the organ followed by centrifugation. The filtered supernatant was repeatedly injected into thymic-deprived mice and increased the number of peripheral blood lymphocytes in these animals. In addition, "wasting syndrome" in newborn thymectomized mice was prevented by treatment with sheep thymus extracts. In 1975, the preparation of THF was modified to produce a heat-labile protein with a molecular weight of approximately 3,200.[33] Fresh calf thymus glands are homogenized with subsequent centrifugations of the supernatants followed by dialysis against distilled water in the cold. The active components are further concentrated and finally purified by gel filtration on a Sephadex G-10 column. Like thymosin fraction V, THF is acidic with an isoelectric point between 5.7 and 5.9. The amino acid composition of THF is reported with 31 residues. Amino acid sequence has not been established.

THYMOPOIETIN AND THYMOPOIETIN PENTAPEPTIDE (TP5)

Thymopoietin was first isolated by Goldstein[34] and was initially termed thymin. In 1974, Goldstein reported the isolation of two closely related polypeptide hormones of the thymus, each with a molecular weight of 7,000, termed thymin I and II. Initially, thymopoietin was isolated because of a presumably secondary effect on neuromuscular transmission that was discovered in the course of studying the human disease myasthenia gravis. Subsequently, thymopoietin was shown to induce the differentiation of mouse lymphopoietic stem cells from prothymocytes to thymocytes.

Thymopoietin has a molecular weight of 5,562, is heat stable, has an isoelectric point of 5.2, and contains 49 amino acid residues without homology to other thymic hormones.[43] Thymopoietin was isolated to homogeneity from calf thymus by saline extraction and heating, molecular sizing on membranes, molecular sieve chromatography, adsorption on hydroxylapatite, and ion exchange chromatography.

Subsequently, amino acid residues 29 to 41 (13 residues) were synthesized and shown to have approximately 3% activity of thymopoietin in inducing the differentiation of T-lymphocytes. Most recently, a pentapeptide containing amino acid residues 32 to 36 of thymopoietin has been isolated and shown to have equivalent activity to thymopoietin in the induction of stem cell differentiation.[37]

SERUM THYMIC FACTOR

In 1972, Bach and associates isolated a factor in human serum that modified the rosette-forming cells present in the spleen of adult thymectomized mice. The serum factor was identified in normal mouse, pig, calf, and rat serums.

Biochemical analysis of the factor characterized it as a polypeptide with a neutral pH and a molecular weight of approximately 1,000. Isolation of the polypeptide was achieved by defibrination of serum, dialysis, concentration on amicon membrane, G-25 Sephadex filtration, cellulose chromatography, and thin-layer chromatographies. The product thus obtained is a pure polypeptide with nine amino acid residues and without homology with other thymic hormones. Following amino acid sequencing, the serum factor was renamed serum thymic factor.[35]

CHEMICAL CHARACTERIZATION OF THYMIC FACTORS: COMPARISON

The thymic hormones discussed are all neutral or acidic polypeptides (see Table 3). They range in molecular weight from 1,000 to 15,000 (thymosin fraction V). With the exception of serum thymic factor, all were originally isolated from bovine thymus glands. In each case, the original investigator prepared a crude isolate from bovine thymus and demonstrated a specific effect on the immune reconstitution of thymus-deprived animals or on differentiation of stem cells to more mature thymocytes. Subsequently, each investigator characterized his product and sought to identify the active amino acid residues within it. In addition to thymosin α-1, five other biologically active polypeptides have been isolated from thymosin fraction V. Within thymopoietin, a pentapeptide has been defined with equivalent biologic activity. Thymic humoral factor remains to be amino acid-sequenced although the amino acid residues have been identified. Serum thymic factor, with the lowest molecular weight at 1,000, is isolated from serum rather than the thymus gland.

Biologic Activities of Thymic Humoral Factors in Animal Models

RECONSTITUTION OF THYMIC-DEPRIVED ANIMALS IN VIVO

During the 1960s and early 1970s, experiments were performed to study the degree to which thymic extracts could prevent or reverse the consequences of thymus deprivation in newborn and adult animals. Trainin[17] used an early preparation of thymic humoral factor (THF) prepared from cell-free extracts of thymus from sheep, calf, and rabbit and observed an increased number of peripheral blood lymphocytes following frequent injections in neonatally or adult thymectomized mice. Normally lymphocyte-depleted areas of the spleen of thymectomized mice were altered by frequent injections of thymic humoral factor. Repeated injections of THF into neonatally thymectomized mice prevented the "wasting syndrome."[17] Thymosin fraction V also was found to reduce "wasting syndrome" in neonatally thymectomized mice and to increase the numbers of lymphoid cells in the peripheral blood, lymph nodes, and spleen when compared to saline-treated neonatally thymectomized controls.[44, 45]

The significance of the changes observed in the lymphoid system after injection of thymic extracts into thymectomized recipients was difficult to evaluate. During the 1960s, as the role of the thymus in the immunocompetence of mammals was established, investigators began to assess the effect of thymic preparations on the integrity of cellular responsiveness rather than on cell numbers and morphology. Neonatally thymectomized mice are unable to reject skin or tumor homographs. Both THF and thymosin fraction V repeatedly injected into these animals restored their ability to reject skin grafts.[17, 46] Graft versus host reactions occur in immunodeficient animals following the injection of immunocompetent lymphocytes from a histoincompatible donor. Mice thymectomized during the neonatal period, following the injection of histoincompatible lymphoid cells, develop splenomegaly and a "wasting syndrome" followed by death. When the histoincompatible lymphoid cells are obtained from a thymectomized but otherwise normal donor, the recipient immunodeficient mouse does not develop graft versus host disease. Trainin and associates[47] demonstrated that, following repeated THF injections, the capacity of lymphoid cells obtained from neonatally thymectomized mice to induce splenomegaly in a recipient mouse is partially restored. Extracts of spleen and mesenteric lymph nodes did not restore the capacity of lymphocytes obtained from neonatal thymectomized mice to induce a graft versus host reaction. Law and associates[48] documented that thymosin fraction V injections would repair the lymphocyte competence of newborn thymectomized mice and cause them to produce GVHR. Goldstein et al.[49] documented that spleen cells obtained from thymus-intact mice prior to age four days did not have the capacity to elicit a graft versus host reaction in a recipient, immunodeficient histoincompatible mouse. However, administration of thymosin fraction V to newborn mice accelerated the development of immunologic competence of their spleen cells, allowing them to induce splenomegaly in recipients when obtained earlier than age three days.

More recently, the effect or effects of injecting thymic factors into mice with documented abnormal cellular immunity has been assessed. The aging process in normal mice and/or thymectomy in adult mice results in decreased circulating serum thymic factor. Lymphocyte-mediated cytotoxicity, a measure of mature T cell function, decreases with aging and after thymectomy in older mice. Injection of serum thymic factor restores lymphocyte-mediated cytotoxicity to these animals.[50] Preservation of this T cell function suggests that serum thymic factor has an effect on the function or functions of mature circulating thymus-derived lymphocytes.

A series of studies involving the injection of thymopoietin and its component TP5 suggest that it affects regulatory T-lymphocytes. Injection of these factors into normal thymus-intact mice enhances the effector cytotoxic lymphocyte splenic cell function. These studies suggest that thymopoietin as well as serum thymic factor affects a mature peripheral blood lymphocyte in addition to its documented effect on early differentiation.[51] Both thymopoietin and TP5, injected intraperitoneally into normal mice, protect these animals from the development of Coombs positivity resulting from the injection of foreign rat erythrocytes. The authors suggest that their studies support the role of thymopoietin and TP5 in the regulation of the immune system and enhancement of suppressor lymphocytes.

The injection of thymosin fraction V into athymic nude mice alters splenic cytotoxic lymphocyte function, induces suppressor T cells, and suggests that the factor has a regulatory function.[52]

Effects of thymosin fraction V and serum thymic factor on the protection of normal mice from Moloney sarcoma virus have been evaluated. Thymectomized and irradiated bone marrow reconstituted mice were injected with Moloney sarcoma virus and subsequently treated with serum thymic factor for 25 days. Without serum thymic factor injections, all mice died. Of those treated, 85% rejected their tumors by day 25. However, the majority had recurrence of tumor after treatment was stopped, whereas normal animals rejected the tumor and had no recurrence.[52] Thymosin fraction V injections likewise increase resistance in mice to Moloney sarcoma virus.[53] Other factors have not been assessed.

Dardenne and Bach reported that in mice a large portion of spontaneous rosette-forming cells (sRFC) depend on the presence of the thymus gland. In both the spleen and thymus, a population of sRFC exist that is sensitive to inhibition of rosette formation in vitro by azathioprine (AZ) or anti-θ serum. A biologic assay quantitates the induction of the θ-antigen on θ-negative T cell precursors after incubation with a specific thymic hormone or with the serum sample supposedly containing thymic extracts.[52] Adult thymectomized and irradiated bone marrow-reconstituted mice and aging mice are deficient in spontaneous rosette-forming cells as defined by this assay. The injection of either THF or thymosin fraction V into these recipients normalizes their splenic rosette forming cells.[54] Subsequent to these experiments, a serum factor was isolated by Bach and associates and termed serum thymic factor, which, as with THF or thymosin fraction V, results in reconstitution of total rosette-forming cells both in bone marrow and spleen of adult thymectomized mice following in vivo injections.[55]

In summary, the in vivo administration of thymic extracts repaired the homograft response, restored the capacity of lymphoid elements from thymectomized recipients to induce cell-mediated responses, or accelerated the natural process of immunologic maturation. Further, the injection of THF or thymosin fraction V protected thymic-deprived animals from Ma-

TABLE 4.—EFFECTS OF ADMINISTRATION OF FACTORS TO THYMUS-DEPRIVED ANIMALS

FACTOR	ALTER "WASTING SYNDROME"	↑ SPLENOCYTE GVH POTENTIAL	↑ HOMOGRAFT REJECTION	↑ LYMPHOCYTE-MEDIATED CYTOTOXICITY	↑ SRFC*	↑ SUPPRESSION T CELL†
Thymosin fraction V	+	+	+	+	+	+
Thymic humoral factor	+	+	+			
Thymopoietin/TP5				+	+	+
Serum thymic factor				+	+	

*Increase S rosette-forming cells by splenocytes; induce θ-antigen.
†Increase suppressor T cells; alter regulatory function.

loney sarcoma virus-induced malignancies. The injection of thymosin fraction V, THF, or serum thymic factor resulted in reconstitution of rosette-forming cells in adult thymectomized mice (Table 4).

RECONSTITUTION OF CELLULAR IMMUNE FUNCTION IN LYMPHOID CELLS FROM THYMIC-DEPRIVED ANIMALS BY IN VITRO INCUBATION WITH THYMIC FACTORS

The effect(s) of thymic factors on the differentiation of T-lymphocytes is associated with their effect(s) on reconstitution of T cell function when incubated with cell populations in the laboratory. Cortical thymocytes, commonly termed T_1 cells, bear the following surface antigens: TL positive, Thy-1 (θ) positive. These same cells respond in vitro to concanavalin A but have only minimal reactivity to other T cell mitogens in comparison to mature circulating T cells (see Table 1). In contrast, T_2 cells, located in the medulla of the thymus gland, have a low concentration of θ-antigen, are TL negative, and respond to phytohemagglutinin, pokeweed mitogen, concanavalin A, and allogeneic cells in a mixed lymphocyte culture and are capable of inducing graft versus host reaction in immunodeficient histoincompatible animals.

Investigators of the biologic effects of serum thymic factor, thymopoietin, thymic humoral factor, and thymosin fraction V generally agree that incubation of putative thymic hormones with mature normal T-lymphocytes affects neither differentiation nor reactivity. Therefore, in vitro assessment of the effects of thymic factors on cellular immunity usually employs splenocytes obtained from thymic-deprived animals. Nude athymic mice have precursor thymocytes but no thymocytes per se.[56] Neonatally thymectomized mice are rendered immunodeficient. Thymectomized mice have abnormal T cell immunity. By incubating splenocytes obtained from these animal models with various thymic extracts and then determining the effect of the extract on cell differentiation and function, investigators have postulated the site of induction (Table 5). That is, studies assess whether a factor matures a prothymocyte to a T_1 thymocyte or reacts primarily by enhancing differentiation of T_1 to T_2 thymocytes. A factor may act at more than one site.

TABLE 5.—EFFECTS OF THYMIC FACTOR INCUBATION WITH CELLS FROM THYMUS-DEPRIVED ANIMALS

FACTOR	↑ TL	↑ THY-1(θ)	↑ TDT*	↑ LYT	↑ CON-A†	↑ PHA‡	↑ MLR§	↑ T HELP‖
Thymosin factor V	+	+	+	+	+			+
Thymic humoral factor		+			+**		+	
Thymopoietin/TP5		+			+	+/−	+**	
Serum thymic factor		+			+	−		

*Terminal deoxynucleotide transferase activity.
†Cell division in response to concanavalin A.
‡Cell division in response to phytohemagglutinin.
§Cell division in response to allogeneic cells.
‖Enhanced production of antibody reflecting increased T help.
**Requires Thy-1 (θ)+ cell.

Serum thymic factor, when incubated with spleen cells obtained from nude athymic mice, enhances the splenocyte response to concanavalin A but has no effect on the splenocyte response to phytohemagglutinin. Likewise, serum thymic factor confers θ-positivity to spleen cells from adult thymectomized, neonatally thymectomized, or nude mice.[52] These results suggest that serum thymic factor promotes the differentiation of prothymocytes to T_1 or cortical thymocytes but has little effect on the differentiation of T_1 to T_2 or medullary thymocytes.

Thymosin fraction V likewise converts splenocytes obtained from nude mice to θ-positivity, suggesting an effect on the differentiation of prothymocytes to T_1 cells.[54] The majority of in vitro studies assessing the effects of thymosin fraction V on cell populations suggest that it also functions to differentiate T_1 to more mature T_2 cells.[57-60] Incubation of murine thymocytes with thymosin fraction V results in an increased mixed lymphocyte responsivity to nondividing allogeneic murine spleen cells.[59] Incubation of prethymic cells obtained from the spleen or bone marrow of normal or nude mice with thymosin fraction V results in increased numbers of cells bearing Lyt antigens in addition to TL and θ. Simultaneous studies suggest that these cells acquire the capacity to provide T cell help in the formation of antibody.[57] Thymectomized and irradiated bone marrow-reconstituted mice have decreased splenic plaque-forming cells following immunization with sheep red blood cells. Spleen cells, when incubated with thymosin fraction V, have enhanced antibody formation reflected by increased numbers of direct plaque-forming cells.[57] If bone marrow cells are pretreated with thymosin fraction V in vitro and subsequently injected with sheep red blood cells into lethally irradiated mice, increased antibody is formed.[59] In the presence of thymosin fraction V, spleen cells from athymic nude mice develop in vitro immune responses to soluble DNP-protein conjugates, to particulate sheep red blood cells, and to allogeneic cells. Thymosin fraction V has no effect on T cell-deprived splenocytes; thus, enhanced antibody formation probably reflects differentiation or activation of T helper cells that then interact with B cells.[61] Finally, thymocytes isolated from NZB/NZW mice, which have an increased incidence of autoimmune disease and abnormal DNA synthesis, have correction of the DNA synthetic rate following treatment with thymosin fraction V.[60] The ability of thymosin to differentiate θ-negative splenocytes to θ-positive rosette-forming cells indicates an effect on prothymocyte to T_1 thymocyte differentiation. Incubation of spleen or bone marrow prethymic cells from normal or nude mice with thymosin fraction V with the subsequent appearance of T_1 thymocyte antigens (TL positive, θ-positive) as well as T_2 antigens (Lyt positive) suggests a second site of action, that is, differentiation of the T_1 cell to T_2 cell. This is supported by the effect of thymosin fraction V on enhancing mixed lymphocyte culture reactivity, specific antibody production, and reconstitution of the graft versus host-producing potential of splenocytes obtained from neonatally thymectomized mice.

Thymic humoral factor (THF) has many effects in common with thymosin fraction V. The majority of its effects are associated with increased intracellular cyclic adenosine monophosphate (AMP).[62-64] Preincubation of murine spleen or thymus cells with THF results in enhancement of mixed lymphocyte culture reactivity along with increased intracellular cylic AMP.[62, 63] Splenocytes obtained from neonatally thymectomized mice, when incubated with THF, are capable of inducing a graft versus host response in splenic explants; reconstitution of the ability to induce a GVHR is associated with an increase in intracellular cyclic AMP.[64, 65] Splenocytes preincubated with THF and obtained from thymectomized mice have an enhanced response to concanavalin A when compared to splenocytes not incubated with THF.[66] In contrast, incubation of splenocytes from athymic nude mice with THF does not enhance responsiveness to concanavalin A; the authors suggest that for THF to differentiate cells, the target cells must already bear the θ-antigen (T_1 cell) on their surface. Athymic nude mice have primarily θ-negative cells. Lymph node cells obtained from normal animals do not have enhanced concanavalin A responsiveness following incubation with THF; the authors postulate that these cells are already differentiated beyond the site at which THF is active.

The majority of studies on thymopoietin assess its ability to induce the differentiation of antigen negative prethymic cells into antigen positive thymocytes. Functional studies support its additional effect on the differentiation of more mature cells. Normal murine spleen and bone marrow cells contain a small proportion of cells that acquire responsiveness to mitogens (concanavalin A, phytohemagglutinin) after incubation with thymopoietin. The precursor, responsive populations are enriched by fractionation on discontinuous gradients of bovine serum albumin (BSA). In these cell populations, a marked enhanced responsiveness to concanavalin A and a minimal increased responsiveness to phytohemagglutinin were observed.[67] Murine cells isolated from lymph nodes and spleen, when incubated with thymopoietin, have an increased response to allogeneic cells in mixed lymphocyte culture. The increased response is associated with enhanced intracellular cyclic GMP and requires the presence of the θ-antigen on the initial cell.[68] θ-Negative cells isolated from athymic nude mice do not have enhanced response to allogeneic cells following incubation with thymopoietin.[68] The authors interpret these findings as evidence for the activity of thymopoietin on a thymic or postthymic lymphocyte. Further evidence for the effect of thymopoietin and its component TP5 on postthymic lymphocytes is the increase in cytotoxic lymphocyte precursor units in spleens of normal thymus-intact mice three days after intraperitoneal injections of TP5. In vitro incubation of splenocytes with TP5 also increases the numbers of cytotoxic lymphocyte precursor units. Both are associated with an increase in intracellular cyclic GMP and probably reflect alteration of the function of mature peripheral blood lymphocytes.[69]

Differentiation of T-Lymphocyte Surface Antigens in Murine Systems Following Incubation with Thymic Factors

The earliest observation that the incubation of murine cells with thymic factors induced specific cell surface antigens was made by Bach and associates.[70] The spontaneous rosette-forming cells (sRFC) present in the normal mouse are found in all lymphoid organs. These sRFC, sensitive to azathioprine or anti-θ serum, are T cells and bear surface θ-antigen. Incubation with thymosin fraction V or THF differentiates θ-negative splenocytes obtained from adult thymectomized mice, aged mice, and nude mice to θ-positive cells.[54] Splenocytes and bone marrow cells obtained from adult thymectomized mice and concentrated on BSA discontinuous gradient contain a relatively homogeneous group of cells that are θ-negative; following in-

cubation with serum thymic factor, these cells acquire θ-positivity.[71]

Levels of serum thymic factor are quantitated by the capacity of serum to render θ-negative rosette-forming cells θ-positive. Serum thymic factor remains stable in most mouse strains
until age six months and then declines. After age 15 months,
levels are not detectable. An early decline is observed in NZB/
NZW mice. Serum thymic factor disappears following thymectomy, is absent in nude mice, and reappears after thymus
graft.[72-74]

Study of the effects of thymosin fraction V on the induction
of murine cell surface antigens in addition to θ-antigen was
begun by Komuro and Boyse.[75] Murine bone marrow cells from
normal animals were obtained. Precursor thymocytes were concentrated following application to a discontinuous BSA gradient. Induction of TL antigen, thy-1 antigen, and Lyt antigens
from bone marrow subpopulations supports the effect of thymosin on differentiation from prothymocyte to a cortical thymocyte and from cortical to medullary thymocyte (see Table 5).
Finally, the incubation of thymocytes with thymosin fraction V
converts TL-positive to TL-negative cells and suggests an effect
of thymosin fraction V on late T cell maturation; that is, on
thymocytes about to be discharged into the periphery.[75] Bone
marrow cells obtained from athymic nude mice can be induced
by incubation with thymosin to express thy-1 positivity and TL
negativity.[76] The induction of Lyt 123-positive cells from bone
marrow subpopulations isolated by discontinuous BSA gradient
and obtained from adult thymectomized and irradiated bone
marrow-reconstituted animals correlates with increased antibody formation to sheep red blood cells.[57] Therefore, differentiation as assessed by cell surface antigenicity supports the functional effect or effects of thymosin fraction V on the conversion
of prothymocytes to thymocytes and the maturation of thymocytes to circulating competent T-lymphocytes. An additional
group of studies, supporting the effect of thymosin fraction V
at an early stage of thymocyte differentiation, assessed the induction of terminal deoxynucleotidyltransferase (TdT), an enzyme present in most thymocytes but very few bone marrow
cells and thought to reflect an early cortical thymocyte. Incubation of thymosin fraction V with TdT negative cells (splenocytes or bone marrow from athymic mice) induces conversion of
these cells to TdT positivity.[77, 78]

The effect of thymopoietin on the differentiation of thymocytes as defined by cell surface antigens has been fully assessed.[79-84] Researchers used murine bone marrow cells obtained from BSA discontinuous gradients and incubated these
cells with thymopoietin to induce antigenic characteristics of
intrathymic T cells. Murine TL negative cells become TL positive and θ-positive.[83] TL positivity, induced by thymopoietin,
occurs along with an abrupt increase in intracellular cyclic
AMP.[85] Although other mediators such as theophylline are capable of altering TL positivity, thymopoietin acts selectively to
induce thymocytes in vitro and does not induce alteration of B
cell antigenicity. Additional studies have documented that precursor cells obtained from mouse bone marrow or spleen incubated with thymopoietin develop a profile of surface antigens
characteristic of thymocytes and associated with an increase in
intracellular cyclic AMP. The precursor cells are not mitogen-
reactive prior to induction, but acquire reactivity after incubation with thymopoietin.[83]

TP5, an isolated amino acid-sequenced component of thymopoietin, has the same capacity as thymopoietin to induce thymocyte differentiation as assessed by cell surface antigens. As
with thymopoietin, TP5 does not alter B cell surface antigenicity.[82] Immature T cells in murine spleen have been quantitated by other markers. Splenocyte-binding to autologous rosettes (A-RFC) and splenocyte-binding with peanut agglutinin
(PNA) are associated with immature T cells and are found in
increased numbers in athymic nude mice. Incubation of splenocytes obtained from aged animals, athymic nude mice, and
adult thymectomized mice with TP5 results in decreased numbers of A-RFC and PNA.[80, 82] In summary, thymopoietin appears to act specifically on T cells to induce thymocytes from
prothymocytes; in all cases, when assessed, induction of new
antigen has been associated with increased intracellular cyclic
AMP.

Proposed Mechanisms of Thymic Factor Activity

The specific thymic origin of the factors discussed above has
not been systematically proved. The majority of studies lead to
the conclusion that thymic humoral factor, thymosin fraction
V, serum thymic factor, and thymopoietin originate in the thymus gland. Careful evaluation of serum thymic factor levels

have shown its rapid disappearance from serum after thymectomy and reappearance after thymus graft.[72-74] No serum
thymic factor is present in the nude athymic mice. The origin
of serum thymic factor in the thymus epithelium is suggested
by its reappearance after grafting a free graft, a graft in cell-
impermeable diffusion chambers, nonlymphoid epithelial thy-
moma, or pure epithelial thymus. All four grafting procedures
result in reconstitution of identical levels of serum thymic factor.[85]

Although the effects of thymic factors on differentiation of
lymphoid cell elements from prothymocytes to mature circulating T-lymphocytes has been established, the molecular events
through which these factors control the differentiation of precursor stem cells to mature T-lymphocytes are not yet fully understood. Murine T-lymphocyte differentiation begins in the
bone marrow, where a prothymocyte is TdT negative and θ-
negative. Cells located both in the bone marrow and the thymus are prethymocytes and are TdT positive but remain θ-negative.

Within the thymus gland, cells obtain surface markers, including θ. They retain their TdT enzyme activity and acquire
the capacity to respond to concanavalin A. Further maturation
from cortical to medullary thymocytes implies the acquisition
of Lyt antigens, loss of TdT activity, and capacity to respond to
phytohemagglutinin and allogeneic cells and to regulate antibody production through a balance between T help and T
suppression (see Table 1). Several questions remain unan-
swered. It is not known whether the pathway is sequential or
whether the cells arise via parallel differentiation. It is not yet
clear whether a single factor or a series of factors is necessary
for complete differentiation of a precursor stem cell to a mature
lymphocyte.

The incubation of thymosin fraction V (see Table 5) with concentrated cell populations obtained from thymic-deprived animals supports its effects on the differentiation of prothymocyte
to thymocyte (acquisition of T1 and Thy-1 (θ)), of maturation to
cortical thymocyte (acquisition of TdT and responsiveness to
concanavalin A), and of maturation to medullary thymocyte
and circulating T-lymphocyte (acquisition of Lyt, responsiveness to allogeneic cells, enhanced antibody production). Goldstein and associates postulate that isolated polypeptides con-

tained within thymosin fraction V act sequentially at various sites of T-lymphocyte differentiation.

Although thymic humoral factor can alter sRFCs in splenocytes and thus induce the θ-antigen in Bach's assay, it can induce splenocyte responsiveness to concanavalin A in cell populations only if the θ-antigen is already present. Therefore, it further differentiates thymocytes into T-lymphocytes capable of altering the "wasting syndrome" and of enhancing homograft rejection (see Tables 4 and 5). THF has no documented effect on prothymocytes. Similarly, thymopoietin differentiates precursor cells most effectively if the Thy-1 (θ) antigen is present. Its role in augmenting splenocyte responsiveness to concanavalin A to a greater extent than to phytohemagglutinin reflects intrathymic differentiation (see Table 5). Serum thymic factor also differentiates intra and postthymic cells.

Since many investigators have documented that T cell differentiation, as described above, results from the interaction of target cells with peptide hormones, this action most likely occurs via second messengers. That is, thymosin fraction V or any other factor that does not enter the cell binds to a specific receptor on the cell surface and induces changes in intracellular signals. These signals could include both cyclic GMP and cyclic AMP and/or ion levels. Naylor and Goldstein[87] have recently reviewed cyclic nucleotides and T cell differentiation. Bach et al. reported in 1973 that cyclic AMP mimicked thymosin in the induction of θ-antigen on murine lymphocytes. Cyclic AMP and agents that elevate cyclic AMP also cause the induction of θ on the same purified stem cell populations as do thymic factors. Cyclic GMP added to the assay system does not mimic thymosin. Trainin and associates found that enhanced MLR reactivity by thymic factors reflected increased intracellular levels of cyclic AMP. On the other hand, thymosin is active in several assays that cyclic AMP inhibits. These assays include lymphotoxin production and the production of migration inhibitory factor.

Trainin has suggested that THF elevates cyclic AMP in cells that are at later stages of T cell development. These statements were based on the observation that thymus and spleen but not bone marrow and lymph node lymphocytes respond to THF with increases in cyclic AMP. Thymosin fraction V elevates cyclic GMP most dramatically in the thymus and to a lesser extent in normal spleen lymphocytes. The complexity of these preliminary results emphasizes the need for careful investigation of the intracellular increases in cyclic AMP and cyclic GMP in relation to cell surface antigenicity and cell function.

Biologic Activities of Thymic Humoral Factors in Man

INTRODUCTION

Until recently, the differentiation of T-lymphocytes in the human system was not as well characterized as that in the murine system. Studies assessing the effects of thymic factors on the differentiation of human T-lymphocytes have relied on: (1) induction of T cell rosette formation following incubation with a specific factor; (2) induction of human T-lymphocyte differentiation antigen (HTLA) on a cell surface of lymphocytes after incubation with a specific factor; (3) alteration of T-lymphocyte response to mitogens such as to phytohemagglutinin or concanavalin A after incubation with thymic factors. Additionally, it has been shown that subpopulations of T-lymphocytes bear surface immunoglobulin G (T-γ) or immunoglobulin M (T-μ) and have been characterized as T suppressor cells or T helper cells; incubation of thymic factors with either pre-T cells or T cells and alteration of populations of T-μ and T-γ cells has been assessed.

Two bioassays have been used to quantitate human "serum thymic factors" in the serum or plasma of normal individuals or patients with various disease entities. In 1972, Bach and associates[88] defined a factor in human serum that modifies the rosette-forming cells present in the spleen of adult thymectomized mice. Modification of the rosette-forming cells in murine spleen reflects induction of the θ-antigen. Human serum levels of θ-antigen-inducing factor are defined by diluting the serum and reporting results as serum titers. The second assay, developed by Lewis and Twomey,[89] assesses the induction of Thy 1.2 antigen on null lymphocytes obtained from athymic nude mice following incubation with human plasma or serum. It is established that thymopoietin is capable of inducing Thy 1.2 antigen on these lymphocytes, and plasma samples from normal individuals and patients, when incubated with null lymphocytes, have a Thy 1.2 inductive capacity equated with a known amount of thymopoietin. Therefore, results are expressed as "inductive activity equivalent to nanograms of thymopoietin/ml."

DIFFERENTIATION OF T-LYMPHOCYTES BY INCUBATION WITH THYMIC FACTORS

Wara and Ammann[90] first documented that incubation of lymphocytes obtained from a subpopulation of patients with primary immunodeficiency disease with thymosin fraction V results in increased T cell rosette formation. T cell rosette formation by lymphocytes obtained from normal individuals is not further increased following incubation with thymosin; lymphocytes obtained from infants with severe combined immunodeficiency disease and, presumably, no stem cell precursors, have no enhancement of T cell rosette formation following incubation with thymosin fraction V. The authors concluded that thymosin fraction V is capable of differentiating a prethymic, E rosette negative cell probably in the "null cell" population, into a T-lymphocyte characterized by its capacity to adhere to sheep red blood cells and to form T cell rosettes. Subsequently, Horowitz and Goldstein[91] obtained peripheral blood mononuclear cells from normal individuals and fractionated these cells on a bovine serum albumin discontinuous gradient. The concentrated putative stem cells were induced to form T cell rosettes following incubation with thymosin. Because there was no change in the number of B cells, monocytes, or cells bearing FC or C3 receptors or in cell viability, the authors concluded that incubation with thymosin induces normal peripheral blood null cells to differentiate to T cells. Other agents that increase intracellular cyclic AMP (DBcAMP) also induce increased T cell rosette formation in null cells obtained from normal individuals.[91]

Further documentation of the effects of thymosin fraction V on the human null cell population was obtained by isolating peripheral blood lymphocytes from normal adult donors; the cells were E rosette negative and surface immunoglobulin negative but still bore the surface antigens HTLA or HBLA (see Table 2). Cells with surface HBLA positivity, when incubated with thymosin fraction V, were not induced to form increased T cell rosettes. In contrast, cells with HTLA positivity, presumed to be precursors of mature T-lymphocytes, had enhanced T cell rosette formation following incubation with thymosin fraction V. The authors conclude that if human T cell differentiation parallels the murine system, then the human thymosin fraction V responsive peripheral blood lymphocyte already possesses T-lymphocyte differentiation antigens.[92, 93]

Bone marrow cells, in addition to peripheral blood lymphocytes, when isolated by discontinuous BSA gradient, have enhanced T cell rosette formation following incubation with thymosin fraction V.[94] In addition, the incubation of thymosin fraction V with bone marrow cells isolated by discontinuous BSA gradient results in the induction of HTLA on the cell surface; the authors concluded that "extracts of human or calf thymus influence the differentiation of human bone marrow cells in vitro."[95]

Therefore, thymosin fraction V has been shown by multiple investigators to induce HTLA antigen positivity on peripheral blood lymphocyte and bone marrow null cells and to enhance T cell rosette formation in the same cell population. The concept that thymosin fraction V effects differentiation of null cells has been supported by results of the incubation of peripheral blood lymphocytes obtained from patients with primary immunodeficiency disease with thymosin fraction V. Several investigators have documented that peripheral blood lymphocytes isolated from patients with DiGeorge syndrome or thymic hypoplasia have enhanced T cell rosette formation following incubation with thymosin fraction V.[90, 91, 96, 97] In theory, peripheral blood lymphocytes from these patients contain putative stem cells that have not undergone thymus processing. In contrast, lymphocytes obtained from patients with severe combined immunodeficiency disease and no putative stem cells have no enhanced T cell rosette formation following incubation with thymosin fraction V.[90, 91]

The effects of thymic factors other than thymosin fraction V on the differentiation of human null cells isolated from the bone marrow or peripheral blood have not been as thoroughly investigated. A thymic factor similar to thymosin fraction V but isolated from young pig thymus by Aiuti and associates[98] does not increase T cell rosette formation by lymphocytes from normal individuals but increases T cell rosette formation by lymphocytes isolated from human cord blood, fetal lymph nodes, fetal thymus gland, and from cells isolated from T cell-deficient patients.[99] Thymopoietin, when incubated with T-lymphocytes isolated from the peripheral blood of healthy donors, increases T-γ (suppressor cells) but has no effect on the proportion of T-μ (helper cells). A single infant, postthymectomy, had decreased percentages of T-γ cells. When the patient's lymphocytes were incubated with TP5, a component of thymopoietin, the proportion of T-γ cells increased.[100] The authors concluded that thymopoietin may enhance the numbers of T suppressor cells and, through this mechanism, affect T cell regulation. Thymic humoral factor, when incubated with peripheral blood lymphocytes of normal individuals, does not increase T cell rosette formation. In a subpopulation of patients with primary cellular immunodeficiency disease, THF did increase T cell rosette formation by peripheral blood lymphocytes; the direct effect of THF on these patients' null cells was not evaluated.[101]

Quantitation of thymopoietin-like activity in human serum is assayed by measuring the induction of Thy 1.2 antigen on lymphocytes from athymic nude mice when incubated with human plasma or serum. Results are expressed as inductive activity equivalent to nanograms of thymopoietin. Utilizing this assay, 19 normal children had thymopoietin activity of 10.6 to 16.2 ng/ml. In contrast, 15 children with severe combined immunodeficiency disease and two infants with DiGeorge syndrome had no measurable plasma thymopoietin-like activity.[89] Plasma thymopoietin-like activity declines with age, is normal in patients with myasthenia gravis younger than 50 years of age, but declines to unmeasurable levels after thymectomy. These studies taken together suggest that thymopoietin-like activity originates in the human thymus gland, disappears after thymectomy and with age and is absent in children with stem cell or thymus abnormalities.[102] Although a radioimmunoassay is available to quantitate serum thymopoietin levels, it measures quantities greater than 5 ng/ml; human serum samples contain less than this amount.[103]

Serum thymic hormone activity, as assessed by the induction of θ-antigen on splenocytes obtained from adult thymectomized mice, disappears after thymectomy in patients with myasthenia gravis with a half-life of six hours.[88] The level of the factor is higher in children than in adults and is not found in persons over age 50.[99] These results agree with those in animals and suggest that there is a thymic hormone in human serum. This same assay showed three patients with severe combined immunodeficiency disease to have individual patterns of circulating serum thymic factor activity. Two patients had nearly normal levels before bone marrow transplantation and normal levels following bone marrow transplantation. One patient lacked serum thymic factor activity before transplantation and had none after two fetal liver transplants. A single patient with DiGeorge syndrome had no circulating serum thymic factor before fetal thymus transplantation but had levels that increased to normal after reconstitution with fetal thymus, a result that again suggests that serum thymic factor originates in the thymus gland and then circulates in the peripheral blood.

ALTERATION OF LYMPHOCYTE FUNCTION BY INCUBATION WITH THYMIC FACTORS

The majority of the information concerning the effect of thymic humoral factors on T-lymphocyte function in man results from incubation of bone marrow cells or peripheral blood lymphocytes from normal individuals with thymosin fraction V. Putative stem cells obtained from normal adult individuals and incubated with thymosin fraction V or other agents that increase intracellular cyclic AMP have enhanced lymphocyte responsiveness to phytohemagglutinin (PHA) and allogeneic cells (in mixed lymphocyte culture—MLC).[91] When thymosin fraction V is maintained in culture throughout the assay, mixed lymphocyte culture reactivity of normal individuals and of patients with thymic hypoplasia is enhanced. Lymphocytes obtained from patients with severe combined immunodeficiency disease are not affected by incubation with thymosin fraction V.[104] Other investigators have shown that incubation of peripheral blood lymphocytes from normal individuals with thymosin fraction V results in decreased responsiveness to PHA, pokeweed mitogen, concanavalin A; in contrast, T suppressor cell activity is enhanced.[105] Thymosin decreases the pokeweed mitogen driven differentiation of B-lymphocytes in culture and results in a decreased synthesis of immunoglobulin when peripheral blood lymphocytes are isolated from healthy adult donors. The authors concluded that thymosin enhances T suppressor activity and, therefore, modulates the production of immunoglobulin in a culture environment.[106]

In Vitro Effect of Thymic Factors on Lymphocytes from Patients with Primary Immunodeficiency Disease, Autoimmune Disease, or Malignancy and Treatment of Patients with Thymic Factors

After documenting that the incubation of null cells obtained from normal individuals with thymosin fraction V were differentiated to T-lymphocytes as documented by enhanced T cell rosette formation and induction of HTLA on the cell surface, patients with primary immunodeficiency disease were investigated. Peripheral blood lymphocytes obtained from patients with combined immunodeficiency disease, DiGeorge syndrome, ataxia telangiectasia, and Wiskott-Aldrich syndrome and incubated with thymosin fraction V had increased T cell rosette formation.[90] Incubation of lymphocytes obtained from a subgroup of children with ataxia telangiectasia or Down's syndrome with thymic humoral factor resulted in increased T cell rosette formation.[101] Incubation of lymphocytes obtained from a single patient with cartilage hair hypoplasia with thymosin fraction V resulted in increased T cell rosette formation.[107] In contrast, lymphocytes obtained from children with severe combined immunodeficiency disease when incubated with thymic humoral factors had no evidence of differentiation to T cells.[90]

Following these initial studies, the effect of thymosin fraction V and other thymic factors on the induction of T cell rosette formation in a variety of pathologic disorders was assessed. Severely burned patients, a subpopulation felt to have a secondary immunodeficiency disease, had increased T cell rosette formation when lymphocytes were incubated with thymosin fraction V.[108] Thymopoietin incubated with peripheral blood lymphocytes from malnourished children with secondary infection resulted in increased T cell rosette formation.[109] Thymosin fraction V increased T cell rosette formation from 26% to 50% in a group of children with kwashiorkor.[110] Children and adults with atopic disease, a subpopulation of whom are felt to have primary or secondary cellular immunodeficiency disease, were assessed by several investigators. Decreased total peripheral blood T cells as assessed by T cell rosette formation was found in a group of children with eczema; the decrease was abolished by in vitro incubation with thymosin fraction V.[111] Likewise, a group of patients with asthma were documented to have decreased total peripheral blood T cells, a condition abolished by in vitro incubation with thymosin fraction V.[112]

Another assay used to investigate T cell function assessed the effect of thymic humoral factor on mononuclear cells obtained from 20 atopic individuals. All individuals had normal numbers of T cells and B cells. Mononuclear cells obtained from the patients investigated were injected intradermally into immunosuppressed rats and failed to induce a local reaction termed graft versus host reaction (GVHR); if the cells were incubated with thymic humoral factor prior to injection into the immunosuppressed rats, a normal, local GVHR resulted.[113] These results indicate that THF affected cell differentiation from less to more competent T cells in atopic individuals. Serum thymic factor activity, assessed by the Bach assay, was decreased in asthmatic patients.[114]

Patients with autoimmune disease and probable abnormal T cell regulation have been evaluated. A group of patients with active systemic lupus erythematosus and decreased T cell rosette formation had enhanced T cell rosette formation following incubation of their cells with thymic humoral factor.[115] Likewise, patients with active systemic lupus erythematosus had increased T cell rosette formation with thymosin fraction V incubation.[116] A further study documented that patients with systemic lupus erythematosus and Sjögren's syndrome and whose T cell rosettes were less than 50% had enhanced rosette formation following incubation with thymosin fraction V.[117]

Recently, 23 patients who received bone marrow transplantation for acute lymphocytic leukemia or aplastic anemia and were treated with chemoradiation therapy were evaluated in terms of cellular responsiveness to thymosin fraction V. Two to seven weeks following transplantation, the patients' lymphocytes when incubated with thymosin fraction V had increased T cell rosette formation. One to eight months following transplantation, incubation of their cells with thymosin fraction V resulted in an enhanced lymphocyte response to phytohemagglutinin and concanavalin A. The authors theorize that patients receiving bone marrow transplantation and immuno-suppression have circulating cells that remain responsive to thymosin fraction V; it is possible that the use of thymosin fraction V in these patients will accelerate a maturational response.[118]

Peripheral blood lymphocytes isolated from patients with a variety of malignancies have been evaluated. Thymic humoral factor when incubated with blood or bone marrow lymphocytes obtained from children with T cell ALL, null cell ALL, or B cell ALL was assessed for its functional capacity to induce a local graft versus host reaction in immunosuppressed rats. Incubation of thymic humoral factor with null cell lymphoblasts from the bone marrow or peripheral blood lymphocytes obtained from patients with null ALL resulted in enhanced local graft versus host reaction in the rat model; the authors concluded that thymic humoral factor in these patients provided differentiation of the null cells.[119] Patients with malignant melanoma have increased T cell rosette formation following thymosin incubation.[120] A variety of patients with solid tumors have been evaluated and subpopulations have been found to respond to thymosin fraction V with increased T cell rosette formation following incubation.[121]

Two groups of patients have been treated with thymic factors, children with primary immunodeficiency disease and patients with malignancies. The first patient to receive thymosin fraction V was a three-year-old girl with combined immunodeficiency disease, 10% T cell rosette formation, but enhancement to 45% when incubated with thymosin fraction V. She had absent T-lymphocyte function, as assessed by response to PHA or to allogeneic cells (MLC). Following treatment with thymosin fraction V, the patient's T cell rosettes increased from 10% to 55%. Her delayed hypersensitivity skin tests to mumps and to *Candida* antigens became positive, and she improved clinically. Therapy was stopped, and T cell rosettes decreased to 20%.[108, 121] This initial success prompted the additional treatment of patients with primary immunodeficiency disease but with variable results (Table 6). Subgroups of patients with chronic mucocutaneous candidiasis, ataxia telangiectasia, Wiskott-Aldrich syndrome, or combined immunodeficiency with or without enzyme defects appeared to respond specifically to treatment with thymosin fraction V.[121-123] Patients with

TABLE 6.—THERAPEUTIC RESPONSE TO THYMOSIN FRACTION
V BY PATIENTS

FINDING	CLINICAL IMPROVEMENT	INCREASED T CELL NOS.	INCREASED T CELL FUNCTION
Severe combined immunodeficiency	0/1	0/1	0/1
DiGeorge syndrome	N.A.*	4/6	4/6
Ataxia telangiectasia	2/4	3/4	2/4
Wiskott-Aldrich syndrome	1/3	2/3	2/3
Chronic mucocutaneous candidiasis	1/4	1/4	1/4
Nezelof's syndrome	2/2	2/2	1/2

*N.A. = not applicable.

DiGeorge syndrome (thymic thypoplasia) had the most consistent response to therapy and in general had an increase in T cell number associated with increased T cell function and clinical stability following therapy.[96, 97, 121, 122] No patient with severe combined immunodeficiency disease responded to therapy.[121, 122] Various authors concluded that patients with putative stem cells and thymic abnormalities responded to treatment with thymosin fraction V because of differentiation of their stem cells. Patients with severe combined immunodeficiency disease and no stem cells lacked the cell that a thymic factor might differentiate. Aiuti and associates[124] using a factor termed thymostimulin and prepared in a manner similar to THF have treated eight patients with combined immunodeficiency disease, one with Wiskott-Aldrich syndrome, and two with severe combined immunodeficiency disease. The patient with Wiskott-Aldrich syndrome had increased T cell numbers and function associated with a positive clinical response. A subgroup of patients with combined immunodeficiency disease responded to treatment, whereas neither patient with severe combined immunodeficiency disease responded. These studies all suggest that combined immunodeficiency disease, or Nezelof's syndrome, represents a heterogeneous population of patients most likely requiring different therapies. In contrast, patients with DiGeorge syndrome represent a more homogeneous group of patients who theoretically lack a thymus and can be reconstituted with either fetal thymus transplant or humoral factors.

Following the initial success in treating patients with primary immunodeficiency disease, several investigators assessed the effect of thymosin fraction V on survival in patients with malignancy. The patients with solid tumors, including melanoma, carcinoma of the breast, dysgerminoma, and lung cancer, received treatment with thymosin fraction V with variable success.[121] Prior to therapy, the most consistent finding was increased T cell rosette formation by peripheral blood lymphocytes isolated from these patients when incubated with thymosin fraction V.[121, 125, 126] Cohen and associates[125] reported a prolonged relapse-free survival of patients with small cell carcinoma of the lung following treatment with thymosin fraction V but no increase in complete response rate. Wara and associates[127] have reported a modest increase in disease-free interval in patients with head and neck cancer treated with thymosin fraction V.

Summary

The central role of the thymus gland in the development and maintenance of the immune system is recognized. Biochemically characterized thymic extracts differentiate murine prethymic cells to functional T-lymphocytes. Thymosin fraction V differentiates prethymocytes to thymocytes, and mature thymocytes to competent T-lymphocytes. Thymopoietin and thymic humoral factor differentiate thymocytes; they have relatively little effect on prethymocytes. Serum thymic factor also affects a cell already at the thymocyte stage. The relative importance of each factor in the differentiation of T-lymphocytes remains unknown. Most likely, they act sequentially to produce a competent circulating T cell.

The site of cellular differentiation in man by thymic factors is less well defined than in the murine system. It is established that thymosin fraction V, thymic humoral factor, and thymopoietin differentiate a subpopulation of isolated peripheral blood null lymphocytes (T cell rosette negative, surface immunoglobulin negative) to form T cell rosettes. In some situations, T cell function as assessed by response to allogeneic cells or plant lectins is enhanced following incubation with the factors.

Peripheral blood lymphocytes isolated from subpopulations of children with primary or secondary immunodeficiency, or from adults with autoimmune disease or malignancy, have been incubated with thymosin fraction V. Enhanced T cell rosette formation has occurred in a subgroup of these patients. Notably, children with severe combined immunodeficiency and without stem cells for thymic factors to differentiate have had no increase in T cell rosette formation.

The most important potential contribution of thymic factor research will be its precise application to the treatment of human disease. As our understanding of the differentiation of the human T cell approaches our understanding of the murine system, a more careful approach to the pathogenesis of human disease should be possible. Monoclonal antibodies capable of identifying human thymocyte and lymphocyte surface antigens have become available. By (1) evaluating the effect or effects of factors on normal human lymphocyte differentiation; (2) understanding the biochemical mechanism or mechanisms through which thymic factor differentiation occurs; (3) identifying specific abnormalities in individual disease entities; and (4) correlating disease pathogenesis with specific thymic factor effect, a logical approach to replacement therapy should be possible.

REFERENCES

1. Owen J.J.T., Ritter M.A.: Tissue interaction in the development of thymus lymphocytes. *J. Exp. Med.* 129:431, 1969.
2. Owen J.J.T., Raff M.C.: Studies on the differentiation of thymus-derived lymphocytes. *J. Exp. Med.* 132:1216, 1970.
3. Janossy G., Thomas J.A., Bollum F.J.: The human thymic microenvironment: An immunohistologic study. *J. Immunol.* 125:202, 1980.
4. McMichael A.J., Pilch J.R., Galfre G., et al.: A human thymocyte antigen defined by a hybrid myeloma monoclonal antibody. *Eur. J. Immunol.* 9:205, 1979.
5. Blomgren H., Anderson B.: Evidence for a small pool of immunocompetent cells in the mouse thymus. *Exp. Cell Res.* 57:185, 1969.
6. Bollum F.J.: Terminal deoxynucleotidyltransferase: Biological studies, in Meiser A. (ed): *Advances in Enzymology.* New York: John Wiley & Sons, 1979, pp 347–374.
7. Touraine J-L., Hadden J.W., Good R.A.: Sequential stages of human T lymphocyte differentiation. *Proc. Natl. Acad. Sci.* 74:3414, 1977.
8. Pahwa R.N., Pahwa S.G., Good R.A.: T-lymphocyte differentiation in vitro in severe combined immunodeficiency. *J. Clin. Invest.* 64:1632, 1979.
9. Reinherz E.L., Schlossman S.F.: Regulation of the immune response: Inducer and suppressor T-lymphocyte subsets in human beings. *N. Engl. J. Med.* 303:370, 1980.
10. Miller J.F.A.P.: Role of the thymus in transplantation immunity. *Ann. N.Y. Acad. Sci.* 99:340, 1962.
11. Ammann A.J., Wara D.W., Golbus M.S.: Thymus transplantation in patients with thymic hypoplasia and abnormal immunoglobulin synthesis. *Transplantation* 20:457, 1975.
12. Osoba D., Miller J.F.A.P.: The lymphoid tissues and immune responses of neonatally thymectomized mice bearing thymus tissue in millipore diffusion chambers. *J. Exp. Med.* 119:177, 1964.

13. Steele R.W., Limias C., Thurman G.B., et al.: Familial thymic aplasia. *N. Engl. J. Med.* 287:787, 1972.
14. Bomskov C., Sladovic L.: Der thymus als innersekretorisches organ. *Dtsch. Med. Wochenschr.* 66:589, 1940.
15. Cantor H., Weissman I.: Development and function of subpopulations of thymocytes and T-lymphocytes. *Prog. Allergy* 20:1, 1976.
16. Stutman O.: Intrathymic and extrathymic T-cell maturation. *Immunol. Rev.* 42:139, 1978.
17. Trainin N.: Thymic hormones and the immune response. *Physiol. Rev.* 54:272, 1974.
18. Comsa J.: Conséquences de la thymectomie totale chez le cobcaye male. *C. R. Soc. Biol. Paris* 127:903, 1938.
19. Good R.A., Dalmasso A.P., Martinez C., et al.: The role of thymus in development of immunologic capacity in rabbits and mice. *J. Exp. Med.* 116:773, 1962.
20. Miller J.F.A.P.: Effect of neonatal thymectomy of the immunological responsiveness of the mouse. *Proc. R. Soc. Lond. [Biol]* 156:415, 1962.
21. Cooper M.D., Gabrielsen M.A., Good R.A.: Role of the thymus and other central lymphoid tissues in immunological disease. *Ann. Rev. Med.* 18:113, 1967.
22. DiGeorge A.M.: Discussion of Cooper, M.D., Peterson, R.D.A., and Good, R.A.: New concept of cellular basis of immunity. *J. Pediatr.* 67:907, 1965.
23. Miller J.F.A.P.: Immunological function of the thymus. *Lancet* 2:748, 1961.
24. Levey R.H., Trainin N., Law L.W.: Evidence for function of thymic tissue in diffusion chambers implanted in neonatally thymectomized mice. *J. Natl. Cancer Inst.* 31:199, 1963.
25. Osoba D., Miller J.F.A.P.: Evidence for a humoral thymus factor responsible for the maturation of immunological faculty. *Nature* 199:653, 1963.
26. Osoba D., Miller J.F.A.P.: The lymphoid tissues and immune responses of neonatally thymectomized mice bearing thymus tissue in millipore diffusion chambers. *J. Exp. Med.* 119:177, 1964.
27. August C.S., Rosen F.S., Filler R.M., et al.: Implantation of fetal thymus, restoring immunological competence in a patient with thymic aplasia. *Lancet* 11:1210, 1968.
28. Cleveland W.W., Fogel B.J., Brown W., et al.: Fetal thymic transplant in a case of DiGeorge syndrome. *Lancet* 2:1211, 1968.
29. Abelous J.E., Billard A.: Recherches sur les fonctions de thymus. *Arch. Physiol. Norm. Pathol.* 28:898, 1896.
30. Gregoire C., Duchateau G.: A study on lympho-epithelial symbiosis in thymus: Reactions of the lymphatic tissue to extracts and to implants of epithelial components of thymus. *Arch. Biol. Liege* 68:269, 1956.
31. Metcalf D.: A lymphocytosis stimulating factor in the plasma of chronic lymphatic leukemia patients. *Br. J. Cancer* 10:169, 1956.
32. Goldstein A.L., Guha A., Zatz M.M., et al.: Purification and biological activity of thymosin, a hormone of the thymus gland. *Proc. Natl. Acad. Sci. U.S.A.* 69:1800, 1972.
33. Kook A.I., Yakir Y., Trainin N.: Isolation and partial chemical characterization of THF, a thymus hormone involved in immune maturation of lymphoid cells. *Cell. Immunol.* 19:151, 1975.
34. Goldstein G.: Isolation of bovine thymin: A polypeptide hormone of the thymus. *Nature* 247:11, 1974.
35. Bach J.F., Dardenne M., Pleau J.M., et al.: *Nature* 266:5597, 1977.
36. Kruisbeek A.M., Astaldi G.C.B.: Distinct effects of thymic epithelial culture supernatants on T-cell properties of mouse thymocytes separated by the use of peanut agglutinin. *J. Immunol.* 123:984, 1979.
37. Goldstein G., Scheid M.P., Boyse D.H., et al.: A synthetic pentapeptide with biological activity characteristic of the thymic hormone thymopoietin. *Science* 204:1309, 1979.

38. Low T.L.K., Goldstein A.L.: The chemistry and biology of thymosin. *J. Biol. Chem.* 254:987, 1979.
39. Low T.L.K., Thurman G.B., McAddo M., et al.: The chemistry and biology of thymosin. *J. Biol. Chem.* 254:981, 1979.
40. Wetzel R., Heynecker H.L., Goeddel D.V., et al.: Production of biologically active N-α-desacetyl-thymosin-α-1 in *Escherichia coli* through expression of a chemically synthesized gene. *Biochemistry*. In press.
41. Klein J.J., Goldstein A.L., White A.: Effects of the thymus lymohocytopoietic factor. *Ann. N.Y. Acad. Sci.* 135:485, 1966.
42. Hooper J.A., McDaniel M.C., Thurman G.B.: The purification and properties of bovine thymosin. *Ann. N.Y. Acad. Sci.* 249:125, 1975.
43. Schlesinger D.H., Goldstein G.: The amino acid sequence of thymopoietin II. *Cell* 5:361, 1975.
44. Goldstein A.L., White A.: The thymus gland: Experimental and clinical studies of its role in the development and expression of immune functions. *Adv. Metab. Disord.* 5:149, 1971.
45. Goldstein A.L., White A.: Role of thymosin and other thymic factors in the development, maturation and functions of lymphoid tissue. *Curr. Top. Exp. Endocrinol.* 1:121, 1971.
46. White A., Goldstein A.L.: The role of the thymus gland in the hormonal regulation of host resistance, in Wolstenholme G.E.W., et al. (eds): Control processes in multicellular organisms. *Ciba Found. Symp.* 210, 1970.
47. Trainin N., Burger M., Lenker-Israeli M.: Restoration of homograft response in neonatally thymectomized mice by a thymic humoral factor (THF), in Dausset J., et al. (eds): *Proc. Intern. Congr. Transplant. Soc.* Copenhagen: Munksgaard, 1967, pp 91–97.
48. Law L., Goldstein A.L., White A.: Influence of thymosin on immunological competence of lymphoid cells from thymectomized mice. *Nature* 219:1391, 1968.
49. Goldstein A.L., Guha A., Howe M.A., et al.: Ontogenesis of cell mediated immunity and its acceleration by thymosin, a thymic hormone. *J. Immunol.* 106:773, 1971.
50. Bach M-A.: Lymphocyte-mediated cytotoxicity: Effects of aging, adult thymectomy and thymic factor. *J. Immunol.* 119:641, 1977.
51. Lau C.Y., Goldstein G.: Functional effects of thymopoietin (TP5) on cytotoxic lymphocyte precursor units (CLP-U). *J. Immunol.* 124:1861, 1980.
52. Marshall G.D., Thurman G.B., Rossio J.L., et al.: In vivo generation of suppressor T cells by thymosin in congenitally athymic nude mice. *J. Immunol.* 126:741, 1981.
53. Zisblatt M., Goldstein A.L., Lilly F., et al.: Acceleration by thymosin in the development of resistance to murine sarcoma-induced tumor in mice. *Proc. Natl. Acad. Sci. U.S.A.* 66:1170, 1970.
54. Dardenne M., Bach J-F.: Studies on thymus products: I. Modification of rosette-forming cells by thymic extracts determination of the target RFC subpopulation. *Immunology* 25:343, 1973.
55. Dardenne M., Charreire J., Bach J-F.: Alterations in thymocyte surface markers after in vivo treatment by serum thymic factor. *Cell. Immunol.* 39:47, 1978.
56. Wortis H.H.: Immunological responses of "nude" mice. *Clin. Exp. Immunol.* 8:305, 1971.
57. Ahmed A., Smith A.H., Wong D.M., et al.: In vitro induction of Lyt surface markers on precursor cells incubated with thymosin polypeptides. *Cancer Treat. Rep.* 62:1739, 1978.
58. Scheid M.P., Hoffmann M.K., Komuro K., et al.: Differentiation of T cells induced by preparations from thymus and by nonthymic agents. *J. Exp. Med.* 138:1027, 1973.

59. Cohen G.H., Hooper J.A., Goldstein A.L.: Thymosin-induced differentiation of murine thymocytes in allogeneic mixed lymphocyte cultures. *Ann. N.Y. Acad. Sci.* 249:145, 1975.
60. Talal N., Dauphinee M., Pillarisetty E., et al.: Effect of thymosin on thymocyte proliferation and autoimmunity in NZB mice. *Ann. N.Y. Acad. Sci.* 249:438, 1975.
61. Armerding D., Katz D.H.: Activation of T and B lymphocytes in vitro: IV. Regulatory influence on specific T cell functions by a thymus extract factor. *J. Immunol.* 114:1248, 1975.
62. Kook A.I., Trainin N.: The control exerted by thymic hormone (THF) on cellular cAMP levels and immune reactivity of spleen cells in the MLC assay. *J. Immunol.* 115:8, 1975.
63. Umiel T., Trainin N.: Increased reactivity of responding cells in the mixed lymphocyte reaction by a thymic humoral factor. *Eur. J. Immunol.* 5:85, 1975.
64. Kook A.I., Trainin N.: Intracellular events involved in the induction of immune competence in lymphoid cells by a thymus humoral factor. *J. Immunol.* 114:151, 1975.
65. Kook A.I., Trainin N.: Hormone-like activity of a thymus humoral factor on the induction of immune competence in lymphoid cells. *J. Exp. Med.* 139:193, 1974.
66. Rotter V., Trainin N.: Effect of thymic hormone on the response of different lymphoid cell populations to T mitogens. *Isr. J. Med. Sci.* 13:363, 1977.
67. Basch R.S., Goldstein G.: Thymopoietin-induced acquisition of responsiveness to T-cell mitogens. *Cell. Immunol.* 20:218, 1975.
68. Sunshine G.H., Basch R.S., Coffey R.G., et al.: Thymopoietin enhances the allogeneic response and cyclic GMP levels of mouse peripheral, thymus-derived lymphocytes. *J. Immunol.* 120:1594, 1978.
69. Lau C.Y., Goldstein G.: Functional effects of thymopoietin (TP5) on cytotoxic lymphocyte precursor units (CLP-U). *J. Immunol.* 124:1861, 1980.
70. Bach J.F., Dardenne M., Goldstein A.L., et al.: Appearance of T cell markers in bone marrow rosette forming cells after incubation with thymosin, a thymic hormone. *Proc. Natl. Acad. Sci. U.S.A.* 68:2734, 1971.
71. Bach J.F., Cantor H., Roelants G., et al.: in *Biological Activities of Thymic Hormones.* Rotterdam: Kooyker Scientific Publications, 1975, p 246.
72. Bach J.F., Dardenne M.: Thymus dependency on rosette-forming cells: Evidence for a circulating thymic hormone. *Transplant. Proc.* 4:345, 1972.
73. Bach J.F., Dardenne M.: Studies on thymus products: V. Demonstration and characterization of a circulating thymic hormone. *Immunology* 25:353, 1973.
74. Bach J.F., Dardenne M., Salomon J.C.: Studies on thymus products: IV. Absence of serum thymic activity in adult NZB F, mice. *Clin. Exp. Immunol.* 14:247, 1973.
75. Komuro K., Boyse E.A.: In vitro demonstration of thymic hormone in the mouse by conversion of precursor cells into lymphocytes. *Lancet* 1:740, 1973.
76. Komuro K., Boyse E.A.: Induction of T-lymphocytes from precursor cells in vitro by a product of the thymus. *J. Exp. Med.* 138:479, 1973.
77. Pazmino N.H., Ihle J.N., Goldstein A.L.: Induction in vivo of terminal deoxynucleotidyl transferase by thymosin in bone marrow cells from athymic mice. *J. Exp. Med.* 147:708, 1978.
78. Pazmino N.H., Ihle J.N., McEwan R.N., et al.: Control of differentiation of thymocyte precursors in the bone marrow by thymic hormones. *Cancer Treat. Rep.* 62:1749, 1978.
79. Goldstein G., Scheid M., Boyse E.A., et al.: Thymopoietin and bursopoietin: Induction signals regulating early lymphocyte differentiation. *Cold Spring Harbor Symp. Quant. Biol.* 41(part 1):5, 1977.
80. Nash L., Good R.A., Hatzfeld A., et al.: In vitro differentiation of two surface

markers for immature T-cells: The synthetic pentapeptide, thymopoietin. *J. Immunol.* 126:150, 1981.
81. Gupta S., Good R.A.: Subpopulations of human T-lymphocytes: II. Effect of thymopoietin, corticosteroids, and irradiation. *Cell. Immunol.* 34:10, 1977.
82. Goldstein G.: A synthesized pentapeptide with biological activity characteristic of the thymic hormone thymopoietin. *Science* 204:1309, 1979.
83. Basch R.S., Goldstein G.: Antigenic and functional evidence for the in vitro inductive activity of thymopoietin on thymocyte precursors. *Ann. N.Y. Acad. Sci.* 249:290, 1975.
84. Scheid M.P., Goldstein G., Hammerling U., et al.: Lymphocyte differentiation from precursor cells in vitro. *Ann. N.Y. Acad. Sci.* 249:531, 1975.
85. Scheid M.P., Goldstein G., Boyse E.A.: The generation and regulation of lymphocyte populations. *J. Exp. Med.* 22:1727, 1978.
86. Dardenne M., Papiernik M., Bach J-F., et al.: Studies on thymus products: III. Epithelial origin of the serum thymic factor. *Immunology* 27:299, 1974.
87. Naylor P.H., Goldstein A.L.: Thymosin: Cyclic nucleotides and T cell differentiation. *Life Sciences* 25:301, 1979.
88. Bach J-F., Dardenne M., Papiernik M., et al.: Evidence for a serum-factor secreted by the human thymus. *Lancet,* November 18, p 1056, 1971.
89. Lewis V., Twomey J.J.: Circulating thymic-hormone activity in congenital immunodeficiency. *Lancet,* September 3, p 471, 1977.
90. Wara D.W., Ammann A.J.: Activation of T cell rosettes in immunodeficient patients by thymosin. *Ann. N.Y. Acad. Sci.* 249:308, 1975.
91. Horowitz S.D., Goldstein A.L.: The in vitro induction of differentiation of putative human stem cells by thymosin and agents that affect cyclic AMP. *Clin. Immunol. Immunopathol.* 9:408, 1978.
92. Kaplan J.: Characterization of thymosin-responsive peripheral blood null cells. *Cancer Treat. Rep.* 62:1757, 1978.
93. Kaplan J., Peterson W.D.: Detection of human T-lymphocyte antigens (HTLA antigens) on thymosin-inducible T cell precursors. *Clin. Immunol. Immunopathol.* 9:436, 1978.
94. Incefy G., Touraine J.L., Touraine F., et al.: In vitro studies on human T-lymphocyte differentiation in primary immunodeficiency diseases. *Trans. Assoc. Am. Physicians* 87:258, 1974.
95. Touraine J.L., Touraine F., Incefy G.S., et al.: Effect of thymic factors on the differentiation of human marrow cells into T-lymphocytes in vitro in normals and patients with immunodeficiencies. *Ann. N.Y. Acad. Sci.* 249:335, 1975.
96. Astaldi A., Astaldi G.C.B., Wijermans P., et al.: Experiences with thymosin in primary immunodeficiency disease. *Cancer Treat. Rep.* 62:1770, 1978.
97. Barrett D.J., Wara D.W., Ammann A.J., et al.: Thymosin therapy in the DiGeorge syndrome. *J. Pediatr.* 97:66, 1980.
98. Aiuti F., Schirrmacher V., Ammirati P., et al.: Effect of thymus factor on human precursor T-lymphocytes. *Clin. Exp. Immunol.* 20:499, 1975.
99. Fiorilli M., Aiuti F., Ammirati P., et al.: Effect of thymic factor on human lymphoid cells of umbilical cord blood and of children with T cell deficiency. *Int. Arch. Allergy Appl. Immunol.* 53:242, 1977.
100. Gupta S., Kapoor N., Goldstein G., et al.: Alterations in circulating T-cell subpopulation and in vitro effects of thymopoietin pentapeptide. *Clin. Immunol. Immunopathol.* 12:404, 1979.
101. Handzel Z.T., Dolfin Z., Levin S., et al.: Effect of thymic humoral factor on cellular immune functions of normal children and of pediatric patients with ataxia telangiectasia and Down's syndrome. *Pediatr. Res.* 13:803, 1979.
102. Twomey J.J., Goldstein G., Lewis V.M., et al.: Bioassay determinations of thymopoietin and thymic hormone levels in human plasma. *Proc. Natl. Acad. Sci. U.S.A.* 74:2541, 1977.

103. Goldstein G.: Radioimmunoassay for thymopoietin. *J. Immunol.* 117:690, 1976.
104. Wara D.W., Barrett D.J., Ammann A.J., et al.: In vitro and in vivo enhancement of mixed lymphocyte culture reactivity by thymosin in patients with primary immunodeficiency disease. *Ann. N.Y. Acad. Sci.* 77:128, 1979.
105. Wolf R.E.: Thymosin-induced suppression of proliferative response of human lymphocytes to mitogens. *J. Clin. Invest.* 63:677, 1979.
106. Wolf R.E., Goldstein A.L., Ziff M.: Suppression by thymosin of pokeweed mitogen-induced differentiation of human B cells. *Clin. Immunol. Immunopathol.* 11:303, 1978.
107. Steele R.W., Britton H.A., Kniker W.T., et al.: Severe combined immunodeficiency with cartilage-hair hypoplasia: In vitro response to thymosin and attempted reconstitution. *Pediatr. Res.* 10:1003, 1976.
108. Goldstein A.L., Wara D.W., Ammann A.J., et al.: First clinical trial with thymosin: Reconstitution of T-cells in patients with cellular immunodeficiency diseases. *Transplant. Proc.* 7(suppl 1):681, 1975.
109. Jackson T.M., Zaman S.N.: The in vitro effect of the thymic factor thymopoietin on a subpopulation of lymphocytes from severely malnourished children. *Clin. Exp. Immunol.* 39:717, 1980.
110. Olusi S.O., Thurman G.B., Goldstein A.L.: Effect of thymosin on T-lymphocyte rosette formation in children with kwashiorkor. *Clin. Immunol. Immunopathol.* 15:687, 1980.
111. Byrom N.A., Staughton R.C.D., Campbell M-A., et al.: Thymosin-inducible "null" cells in atopic eczema. *Br. J. Dermatol.* 100:499, 1979.
112. Byrom N.A., Caballero F., Campbell M-A., et al.: T cell depletion and in vitro thymosin inducibility in asthmatic children. *Clin. Exp. Immunol.* 31:490, 1978.
113. Shohat B., Metzker A., Trainin N.: Cell-mediated immunity and the in vitro effect of thymic humoral factor (THF) on blood lymphocytes of children with atopic dermatitis. *Clin. Immunol. Immunopathol.* 15:646, 1980.
114. Garaci E., Ronchetti R., Gobbo V.D., et al.: Decreased serum thymic factor activity in asthmatic children. *J. Allergy Clin. Immunol.* 62:357, 1978.
115. Michalevicz R., Many A., Ramot B., et al.: The in vitro effect of thymic humoral factor and levamisole on peripheral blood lymphocytes in systemic lupus erythematosus patients. *Clin. Exp. Immunol.* 31:111, 1978.
116. Scheinberg M.A., Cathcart E.S., Goldstein A.L.: Thymosin-induced reduction of "null cells" in peripheral blood lymphocytes of patients with systemic lupus erythematosus. *Lancet,* February 22, p 424, 1975.
117. Moutsopoulos H., Fye K.H., Sawada S., et al.: In vitro effect of thymosin on T-lymphocyte rosette formation in rheumatic diseases. *Clin. Exp. Immunol.* 26:563, 1976.
118. Elfenbein G.J., Goldstein A.L., Adams J.S., et al.: Thymosin-induced T cell marker expression and enhanced mitogen responsiveness in allogeneic marrow transplant recipients. *Transplantation* 29:113, 1980.
119. Shohat B., Wolach, B., Trainin, N.: Effect of thymic humoral factor in vitro on human bone marrow and blood cells from B-, T-, and null-cell acute lymphatic leukemia. *Cell. Immunol.* 45:255, 1979.
120. Byrom N.A., Campbell M.A., Dean A.J., et al.: Thymosin-inducible lymphocytes in the peripheral blood of patients with malignant melanoma. *Cancer Treat. Rep.* 62:1769, 1978.
121. Goldstein A.L., Cohen G.H., Rossio J.L., et al.: Use of thymosin in the treatment of primary immunodeficiency diseases and cancer. *Med. Clin. North Am.* 60:591, 1976.
122. Wara D.W., Ammann A.J.: Thymosin treatment of children with primary immunodeficiency disease. *Transplant. Proc.* 10:203, 1978.
123. Rubinstein A., Hirschhorn R., Sicklick M., et al.: In vivo and in vitro effects of

thymosin and adenosine deaminase on adeonosine-deaminase-deficient lymphocytes. *N. Engl. J. Med.* 300:387, 1979.
124. Aiuti F., Ammirati P., Fiorilli M., et al.: Immunologic and clinical investigation on a bovine thymic extract: Therapeutic applications in primary immunodeficiencies. *Pediatr. Res.* 13:797, 1979.
125. Cohen M.H., Chretien P.B., Ihde D.C., et al.: Thymosin fraction V and intensive combination chemotherapy. *J.A.M.A.* 241:1813, 1979.
126. Rossio J.L., Goldstein A.L.: Immunotherapy of cancer with thymosin. *World J. Surg.* 1:605, 1977.
127. Wara W., Neely M., Ammann A.J., et al.: Thymosin adjuvent therapy in advanced head and neck cancer, in Salmon S.E., et al.: *Third International Conference on Adjuvent Therapy of Cancer.* New York: Grune & Stratton. In press.

Anatomical Asymmetries in the Adult and Developing Brain and their Implications for Function

ALBERT M. GALABURDA, M.D.

AND

NORMAN GESCHWIND, M.D.

*The Neurological Units of Beth Israel Hospital and Boston City Hospital,
The Department of Neurology of Harvard Medical School, and
Charles A. Dana Research Institute, Beth Israel Hospital
Boston, Massachusetts*

AFTER THE DISCOVERY IN THE MID 19TH CENTURY of language disturbances in adults following acquired localized injury to the left hemisphere of the brain, reports began to appear of delayed development of language skills[25, 40] as well as of acquired lesions in the brains of children resulting in language and/or cognitive loss.[37] Soon publications containing reports of cases with exquisitely isolated language disturbances in children were numerous, and distinct aphasic syndromes and specific learning disabilities could be identified. Anatomical correlates were sought and described, often with a high degree of success for aphasias and related disturbances recurring in adult life. Yet anatomical analysis of these disturbances in children was much less fruitful, partly because the brains of children with developmental and acquired language disorders were not as readily available as those of adults.[20, 28, 44] Evidence from acquired lesions in children indicates that the left hemisphere of

Work supported in part by NIH grant NS14018, by a Biomedical Research Support grant to the Beth Israel Hospital, and by a grant from the Underwood Company to the Orton Society for research on the neurologic foundations of childhood dyslexia.

children, as in adults, is usually dominant for language function and that within the left hemisphere areas typically associated with language deficits are the same as those in adults.
A major difference, however, is the ability of children to recover more often and more thoroughly from unilateral (usually
left-sided) lesions leading to language disorders.[68, 80] Thus, the
juvenile brain shares with the adult brain some aspects of lateralization and localization of language function but has its
own capability to compensate, often extremely well, for the effects of unilateral and occasionally bilateral lesions that cause
language deficits. Although it is outside the scope of this chapter to review completely the factors leading to recovery after
language disturbances in the child, we will review aspects of
language localization and lateralization relevant to both adults
and children, as well as some aspects of plasticity in childhood.

Localization

LESION DATA

Lesions resulting in language disturbance most often involve
the left hemisphere.[80] The most striking abnormalities occur
when the entire middle cerebral artery territory is involved.[6]
Thus an occlusion of this vessel may produce a cortical infarction involving the whole perisylvian region (Fig 1): the inferior
frontal gyrus, the hand and face representations of the precentral and postcentral gyri, the parietal operculum, the supramarginal and angular gyri, the superior and middle temporal
gyri, and the temporal pole. Lesions involving a major portion
of this territory are likely to produce a global language disturbance affecting production and comprehension of spoken and
written language. When the lesion occupies only a portion of
the total territory more delimited syndromes may be seen.
Thus a large lesion in the area of the inferior frontal gyrus
produces the syndrome of Broca's aphasia, characterized by decreased and abnormal verbal output, both spoken and written,
and poor repetition, but in which comprehension of language is
much less affected.[6] A major portion of the pars opercularis of
the inferior frontal gyrus and of the inferior precentral gyrus
probably must be destroyed before a long-lasting Broca's
aphasia will result.[53]

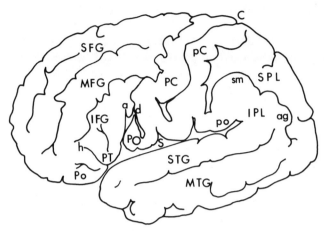

Fig 1.—Diagram of lateral surface of brain shows major gross anatomical landmarks with special emphasis on perisylvian language areas. Posterior speech area is located in posterior third of superior temporal gyrus *(STG)*. Anterior speech area contains pars opercularis *(PO)* and a variable portion of pars triangularis *(PT)* and inferior precentral region *(PC)*. Note that PO and inferior portion of PC form a unit separated from anterior opercular portions PT and pars orbitalis *(Po)* by a deep furrow known as the ascending limb *(a)* of the sylvian fissure *(S)*. This furrow often has a branch known as the diagonal sulcus *(d)*, more often present on the left side. The inferior parietal lobule *(IPL)* contains parietal operculum *(po)*, supramarginal gyrus *(sm)* and angular gyrus *(ag)*, all part of the posterior language representation. The supplementary speech areas on medial surface of hemisphere are not shown. Other abbreviations: c, central sulcus; h, horizontal limb of sylvian fissure; *IFG*, inferior frontal gyrus; *MFG*, middle frontal gyrus; *MTG*, middle temporal gyrus; *pC*, postcentral gyrus; *SFG*, superior frontal gyrus; *SPL*, superior parietal lobule.

Conversely, a lesion in the posterior portion of the middle cerebral artery bed territory that specifically destroys most of the posterior third of the superior temporal gyrus and adjacent parietal operculum (Wernicke's area) usually results in an aphasic disturbance in which comprehension of spoken and written language is impaired in the face of a fluent but abnormal speech output, both in spontaneous speech and repetition.[6] There is usually no hemiplegia. A lesion in either the white matter of the parietal operculum or white matter underlying the insula may result in still another syndrome, conduction aphasia. Patients with this disorder (who usually have no hemiplegia) have fluently abnormal speech but relatively intact comprehension together with poor repetition of sentences.[6,7] In children fluently abnormal, speech is not seen and children with posteriorly located lesions in the brain usually have a paucity of speech.[4]

Anomia, the difficulty in naming objects on confrontation tasks, is a common accompaniment of all aphasias and of several nonaphasic language disorders as well. The syndrome of anomic aphasia consists of word-finding difficulty in speech without articulatory disorder or problems in comprehension or repetition. In the absence of confusion the lesion in these patients may be found in the angular gyrus, i.e., in the posterior inferior parietal region (see Fig 1), or in the border zone between the second and third temporal gyri and the occipital lobe.[5] Lesions in the left supplementary motor region, located near the anterior portion of the cingulate gyrus, as well as subcortical lesions surrounding the lateral superior aspect of the frontal horns of the left lateral ventricle, may be accompanied by the so-called transcortical motor aphasia,[64] a relatively benign form of disordered language characterized by limited spontaneous output in the presence of intact comprehension and repetition. Conversely, a lesion more posteriorly surrounding the cingulate gyrus, as well as lesions involving the cortex lying in the posterior border zone of anterior and middle cerebral artery bed territories, can result in a language disturbance known as transcortical sensory aphasia, characterized by the remarkable preservation of the ability to repeat sentences in the face of a severe language comprehension deficit.[64]

A combination of the two pericingulate lesions or of the anterior and posterior border zone lesions can be associated with a language disorder of striking appearance in which the patient exhibits no spontaneous speech and no comprehension of language but has a tendency to echo the examiner's speech and thus demonstrates perfect repetition ability.[33] Thus, the syndrome of the isolated speech area might result from the disconnection of supplementary regions on the medial hemisphere from perisylvian speech areas on the left side, since border zone lesions probably interrupt fiber connections between supplementary and perisylvian language areas.

NEUROPHYSIOLOGICAL DATA

It was also during the second half of the nineteenth century that neurophysiological manipulation of the brain had its beginnings. Most data of this type have been obtained by cortical stimulation during surgery,[60] but additional information has been made available through techniques of evoked potentials[54] and measurements of regional blood flow[41] and regional glucose consumption.[70] Areas thus outlined correspond to a surprising degree to areas identified by the analysis of lesions (see above). For instance, speech arrest and errors in naming have been obtained after stimulation of most of the posterior half of the inferior frontal gyrus[60] (see Fig 1). Furthermore, an area of special sensitivity to low amplitude stimulation, which produces aphasic disturbances in nearly all patients tested, is found specifically on the pars opercularis region of the left hemisphere[77] (see "Architectonic Asymmetries" below). Other areas of the left cerebral cortex involved with language as disclosed by stimulation experiments are located in the posterior half of the superior temporal gyrus, especially its posterior third; in the inferior parietal lobule; and on the physiologically parcellated supplementary motor area on the medial portion of the hemisphere.[60] Studies of regional blood flow and regional glucose metabolism, especially in younger individuals, tend to confirm the findings of the older stimulation techniques.

GROSS ANATOMICAL LANDMARKS

Lesions resulting in aphasia and language areas outlined physiologically can both be superimposed on gross anatomical substrates that possess distinct characteristics (see Fig 1). Some of the difficulties of confirming the localization of aphasia-producing lesions in the literature are the consqeuence of overlooking the relationship of the lesions to the underlying gross anatomical landmakrs. Most of Broca's area lies in the inferior frontal gyrus, which is separated superiorly from the middle frontal gyrus by a deep furrow (deeper than the one that separates the superior and middle frontal gyri) and which is known as the inferior frontal sulcus. Data from comparative neuroanatomy studies appear to support the view that this sulcus separates two regions of the frontal lobe of different origin, architecture, and function.[65] The inferior frontal gyrus, which contains on its inferior margin the frontal operculum, is bordered inferiorly by the Sylvian fissure. The operculum is divided into three distinct sections: the pars orbitalis anteriorly; the pars triangularis in intermediate position; and the pars opercularis posteriorly. Posterior to the pars opercularis, the inferior precentral region also plays a role in language (see above). Although numerous vertical sulci divide and subdivide the opercular portions, they tend to be extremely variable among individuals, except for a deep vertical furrow separating the pars triangularis from the pars opercularis and known as the ascending limb of the sylvian fissure. This furrow may be branched, and the branch often takes a diagonal backward direction under the name of the diagonal sulcus. The center of the lesion producing Broca's aphasia tends to lie behind the ascending limb of the Sylvian fissure.[44] Furthermore, the area demonstrated in stimulation experiments by Whitaker and Ojemann[77] to be particularly sensitive to aphasic production also lies behind the ascending Sylvian limb. Medially, the operculum rises to join the upper margin of the insula, and fibers entering and exiting from the opercular portions flow over this rim.

The gross anatomical landmarks of Wernicke's area bear a close relationship to the posterior third of the superior temporal gyrus and the upper surface of the temporal lobe buried within the Sylvian fossa (see Fig 1 and "Gross Asymmetries" below). On the upper surface one or more transversely oriented gyri can be found. These gyri, of which the most anterior bears the name of Heschl, arise behind the insula medially, proceed in a rostralateral direction, and flatten out by the time they reach the convexity of the brain. Behind the most anterior of the transverse gyri (Heschl's gyrus proper) lies a triangular surface known as the planum temporale. The superior temporal gyrus is not separated from the posteriorly adjacent inferior parietal lobule by a sulcus, but rather continues smoothly into the parietal lobe. Additional landmarks of relevance to language localization are the parietal operculum immediately behind the inferior postcentral region, and the supramarginal gyrus cupping the posterior end of the Sylvian fissure and bounded superiorly by the intraparietal sulcus. The angular gyrus cupping the posterior end of the superior temporal sulcus is also bounded superiorly by the intraparietal sulcus (see Fig 1). The parietal operculum, supramarginal gyrus, and angular gyrus comprise what is known as the inferior parietal lobule. The supplementary motor area corresponds to the pericingulate region anteriorly but has no clear gross anatomical boundaries.

Likewise, the supplementary sensory area is not clearly bounded by anatomical landmarks, although it appears to be just caudal to the paracentral lobule, behind the sensory representation of the foot.

The course of the fiber pathways relating the various cortical areas concerned with language function is poorly understood; our knowledge is still based on studies from the 19th and early 20th centuries, when early investigators laboriously traced these connections by blunt dissection and after painstaking staining of fibers in normal and lesioned brains. Additional information followed the pioneering work of Flechsig,[26] who demonstrated the time course of myelination of distinct fiber systems during antenatal and postnatal brain development. The most important fiber bundle of the language areas is the superior longitudinal (arcuate) fasciculus.[31] This group of fibers, compact only in the parietal operculum, arises in the superior, middle, and in portions of the inferior temporal gyri, runs around the back end of the Sylvian fissure and then forward in the parietal operculum and toward the inferior precentral and opercular portions of the frontal lobe. It is assumed that in man some of the fibers that make up the arcuate fasciculus serve to connect Wernicke's to Broca's areas. Recently, more refined connectional work possible only in experiments on animals has, in fact, demonstrated a similar connection in the rhesus monkey.[58] Furthermore, in the macaque, the posterior and anterior pericingulate regions have been shown to be connected to each other[57]; the supplementary motor and supplementary sensory regions are connected to Broca's area and Wernicke's area, respectively.[59]

Anatomical Lateralization

Gross Asymmetries

Interest in cerebral lateralization, judging from large numbers of journal articles and books, has grown enormously over the past fifteen years. In adult man, lesions in the left hemisphere can produce irreversible disturbances in language function. Similar lesions in children tend to produce much less severe disorders.[80] It is probably the case, however, that under

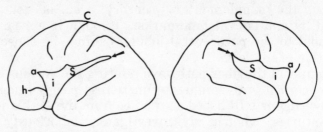

Fig 2.—Diagram of left and right hemispheres of the brain of a human fetus shows asymmetry of Sylvian fissures *(S) (arrows)*. At this stage the insula *(i)* is not fully covered. Note that the left Sylvian fissure is longer and more horizontal than the right. This asymmetry is accompanied by a larger planum temporale and parietal operculum on the left side. (See also Figure 3 and accompanying text.) *C*, central sulcus; *a*, ascending limb of Sylvian fissure; *h*, horizontal limb of Sylvian fissure.

the appropriate testing conditions children remain permanently though subtly affected by unilateral lesions producing aphasia.[18, 38] Attempts to demonstrate anatomical asymmetries to explain functional lateralization followed shortly after the discoveries by Broca[10] and Wernicke[76] of lesions producing aphasia. Eberstaller[21] and Cunningham[17] first reported asymmetries in the Sylvian fissures (Fig 2). They found that the left fissure tended to be longer and more horizontal than its mate, which usually showed an upward turn in its posterior end. More recently, LeMay and Culebras[47] have reported the distribution of this Sylvian asymmetry in large numbers of patients undergoing cerebral angiography. Their data show that in right-handers the above asymmetry is found in 67% of brains, while only 8% show a reversal of this asymmetry; 25% show symmetrical Sylvian fissures. In left-handers the proportion of patients who show symmetrical fissures is much larger. Thus 71% of 28 left-handers showed no asymmetry, while 22% showed the same asymmetry as most right-handers and 7% showed the reversed pattern. Similar asymmetries have been described in children and fetal brains[15, 46] (see Fig 2). It is also of interest to note that some of the nonhuman primates, especially the orangutan, appear to exhibit Sylvian asymmetries as well,[48] and that a similar asymmetry was shown in the endocast of the skull of a Neanderthal man.[46]

Asymmetries are also seen in a part of the temporal lobe known as the planum temporale (Fig 3). This region lies on the posterior upper surface of the temporal lobe, where lesions are

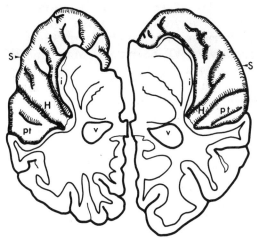

Fig 3.—Diagram of left and right human cerebral hemispheres shows superior temporal surfaces. Sylvian fissures *(S)* have been unroofed in order to allow a view of the superior temporal planes from above. The temporal poles are up on the figure. It is possible to see Heschl's gyrus *(H)* and, behind it, the planum temporale *(pt)*. As is the case in 65% of normal brains, the left pt is larger than the right in this example. Other abbreviations: *i,* insula; *v,* lateral ventricle.

apt to result in Wernicke's aphasia in children and adults. Following up the observations by Pfeifer[62] (a student of Flechsig), Geschwind and Levitsky[32] found that the planum temporale was larger on the left in 65% of human brains, equal on the two sides in 24%, and larger on the right in 11%. Similar asymmetries have been found in children and fetal brains.[15, 74] A second transverse gyrus is, on the other hand, more common on the right side.[14, 15, 22]

Gross anatomical asymmetries in and around the anterior speech area have been the subject of study as well. Eberstaller[21] noted that this area is more often highly folded on the left than on the right. On the other hand, Wada and colleagues[74] have reported that the surface extent of the posterior half of the inferior frontal gyrus is larger on the right. Another more recent study, however, which takes into account the extent of buried cortex, finds the opposite result.[73]

Asymmetries other than the Sylvian fissure may be seen in living persons undergoing radiological procedures. For instance, normally occurring asymmetries in the ventricular system can be seen on pneumoencephalography.[52] The left lateral ventricle tends to be larger and the left occipital horn is usually longer. Similar asymmetries have been demonstrated in children.[72] Furthermore, asymmetries are disclosed by computerized tomography (CAT scans). LeMay and Kido[46, 49] have shown the asymmetries in the frontal lobe and temporo-occipital region. The right frontal lobe tends to be wider than the left, while in right-handers the left temporo-occipital region is more often longer and wider than the right. These findings, however, may depend in part on the scanning angle and one should be cautious about these findings until more reliable methods of measurement are developed.

ARCHITECTONIC ASYMMETRIES

Architectonics refers to the study of the cellular arrangement in layers and columns in the cortex, and to general cell-packing density and cell size in cortical and subcortical structures. This type of analysis allows one to distinguish subdivisions within the cortex and subcortical nuclei. Patterns of subdivisions are seen in architectonic maps. The best known maps of the cortex are those of Brodmann[11] and Economo and Koskinas.[23] The main advantage of this type of analysis over gross anatomical study of the brain is that architectonic areas, unlike gross anatomical landmarks, probably correspond much more closely to regions of special functional differentiation of the brain and to regions with different connections.[58, 65]

The architectonic mapping of the superior temporal gyrus and planum temporale provides a means to study in greater detail the asymmetries disclosed by gross examination of the Sylvian fissures and planum temporale. Furthermore, an asymmetry discovered by architectonic means is probably more likely to reflect the functional asymmetries associated with these regions. Asymmetries at an architectonic level were reported by Economo and Horn[22] in the planum temporale: they described the primary areas to be larger on the right, while the left side had larger association areas. This study, however, did not measure the full extent of the areas, but only those portions lying within the boundaries of the planum temporale. The auditory fields, however, do extend outside the planum temporale,[11, 23, 29] and measurement of the full extent of these areas is required to confirm the presence or absence of asymmetries in this region. We have carried out this study and have shown that one of the auditory association areas, area Tpt (Fig 4), is larger on the left in brains in which the left planum is grossly larger.[30] Area Tpt is of particular importance because it lies on the outer, posterior corner of the planum temporale and the posterior third of the superior temporal gyrus, a region in which lesions are apt to cause Wernicke's aphasia. Tpt is thus almost certainly an important part of language representation in the left hemisphere.

Architectonic studies of asymmetry in the anterior speech area are more difficult to interpret. The exact extent of lesions resulting in Broca's aphasia is not well established. The classical teaching is that the lesion must involve the pars opercularis and at least a portion of the pars triangularis of the frontal operculum,[6] i.e., area 44 and part of area 45 of Brodmann.[11] Previous studies of architectonic asymmetry in this region were carried out by workers in the Vogt School (a prominent German architectonic research center headed by Oscar and Cecile Vogt, of which Brodmann was one of the most illustrious early members and Sanides one of the most recent). Strassburger[71] divided the opercular area into architectonic subdivisions

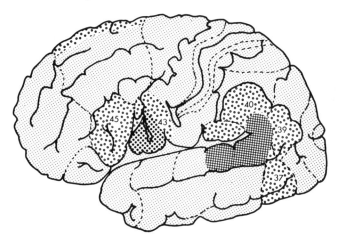

Fig 4.—Diagram of lateral surface of left hemisphere in man shows architectonic areas implicated in language localization. Asymmetries have been demonstrated in an area lying on the pars opercularis *(closed circles)*, and in area Tpt on the posterior third of the superior temporal gyrus *(cross-hatched)*. *Open circles* denote additional architectonic areas important for language. The supplementary speech area is mostly medial, but a portion of it extends to the lateral surface high in the frontal lobe.

based on myeloarchitectonic appearance (This refers to the pattern of radial and tangential fibers of a given area of cortex. Maps obtained in this manner correspond closely to those obtained by analyzing cell stains (cytoarchitectonics). See also Sanides.[65]) and found no consistent left-right asymmetries. Analysis of Strassburger's divisions, however, discloses that they bear little similarity to other maps of this region[9, 43, 63] and places his findings in doubt. On the other hand, we have carried out a pigmentoarchitectonic analysis* of the frontal opercular zone based on Braak's criteria[8] that demonstrates that an area in the pars opercularis is larger on the left[27] (see Fig 4). Thus, in ten adult and juvenile brains, a pigmentoarchitectonic area characterized by large pyramidal cells with characteristic clumping of lipofuscin in their cytoplasm, lying over most of the pars opercularis, is more than 30% larger on the left in six specimens, less than 30% larger on the left in three specimens, and larger on the right in only one specimen (p <0.01). This area is located in the heart of the region in which lesions can produce Broca's aphasia.[42] In addition, the homologous field in the monkey is the only granular area of the inferior frontal region that receives direct connections from the posterior temporal area, and it is this connection that has been suggested to be the basic unit for the temporofrontal organization of language in man.[31] Therefore, it seems that, parallel to the situation in the posterior language region, an area that is an important part of the anterior speech zone is also larger on the left.

We have found recently asymmetries in the human thalamus.[24] The lateralis posterior nucleus is larger on the left side in eight out of nine brains of children and adults. Although the thalamus appears to evolve in conjunction with the cerebral cortex[79] and seems to play a role in language function,[55] there has been no earlier evidence that anatomical lateralization in the cortex will be reflected in thalamic asymmetries. On the other hand, it is possible that thalamic nuclei projecting to asymmetrical cortical areas may be asymmetrical as well, albeit to a lesser extent. Discrete nuclear thalamic projections to areas Tpt and to the asymmetric inferior frontal granular field (see above) are not found, although regions in the pulvinar con-

---

*This is based on the staining characteristics of lipofuscin deposits in cells, and constitutes an efficient way of architectonic division of the brain.

tain diffuse projections from these areas.[3, 13, 75] On the other hand, the inferior parietal lobule of rhesus monkey appears to be discretely connected to the lateralis posterior nucleus,[13] and architectonic asymmetries for these cortical areas in man are suggested by the findings of Diamond and colleagues.[19] A volumetric analysis of ten adult and juvenile brains has disclosed no significant asymmetry in any thalamic nucleus except for the nucleus lateralis posterior. The pulvinar is perhaps slightly larger on the right, although the difference is only at the 10% confidence level. The left lateralis posterior nucleus, on the other hand, is larger in all the brains ($p < 0.01$).[24] In view of the findings in the thalamus, further work needs to be done on the asymmetries of areas 39 and 40 (of Brodmann[11]) lying on the inferior parietal lobule, since lesions in this area on the left are often accompanied by disorders of spoken and written language.[6]

PATHOLOGIC MANIFESTATIONS OF CEREBRAL ASYMMETRY

The exact developmental mechanism leading to the formation of cerebral asymmetries is unknown. That the mechanism is at least partially determined by genetic factors is suggested by data on handedness that clearly point out that right-handedness and left-handedness tend to run in families.[1, 2, 34, 50] Furthermore, genetic theories can be constructed to explain the distribution of handedness in the general population (see Annett[2]). In addition, the presence of certain cerebral asymmetries in the fetus and at birth (see above) supports a genetic theory, and at least it excludes purely postnatal environmental influences on asymmetry. On the other hand, there are data to suggest that lateralization is partly under environmental influence, as illustrated by the well-known fact that children born left-handed are capable of shifting hand dominance with encouragement.[16] The effect of this shift of functional lateralization on cerebral asymmetry, however, is unknown. It appears that while rats reared in the usual laboratory setting do not show lateralization on maze tests, handling them and general enrichment of the environment during the first few days of life now results in lateralized behavior in the same tests.[67] Therefore it may follow that disorders in lateralization may also be jointly genetically and environmentally mediated.

DEVELOPMENTAL DYSLEXIA: ANATOMICAL FINDINGS IN ONE CASE*

The brain of a deceased 20-year-old man was analyzed in whole brain serial sections. During his life the patient had been carefully followed in a language disabilities clinic because of severe difficulty with reading. Despite a normal level of intelligence and more than adequate cultural opportunities, the patient had been unable to progress in his reading beyond the fourth-grade level. In addition to his reading difficulties, he had a speech delay and later showed deficits in arithmetic and right-left orientation. Several years before his death, which was due to an accidental fall, he developed a seizure disorder that was easily controlled with anticonvulsant medication. His brain showed no gross abnormalities. On microscopic examination a striking disorder of cortical organization characterized by micropolygyria (the excessive folding of the cortical plate into architectonically disorganized small gyri) was found to involve predominantly the region in which area Tpt is usually found on the left side (Fig 5). Only fragments of the normal area could be identified. Additional abnormalities, characterized by ectopic cell collections, disordered layering, and primitive-appearing cells were found throughout the left hemisphere, but more frequently in the posterior half. The inferior parietal lobule contained a particularly large collection of these lesions. In addition, there was an asymmetric amount of subcortical white matter on the two hemispheres; the left side contained more of it throughout the hemisphere. The planum temporale was equal in size on the two sides, and the Sylvian fissures were minimally asymmetric, with the left one slightly lower than the right. The brain of the dyslexic patient showed abnormalities relevant to the data on normally occurring cerebral asymmetries. First, the abnormalities in cortical structure were restricted to the left, i.e., the language hemisphere. Second, the abnormalities were most striking in areas concerned with language function in the normal person, especially in an area (Tpt) known to be asymmetrical on the two sides (see above). Third, there is an abnormal asymmetry in the width of the hemisphere, so that the left hemisphere is wider through

---

*A detailed account of the findings has been presented elsewhere.[28]

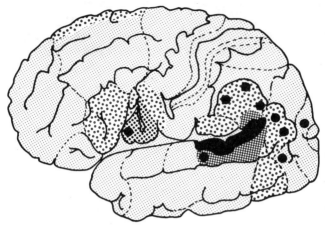

Fig 5.—Diagram of lateral surface of left hemisphere shows lesions in patient with developmental dyslexia and their relation to language-relevant architectonic areas (see Fig 4). There is a large area of micropolygyria *(blackened area)* in area Tpt *(crosshatched)* and several foci of cortical dysplasia in other areas *(black dots)*.

its total rostrocaudal extent, while the normal brain is torqued, i.e., it is wider in the front on one side (usually the right) and in the back on the opposite side (usually the left).

That cortical abnormalities of the sort exhibited by the above patient can occur in families is well known,[12] although the exact inheritance pattern has not been described. Other male members of the patient's family were affected by dyslexia, which also suggests a genetic relationship. Recent work by Shelly Smith and co-workers[69] has disclosed a strong linkage of the familial dyslexia phenotype to a highly fluorescent satellite on the 15th chromosome. The satellite is found in affected members and is absent in unaffected members of the same family in six of eight families. Since the neuropathology of clinical entities showing chromosomal alteration has not been worked out in detail, even for the common disorders, it is not known what possible effect on cortical organization a lesion in the 15th chromosome could have, although it is tempting to speculate about the possible effect of this chromosome on cerebral lateralization and malformations. Other examples of lateralized brain anomalies are found in the literature. For example, megalencephaly can be restricted to the right side.[51]

Lateralized limb anomalies have been described to occur in

both animals and man and may result from effects early in development. For instance, the normally occurring asymmetry in the habenula of newts can be reversed by lesions placed in the gastrula.[78] When pregnant rats are exposed to high concentrations of acetozolamide in their diet, nearly a third of their newborn pups exhibit an abnormal formation of one of the limbs, which is called paraxial hemimelia.[45] Most of the malformations occur in the right upper limb. Spontaneous occurrence of paraxial hemimelia in man also shows a tendency to affect the right upper limb much more frequently than the left, and in humans the disorder is more common in males.[56] There is no evidence that the brains of malformed rats or of patients with hemimelia have been examined, and it thus remains to be shown whether or not the developmental limb abnormalities reflect a lateralized disorder in the development of the cerebral hemispheres. Although the situation in the rat clearly demonstrates an environmental influence on the malformation, some rats may still be genetically more susceptible; genetic studies are needed to clarify this point.

The abnormal asymmetry of the width of the hemispheres in the dyslexic patient deserves additional comment. The distribution of asymmetry in the width and length of the hemispheres (see above) is reportedly different in dyslexic patients with delayed speech. Thus, a wider right temporo-occipital region, which occurs in only approximately 10% of normal patients,[49] is said to be more common in dyslexics, and particularly in those dyslexics with speech delay and lower verbal IQ. The finding of a wider left hemisphere both anteriorly and posteriorly in the brain of the dyslexic patient described raises the possibility that some dyslexics have brains with anatomical lateralization altogether different from the usual pattern. The increased number of subcortical fibers on the left may be dictated by abnormal genetic information or may result from the anomalous pattern present in the cortex. It has been shown in the rhesus monkey that lesions placed in the brains of fetuses at the appropriate time can result in the formation of connections not found in the unlesioned animal or in the animal receiving a lesion at a later date.[36] Thus prefrontal lesions may produce changes in the normal architecture and connectivity of the cortex not produced when the lesions are placed later. Furthermore, partial lesions in the hamster brain early in life may lead to compensatory overgrowth of fibers. Schneider[66] argues that such lesions in the visual system of the newborn hamster result in an overgrowth of fibers that worsens rather than normalizes visual behavior; the surgical disruption of these anomalous fibers tends to reverse the deficit toward normal. It is conceivable that the cortical malformations in the dyslexic brain have also produced the increased number of subcortical connections, thus resulting in a larger left hemisphere, albeit a left hemisphere still incapable of carrying out fully normal language function. It is even conceivable that interruption of appropriate fibers might improve left hemisphere capabilities.

On the other hand, early *complete* destruction of the left-sided language areas will not result in fiber overgrowth and will have the effect of releasing language function to the right hemisphere. Data from early hemispherectomy in humans have shown a remarkable, although not complete, preservation of language function carried out by the right hemisphere.[18, 68]

SUMMARY AND CONCLUSIONS

The left cerebral hemisphere is dominant for language function. Thus, lesions involving this hemisphere in children and adults are more likely to cause disorders in language function than the same or even larger lesions in the opposite hemisphere. Lesions that interfere with language tend to be clustered around the Sylvian fissure. Two regions appear to be especially important: one in the posterior frontal opercular area, the other in the posterior third of the superior temporal gyrus and adjacent parietal operculum. Lesions in other language regions that occupy more posterior portions of the inferior parietal lobule appear to result in disorders of written language; supplementary motor and sensory areas located on the medial portion of the left hemisphere surrounding the cingulate gyrus appear to influence spontaneous language activity. Finally, lesions in the left posterior pulvinar may also produce short-lived aphasic disturbances.

The brain exhibits both gross anatomical and microscopic asymmetries in the region of the language areas. Sylvian fissure asymmetries suggest a greater development of the posterior temporal region and of the parietal operculum on the left. The greater development of the left posterior temporal region is also illustrated by a larger posterior upper surface (planum temporale) on that side. Furthermore, the anterior speech area on the frontal operculum may be more convoluted and therefore larger on the left. Asymmetries in the Sylvian fissures and in the relative widths of portions of the hemispheres can be demonstrated during life by radiologic means.

Gross anatomical asymmetries appear to reflect side differences in areas of distinctive microscopic structure (architectonic areas) and function. Thus, in the posterior speech area the auditory field Tpt is larger on the left, and in the frontal lobe an opercular motor field is also larger on the left. Area 39, an inferior parietal association cortex, may be thicker on the left side, and its corresponding thalamic projection nucleus, nucleus lateralis posterior, is also larger on the left.

The normally occurring asymmetry may be altered in pathology and pathological lesions may be asymmetrically distributed. Thus, the analysis of a brain of a dyslexic patient has disclosed an abnormally large left hemisphere as well as cortical malformations restricted to the left side of the brain. Lateralized abnormalities may occur in other disease entities and may be linked to genetic abnormalities, as evidenced by the familial occurrence of some dyslexias as well as of similar brain malformations. On the other hand, lateralized abnormalities may result from early lesions, as illustrated by limb malformations in rats and reversals of habenular asymmetries in newts. Lateralized limb malformations with a male preponderance also occur in man, although genetic or environmental factors have not been identified. Finally, lateralized malformations in fiber connectivities may be the result of early lesions in the brain, as shown by experimental data from fetal monkeys and newborn hamsters.

Thus, knowledge of functional and structural lateralization of the human brain has begun to play an increasingly important role in our understanding of the neurologic bases of normal language function and of some disorders of functional lateralization of which developmental dyslexia is an example. Future improvements in the anatomical model of language and related functions will come from additional studies of anatomical lateralization. It is likely that anatomical lateralization results from genetic and prenatal environmental influences, and that a clearer picture of the factors leading to normal and abnormal manifestations of asymmetry will come from animal models of lateralization. Until recently, lateralization in function has been thought to be an exclusively human trait. However, animal models appear to be emerging with the discovery of functional lateralization in rats[35, 67] and monkeys.[61] Furthermore, the effects of early lesions on recovery and laterality are under current investigation in these animal models.[36, 66] Finally, the possible identification of intrauterine environmental insults leading in some manner to abnormalities in lateralization of structure and function provide additional hope for improvement of our ability to prevent and treat disorders of brain asymmetry.

BIBLIOGRAPHY

1. Annett M.: The distribution of manual asymmetry. *Br. J. Psychol.* 63:343, 1972.
2. Annett M.: Genetic and nongenetic influences on handedness. *Behav. Genet.* 8:227, 1978.
3. Benevento L.A., Rezak M.: The cortical projections of the inferior pulvinar and adjacent lateral pulvinar in the rhesus monkey (Macaca mulatta). *Exp. Neurol.* 57:849, 1976.
4. Benson D.F.: *Aphasia, Alexia, and Agraphia.* New York: Churchill Livingstone, 1979.
5. Benson D.F.: Neurologic correlates of anomia, in Whitaker H., et al (eds): *Studies in Neurolinguistics.* New York: Academic Press, 1979.
6. Benson D.F., Geschwind N.: Aphasia and related cortical disturbances, in Baker A.B., et al. (eds): *Clinical Neurology.* New York: Harper & Row, 1971.
7. Benson D.F., et al.: Conduction aphasia. *Arch. Neurol.* 28:339, 1973.
8. Braak H.: On the pigment architectonics of the human telencephalic cortex, in Brazier M.A.B., et al. (eds): *Architectonics of the Cerebral Cortex.* New York: Raven Press, 1978.
9. Braak H.: The pigment architectonics of the human frontal lobe: I. Precentral, subcentral and frontal region. *Anat. Embryol.* 157:35, 1979.
10. Broca P.: Remarques sur le siège de faculté de langage articulé suivies d'une observation d'aphémie (Perte de la parole). *Bull. Soc. Anat. Paris* 2:330, 1861.
11. Brodmann K.: *Vergleichende Lokalisationslehre der Grosshirnrinde.* Leipzig: Barth, 1909.
12. Brun A.: The subpial granular layer of the foetal cerebral cortex in man. *Acta Pathol. Microbiol. Scand. (Suppl)* 179:40, 1965.
13. Bruton H., Jones E.G.: The posterior thalamic region and its cortical projections in new world and old world monkey. *J. Comp. Neurol.* 168:249, 1976.
14. Campain R., Minckler J.: A note on the gross configuration of the human auditory cortex. *Brain Language* 3:318, 1976.
15. Chi J.G., et al.: Gyral development of the human brain. *Ann. Neurol.* 1:86, 1977.
16. Clark M.M.: *Left-Handedness.* London: University of London Press, 1957.
17. Cunningham D.J.: Contribution to the surface anatomy of the cerebral hemispheres. *Cunningham Memoirs (R. Irish Acad.)* 7:372, 1892.
18. Dennis M., Whitaker H.A.: Language acquisition following hemidecortication: Linguistic superiority of the left over the right hemisphere. *Brain Language* 3:404, 1976.

19. Diamond M.C., et al.: A search for morphological asymmetries in areas 9 and 39 in human male cerebral cortex. *Neurosci. Abstr.* 6:195, 1980.
20. Drake W.E.: Clinical and pathological findings in a child with a developmental learning disability. *J. Learn. Dis.* 1:9, 1968.
21. Eberstaller O.: Zür oberflachen anatomie der grosshirn hemisphaeren. Wien *Med. Bl.* 7:479, 642, 644, 1884.
22. Economo C.v., Horn L.A.: Ueber windungsrelief masse und rindenarchitektonik der supratemporalfläche, ihre individuellen und ihre seintenunterschiede. *Z. Neurol. Psychiatr.* 130:678, 1930.
23. Economo C.v., Koskinas G.N.: *Die Cytoarchitektonik der Hirnrinde des erwachsenen Menschen.* Berlin: Springer, 1925.
24. Eidelberg D., Galaburda A.M.: Unpublished data.
25. Ewing A.W.G.: *Aphasia in Children.* London: Oxford University Press, 1930.
26. Flechsig P.: *Anatomie des menschlichen Gehirns und Rückenmarks auf Myelongenetischer Grundlage.* Leipzig: Thieme, 1920.
27. Galaburda A.M.: La région de Broca: Observations anatomiques faites un siècle après la mort de son découvreur. *Rev. Neurol.* 136:609, 1980.
28. Galaburda A.M., Kemper T.L.: Cytoarchitectonic abnormalities in developmental dyslexia: A case study. *Ann. Neurol.* 6:94, 1979.
29. Galaburda A.M., Sanides F.: Cytoarchitectonic organization of the human auditory cortex. *J. Comp. Neurol.* 190:597, 1980.
30. Galaburda A.M., et al.: Human brain: Cytoarchitectonic left-right asymmetries in the temporal speech region. *Arch. Neurol.* 35:812, 1978.
31. Geschwind N.: The organization of language and the brain. *Science* 170:940, 1970.
32. Geschwind N., Levitsky W.: Human brain: Left-right asymmetries in temporal speech region. *Science* 161:186, 1968.
33. Geschwind N., et al.: Isolation of the speech area. *Neuropsychologia* 6:327, 1968.
34. Gesell A., Ames L.B.: The development of handedness. *J. Genet. Psychol.* 70:155, 1947.
35. Glick S.D., et al.: Multiple and interrelated functional asymmetries in rat brain. *Life Sci.* 25:395, 1979.
36. Goldman P.S., Galkin T.W.: Prenatal removal of frontal association cortex in the fetal rhesus monkey: Anatomical and functional consequences in postnatal life. *Brain Res.* 152:451, 1978.
37. Guttman E.: Aphasia in children. *Brain* 65:205, 1942.
38. Hecaen H.: Acquired aphasia in children and the ontogenesis of hemispheric functional specialization. *Brain Lang.* 3:114, 1976.
39. Hier D.B., et al.: Developmental dyslexia. *Arch. Neurol.* 35:90, 1978.
40. Hinshelwood J.: *Congenital Word-Blindness.* London: Lewis, 1917.
41. Ingvar D.H.: Localization of cortical functions by multiregional measurements of cerebral blood flow, in Brazier M.A.B., et al. (eds): *Architectonics of the Cerebral Cortex.* New York: Raven Press, 1978.
42. Kertesz A., et al.: Isotope localization of infarcts in aphasia. *Arch. Neurol.* 34:590, 1977.
43. Kreht H.: Cytoarchitektonik der felder der Brocaschen region. *J. Psychol. Neurol.* 42:496, 1931.
44. Landau W.M., et al.: Congenital aphasia: A clinicopathologic study. *Neurology* 10:915, 1960.
45. Layton W.M., Hallesy D.W.: Deformity of forelimbs in rats: Association with high doses of acetozolamide. *Science* 149:306, 1965.
46. LeMay M.: Morphologic cerebral asymmetries in modern man, fossil man, and nonhuman primates. *Ann. N.Y. Acad. Sci.* 280:349, 1976.
47. LeMay M., Culebras A.: Human brain: Morphologic differences in the hemispheres demonstrable by carotid arteriography. *N. Engl. J. Med.* 287:168, 1972.

48. LeMay M., Geschwind N.: Hemispheric differences in the brains of great apes. *Brain Behav. Evol.* 11:48, 1975.
49. LeMay M., Kido D.K.: Asymmetries of the cerebral hemispheres on computed tomograms. *J. Comp. Assist. Tomogr.* 2:471, 1978.
50. Levy J., Nagylaki T.: A model for the genetics of handedness. *Genetics* 72:117, 1972.
51. Manz H.J., et al.: Unilateral megalencephaly, cerebral cortical dysplasia, neuronal hypertrophy and heterotopia: Cytomorphometric, fluorometric, cytochemical, and biomedical analysis. *Acta Neuropathol. (Berl.)* 45:97, 1979.
52. McRae D.L., et al.: The occipital horns and cerebral dominance. *Neurology* 18:95, 1968.
53. Mohr J.P., et al.: Broca aphasia: Pathologic and clinical aspects. *Neurology* 28:311, 1978.
54. Molfese D.L., et al.: Neuroanatomical correlates of semantic processes, in Begleiter H. (ed): *Evoked Brain Potentials and Behavior.* New York: Plenum Press, 1979.
55. Ojemann G., Ward A.: Speech representation in the ventrolateral thalamus. *Brain* 94:669, 1971.
56. O'Rahilly R.: Morphological patterns of limb deficiencies and duplications. *Am. J. Anat.* 89:135, 1951.
57. Pandya D.N.: Personal communication.
58. Pandya D.N., Galaburda A.M.: Role of architectonics and connections in the study of primate brain evolution. *Am. J. Phys. Anthropol.* 52:197, 1980.
59. Pandya D.N., et al.: Intra- and interhemispheric connections of the neocortical auditory system in rhesus monkey. *Brain Res.* 14:49, 1969.
60. Penfield W., Roberts L.: *Speech and Brain Mechanisms.* Princeton, N.J.: Princeton University Press, 1959.
61. Petersen M.R., et al.: Neural lateralization of species-specific vocalizations by Japanese macaques. *Science* 202:324, 1978.
62. Pfeifer R.A.: Pathologie der horstrauhlung und der corticalen horsphäre, in Bumke O., et al. (eds): *Handbuch der Neurologie.* Berlin: Springer, 1936.
63. Riegele L.: Die cytoarchitektonik der felder der Brocaschen region. *J. Psychol. Neurol.* 42:496, 1931.
64. Ross E.: Left parietal lobe and receptive language functions: Mixed transcortical aphasia after left anterior cerebral artery infarction. *Neurology* 30:144, 1980.
65. Sanides F.: Representation in the cerebral cortex and its areal lamination patterns, in Bourne G.H. (ed): *The Structure and Function of Nervous Tissue.* New York: Academic Press, 1972, vol. V.
66. Schneider G.E.: Is it really better to have your brain lesion early? A revision of the "Kennard principle." *Neuropsychologia* 17:557, 1979.
67. Sherman G.F., et al.: Brain and behavioral asymmetries for spatial preference in rats. *Brain Res.* 192:61, 1980.
68. Smith A.: Speech and other functions after left dominant hemispherectomy. *J. Neurol. Neurosurg. Psychiatry* 29:467, 1966.
69. Smith S.: Personal communication.
70. Sokoloff L.: Circulation and energy metabolism of the brain, in Siegel G.J., et al. (eds): *Basic Neurochemistry,* ed 2. Boston: Little, Brown & Co., 1976.
71. Strassburger E.H.: Vergleichende myeloarchitektonische studien und der erweiterten Brocaschen region des menschen. *J. Psychol. Neurol. (Leipzig)* 48:477, 1938.
72. Strauss E., Fitz C.: Occipital horn asymmetry in children. *Ann. Neurol.* 8:437, 1980.
73. Vignolo L.: Personal communication.
74. Wada J.A., et al.: Cerebral hemispheric asymmetry in humans. *Arch. Neurol.* 32:239, 1975.
75. Walker A.E.: *The Primate Thalamus.* Chicago: University of Chicago Press, 1938.

76. Wernicke C.: *Der aphasische Symptomencomplex*. Breslau: Cohn & Weigart, 1874.
77. Whitaker H.A., Ojemann G.A.: Graded localization of naming from electrical stimulation of left cerebral cortex. *Nature* 270 (5362):50, 1977.
78. Woellworth C.V.: Auslörung von Situs inversus durch materialdefekte in lateralen ektoderm der grastrula bei triturus alpestris. *Roux Arch. Entwicklungsnech. Organ.* 162:336, 1969.
79. Yakovlev P.I.: Localization of lesions of the thalamus, in Haymaker W. (ed): *Bing's Local Diagnosis in Neurological Diseases*. St. Louis: C.V. Mosby Co., 1969.
80. Zangwill O.L.: *Cerebral Dominance and its Relation to Psychological Function*. Springfield, Ill.: Charles C Thomas, Publisher, 1960.

The Somatomedins

RAYMOND L. HINTZ, M.D.

*Associate Professor of Pediatrics and
Head, Division of Endocrinology
Stanford University Medical Center
Stanford, California*

Introduction

SINCE THE BEGINNINGS OF PEDIATRICS one of the major focuses of
its scientific interest has been on the problems of growth and
the physiologic mechanisms controlling growth. In the last two
decades a series of discoveries have been made about the cellular control mechanisms of growth that provide a brand new
viewpoint from which to examine the pediatric interests of
growth and its derangements. These new discoveries relate to
the peptide growth factors and more particularly to the group
of interrelated growth factors known as the somatomedins
(SMs). The SMs appear to play a crucial role in GH-dependent
growth in postnatal life, and the clinical measurement of somatomedin aids in the diagnosis of growth disorders. There is
also reason to believe that the SMs are intimately involved in
fetal growth, in the metabolic changes associated with malnutrition, cirrhosis, and renal failure, and in the feedback control
of GH secretion. Like many rapidly developing fields of science,
multiple lines of evidence that originally seemed unrelated can
now be seen as segments of an integrated whole. However, because the origin of the initial observations in different laboratories were from different points of view, the terminology has
become forbiddingly complex. To understand the field it is

This study was supported in part by grants AM 21058 and AM 24085 from the
Department of Health, Education and Welfare.

therefore important that we first review the history of discoveries leading to our present knowledge about the somatomedins. Once the history is understood, the terminology becomes clearer, and we can then review the physiologic and clinical correlates of the SMs.

Historical Background: Sulfation Factor and Nonsuppressible Insulin-Like Activity

Two lines of research contributed the major portion of knowledge to our present understanding of the SMs. Most of the pioneering work that was published used two terms now abandoned: sulfation factor (SF) and nonsuppressible insulin-like activity (NSILA). The history of SF can be traced to pioneering work done on the action of GH on rats,[1] work that demonstrated that one of the in vivo actions of GH was on cartilage growth, as measured by $^{35}SO_4$ incorporation into cartilage. It was then a logical step to see if this GH effect could be duplicated in vitro. When Salmon and Daughaday[2] investigated this question, they were completely unable to show any direct effect of growth hormone (GH) on cartilage. However, they were able to demonstrate that (1) there was a substance in normal plasma that did stimulate cartilage metabolism, and (2) this substance was absent in hypopituitary plasma and reappeared if the hypopituitary subject was treated in vivo with GH. Direct addition of GH to hypopituitary plasma did not cause the appearance of the cartilage-stimulating activity. They therorized that GH acted to cause growth of cartilage epiphyseal plates by way of another factor (Fig 1). They called this substance sulfation factor, since the metabolic parameter they were monitoring was the sulfation of glycosaminolglycans. Work in the succeeding years showed that this name was too limited, since the same type of GH-dependent factor could be shown to be stimulating a wide variety of metabolic parameters in cartilage and in other tissues. Furthermore, partial purification studies showed a close similarity to another plasma factor, NSILA. It was therefore decided to adopt a new, broader, and more ambitious name that would include all the work on sulfation factor and annex into it the work on NSILA. The name chosen, somatomedin,[3] implied that this factor or factors mediated somatic growth. Further work demonstrated that there was ap-

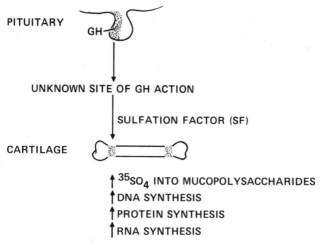

PITUITARY

UNKNOWN SITE OF GH ACTION

SULFATION FACTOR (SF)

CARTILAGE

↑ $^{35}SO_4$ INTO MUCOPOLYSACCHARIDES
↑ DNA SYNTHESIS
↑ PROTEIN SYNTHESIS
↑ RNA SYNTHESIS

Fig 1.—The original sulfation factor concept.

parently more than one SM present in serum. SM-A was characterized as a neutral peptide.[4] SM-C was a biologically similar peptide with a basic isoelectric point.[5] Another plasma peptide with growth-promoting action on glial cells was designated as SM-B.[6] However, because of its apparent lack of relationship to the other somatomedin peptides, SM-B is no longer considered part of this family. Since the original distinction of SM-A and SM-C, several other peptides have been described under the designation somatomedin. SMs purified from bovine[7] and rat[8] serums appear to be similar in actions, size, and isoelectric point to human SM-C. A slightly acidic peptide has been purified from human plasma and designated ILAs, which may be the same as or very similar to SM-A.[9] Recently Bala and Bhaumick[10] have purified a human SM peptide to homogeneity and called it basic somatomedin. According to published data it appears to be the same as SM-C. Future direct comparisons will be needed before we can be certain just how much of the apparent multiplicity of SM peptides is due to different gene products.

The work on nonsuppressible insulin-like activity originated from an entirely different area of science. The original methods for measuring insulin in blood were bioassay techniques using rat muscle or adipose tissue.[11, 12] When the specific and sensitive radioimmunoassay for insulin became available,[13] it was clear that this assay measured only a small proportion of the insulin-like activity in serum detected by the bioassays. In addition, anti-insulin antibody added to serum was able to neutralize only a small amount of the insulin-like activity. The term nonsuppressible insulin-like activity (NSILA) was coined to designate this insulin activity in serum that was not due to insulin itself[14] (Fig 2). Further characterization and partial purification of NSILA revealed that part of it is soluble in acid-ethanol, as is insulin itself (NSILA-S), and part of it is precipitated by acid ethanol (NSILA-P).[15] The major effort of those who worked on NSILA was concentrated on the soluble form (NSILA-S) because this appeared to be a small peptide separable from the bulk of plasma proteins. The viewpoint and work

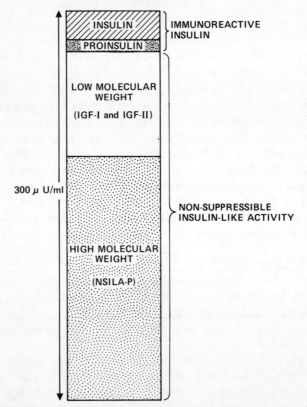

Fig 2.—Schematic diagram of the different forms of insulin-like activity in plasma.

in this field was to characterize the carbohydrate metabolism effects of this substance, and no work was done on its possible anabolic effects. When those working on sulfation factor proposed a new name that included NSILA-S,[3] it was understandable that the group working on NSILA-S did not immediately welcome this change imposed on their terminology, although they did then recognize the important GH-dependent anabolic role of NSILA-S. When they were successful in purifying to homogeneity and sequencing two forms of NSILA-S they decided to change their terminology to insulin-like growth factor (IGF) I and II to highlight the structural and biologic relationships to insulin and to point up their anabolic role as growth factors. There is now strong evidence, reviewed later, that at least IGF-I is identical to one of the SMs (SM-C). It is too early to tell whether the IGF or SM terminology will prevail, or whether an entirely new name will supplant both. In this review, "the somatomedins" (SM) is used to designate the entire group of peptides that share growth-stimulating properties in vitro, insulin-like action, and evidence of homology to insulin. The other terms, such as SM-C and IGF-II, are used to designate peptides within the SMs. Some of these peptide designations may turn out to be superfluous as the peptides become better characterized, but the concept of the SMs as a group of related growth factors seems likely to stand the test of time.

There is one other group of peptides that are members of the SM family that had still a different historical origin. Dulak and Temin[16] purified a group of peptides originally from fetal calf serum and later from rat liver cell-conditioned medium, that stimulated multiplication in embryonic fibroblasts. They designated this activity multiplication stimulating activity (MSA) and proposed that it was similar to NSILA-S and SM. Although

TABLE 1.—THE
SOMATOMEDINS

Human peptides
  SM-C/IGF-I
  IGF-II
  SM-A (ILAs)
Rat peptides
  Rat SM
  MSA
Bovine peptides
  Bovine SM

---

the exact relationships of these peptides to SMs in rat and human plasma remain undefined, it is clear that MSAs are closely related to the SMs[17] and we will consider them part of SM peptides.

This multiplicity of terms used to designate the purified SMs is summarized in Table 1. IGF-I and SM-C are well characterized and appear to be functionally interchangeable terms. IGF-II is clearly distinct in structure and physiology from IGF-I/SM-C, so that there are at least two SMs circulating in human plasma. The understanding of the true relationship of SM-A to the other human SMs and the relationship of the nonhuman SMs to SM-C/IGF-I and IGF-II await more careful structural and antigenic comparisons.

Purification and Structure

There have been almost as many purification methods used as there are investigators involved in the work. However, almost all of the methods used share common philosophies and problems. The basic problem is that unlike the classical hormones, there does not appear to be an organ storing the somatomedins. Therefore, unlike insulin or GH, the purification has had to be done starting from relatively dilute sources of hormone, in most cases plasma itself. Since a milliliter of plasma contains nanogram quantities of peptide hormones, and milligram amounts are needed for complete characterization, it is obvious that large volumes of starting material are needed. In addition, the large numbers of other proteins in plasma complicate the task of obtaining truly pure material. All of the purification methods have used an acidification step early in the process, making use of the fact that the SM peptides can be dissociated from the larger proteins to form small (about 7,000 daltons) peptides under severely acid conditions, and that the overwhelming bulk of plasma proteins are larger than this. Following the acid step, investigators have used a variety of methods of separation on the basis of size, charge, isoelectric point, hydrophobicity, or combinations of these fundamental properties.

Because of the practical difficulties in purifying the SM peptide "needles" from the "haystack" of plasma proteins, only two SM peptides have been purified in large enough quantities to

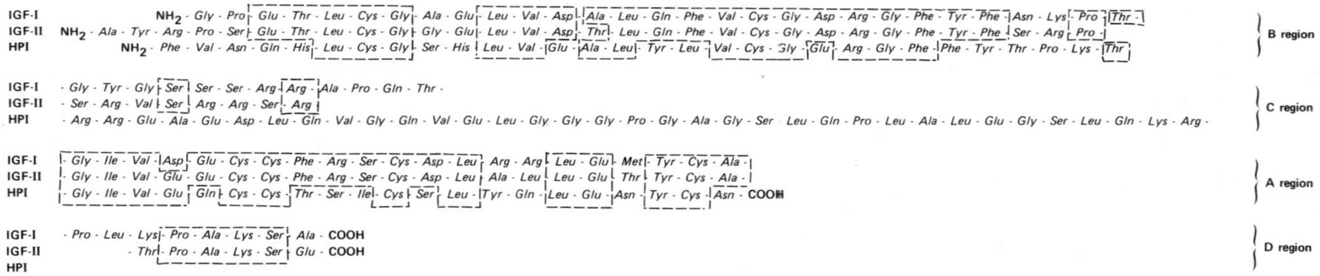

B region

IGF-I   NH₂-Gly-Pro-|Glu-Thr-Leu-Cys-Gly|-Ala-Glu-|Leu-Val-Asp|-|Ala-Leu-Gln-Phe-Val-Cys-Gly|-Asp-Arg-Gly-|Phe-Tyr|-Phe-|Asn-Lys|-Pro-|Thr|
IGF-II NH₂-Ala-Tyr-Arg-Pro-Ser-|Glu-Thr-Leu-Cys-Gly|-Gly-Glu-|Leu-Val-Asp|-Thr-|Leu-Gln-Phe-Val-Cys-Gly|-Asp-Arg-Gly-Phe-|Tyr|-Phe-Ser-Arg-Pro
HPI   NH₂-Phe-Val-Asn-Gln-His-|Leu-Cys-Gly|-Ser-His-|Leu-Val-Glu|-|Ala-Leu|-|Tyr-Leu-Val-Cys-Gly|-|Glu|-Arg-Gly-Phe-|Phe-Tyr|-Thr-Pro-Lys-|Thr|

C region

IGF-I   -Gly-Tyr-Gly-|Ser|-Ser-Ser-Arg-|Arg|-Ala-Pro-Gln-Thr-
IGF-II -Ser-Arg-Val-Ser-|Arg|-Arg-Ser-|Arg|
HPI   -Arg-Arg-Glu-Ala-Glu-Asp-Leu-Gln-Val-Gly-Gln-Val-Glu-Leu-Gly-Gly-Gly-Pro-Gly-Ala-Gly-Ser-Leu-Gln-Pro-Leu-Ala-Leu-Glu-Gly-Ser-Leu-Gln-Lys-Arg-

A region

IGF-I   -Gly-Ile-Val-|Asp|-|Glu-Cys-Cys|-Phe-Arg-Ser-Cys-Asp-|Leu|-Arg-Arg-|Leu-Glu|-Met-|Tyr-Cys-Ala|
IGF-II -Gly-Ile-Val-Glu-|Glu-Cys-Cys|-Phe-Arg-Ser-Cys-Asp-Leu-Ala-Leu-|Leu-Glu|-Thr-|Tyr-Cys-Ala|
HPI   -Gly-Ile-Val-Glu-|Gln-Cys-Cys|-|Thr-Ser-Ile|-Cys-|Ser|-Leu-|Tyr-Gln-Leu-Glu|-Asn-|Tyr-Cys-Asn|-COOH

D region

IGF-I   -Pro-Leu-Lys-|Pro-Ala-Lys-Ser|-Ala-COOH
IGF-II -Thr-Pro-Ala-Lys-Ser-Glu-COOH
HPI

Fig 3.—Homologies between amino acid sequences of insulin-like growth factor I (IGF-I), insulin-like growth factor II (IGF-II), and human proinsulin (HPI). Dashed lines enclose the amino acids that are exactly the same in the three molecules. For compactness the B,C,A, and D regions are lined up separately.

have been completely sequenced: IGF-I[18] and IGF-II.[19] As shown in Figure 3, these SM peptides have close homology to each other and to proinsulin. This explains the close biologic relationships of the SM peptides to insulin and implies that there was a common ancestral hormone in the distant past.[20] The IGF-I and IGF-II molecules have been divided into four regions. The B and A regions are homologous to the B and A chains of insulin. Of the 51 amino acids of insulin, 20 are exactly the same in IGF-I and IGF-II, including all of the disulfide bond-forming cysteines. The C region is in an analogous position to the C peptide of proinsulin, but there is no obvious homology between IGF-I, IGF-II, or proinsulin in this region. The D region of IGF-I and II has no counterpart in any known insulin, but there is a strong homology in this region between IGF-I and IGF-II.

SM-C seems almost certain to be functionally identical to IGF-I. In addition to having a similar isoelectric point, it has been shown to be indistinguishable from IGF-I by radioreceptor (RRA) and RIA,[21] and immunologically identical by region-specific antibodies directed against the synthetic IGF-I C-peptide[22] and D-peptide regions.[23] In addition, partial sequence data of SM-C has shown that the nine N-terminal amino acids are identical to IGF-I.[24] The minor differences in total amino acid composition data remain to be resolved. In addition the basic SM of Bala and Bhaumick[10] has the five N-terminal amino acids exactly the same as IGF-I. Thus it seems that all the basic human SM peptides are one and the same molecule, for which the terminology IGF-I/SM-C (or SM-C/IGF-I) has been proposed.[21]

The amino acid composition of SM-A has been published.[25] It seems that its structure must be quite different from IGF-I or IGF-II. However, no amino acid sequence data are as yet available for SM-A. The functional similarities of SM-A to the structured SM peptides in radiologic assays make it seem likely that there will be a structural kinship too. It is even possible that SM-A will be shown to be a mixture of IGF-I/SM-C and IGF-II, as has been proposed recently.[26] The neutral SM peptides, the ILAs of Posner et al.,[9] and a similar peptide partially purified by Ginsberg et al.,[27] have not yet been obtained in sufficient purity or quantities for structural studies.

Of the nonhuman SM peptides, none has yet been structured.

MSA has been resolved into six individual peptides[28] and it is hoped that structural data will soon be available on at least one of the MSA peptides. Rat SM[8] and bovine SM[7] may both be close to having sequence data for comparison to the human peptides. Somatomedins of all other species are far from that stage. It seems likely, however, that as in other peptide hormones there will be broad structural homology within the SM peptides of different species.

Assay Techniques

Many assay techniques have been used to assay the SM/IGF activities of plasma. As is true of most hormones, the original techniques used were bioassays. These techniques have the advantage of measuring a biologic action, thus something "real." However, they tend to have rather poor reliability, and many of them do not have clear specificity for SM peptides. The first assays used the biologic system of discovery. Thus, for SF it was the hypophysectomized rat bioassay,[2] and for NSILA (IGF) it was the rat adipose tissue assay.[7] Both of these assays with modifications are still in use today. In addition, technically easier and/or more reproducible assays have been developed with embryonic chicken cartilage,[29] porcine cartilage,[30] and chick embryo fibroblasts.[16] With these bioassays a great deal of information has been amassed. However, it is still unclear whether any of these assays is absolutely specific for SM peptides, and to what extent other non-SM factors in plasma are active. It is clear that insulin (in nonphysiologic amounts) is detected in the hypophysectomized (hypox) rat bioassay,[2] and that triiodothyronine (T_3) is important to the response of chick cartilage.[31] In addition, some plasmas have inhibitor(s) of the bioassays. This has been shown clearly for both the hypox rat[32] and porcine[33] bioassays. The inhibitor is not present in all plasmas. It has been specifically found in plasma in malnutrition, both in human beings[34] and rats[32] and in severely diabetic rats.[35] The inhibitor(s) may be an important factor in net somatomedin biologic activity in vivo or a relatively nonspecific cytotoxic factor that is not of import in vivo. Only further work will resolve this question. One hypothesis that needs to be tested is that the inhibitor is at least in part the unsaturated SM binding protein (see below).

When SM peptides pure enough to be useful as radioligands became available, radioreceptor assays were developed by using human placental membranes[36] or rat liver membranes.[37] These assays provided an advance in ease of performance, reproducibility, and potential specificity. The exact specificity of these radioreceptor assays is still unclear. In our hands it seems that the placental membrane RRA favors SM-C/IGF-I tenfold compared to IGF-II, but there may also be another SM species detected in this RRA.[38] The placental membrane radioreceptor assay using 125-I-SM-A gives quantitatively similar results to those of the SM-C RRA.[39] It seems very likely that both the placental membrane RRA using 125-I-SM-A and the placental membrane RRA using 125-I-SM-C detect very nearly the same mixture of SM/IGF peptides in plasma. However, this remains to be tested in an unequivocal way. It is also a subject of debate whether or not the plasma needs to be acid separated prior to assay in the RRA.[40] The rat liver membrane RRA preferentially detects IGF-II[41] and this may well explain the different results obtained with this assay in clinical states.

Unlike any other peptide hormone, the SMs have a specific plasma-binding protein.[42] (This phenomenon is described in detail under "Physiology" below.) This plasma-binding protein has been partially purified and used as the basis of an RRA.[43, 44] This RRA appears to detect IGF-II about fivefold better than IGF-I when 125-I-IGF-I is used as radioligand and about 12-fold better than IGF-I when 125-IGF-II is used. It is thus much more of an "IGF-II RRA" than is either the SM-C or SM-A placental membrane RRAs.

Over the last few years, several RIAs have been developed for SM/IGF peptides. These include RIAs for SM-C,[45] IGF-I[22, 46] SM-A,[47] and basic SM.[48] All of these assays show specificity for the IGF-I/SM-C group of SMs and are much less sensitive to IGF-II. The discrimination factor ranges from 30-fold[46] to 300-fold or greater.[22, 45] The SM-A RIA actually prefers IGF-I to SM-A. This broad agreement using many different antiserums is one of the strong reasons for considering SM-C/IGF-I to be functionally identical.[20, 22] There is some evidence that SM-A may be different,[21] but this must await more structural data. The RIAs thus represent an advance in specificity over the RRAs and bioassays, and in general they are more sensitive than the other assays. It is clear that these RIAs are going to have a major impact on the usefulness and availability of SM determinations clinically. One of these RIAs is commercially available; others will doubtless follow. It is clear, however, that the specificity of the RIA is such that only a part of the plasma SM/IGF is being measured.[46, 49] Whether this is of any clinical significance is dubious, since it appears that SM-C/IGF-I is the most GH-responsive of the SM peptides.

Specific radioimmunoassays for the other well-characterized SM peptide, IGF-II, have been recently developed by Zapf et al.[46] and Hintz and Liu.[50] So far there appears to be broad agreement between the two assays that hypopituitary patients are lower than normal but that acromegalic patients are not higher than normal in IGF-II content. They also both find that normally there is a higher content of IGF-II in plasma than of SM-C/IGF-I. These broad outlines are also confirmed by the specific RRA for IGF-II utilizing rat placental membranes that has been developed by Daughaday et al.[51] It is too soon to predict in what clinical circumstances (if any) an IGF-II assay will be important.

Physiology

PRODUCTION

As with any hormone, the physiology can be viewed as the processes of production of the hormone, modulation of production and release of the hormone, plasma transport of the hormone, and cellular action. The SMs are unique among the peptide hormones in several of their characteristics. First, there does not appear to be a concentrated form of the hormone in a discrete organ, unlike all the well-known hormones. We have already mentioned the difficulties this presented to those purifying SM. However, a number of observations suggest that the liver is at least one site of SM production. If one perfuses a whole rat liver[52, 53] or liver slices,[54] GH-dependent release of SM activity occurs. In addition, partially hepatectomized rats show a marked drop in SM levels with recovery parallel to the regrowth of hepatic tissue,[55] and fetal liver has been shown to produce MSA, a rat SM peptide.[56] However, no one has been able to extract a high concentration of SM from liver, and even using immunofluorescent techniques there does not appear to be any significant storage of SM in liver. Furthermore, there is evidence that SM may be produced in tissues other than liver. Kidney[57] has been suggested as another site of SM production. More recently, mouse limb bud mesenchymal tissue,[58] human fetal lung fibroblasts,[59] and fibrosarcoma and osteosarcoma cells[60] have all been shown to release SM-like peptides. Thus SM appears not to be stored for quick release, but to be synthesized on demand. This arrangement makes sense, since the half-life of SM in serum is very long and there appears to be no need for producing quick increases of hormone concentration. Rather, the levels throughout the day appear to be remarkably constant, and the plasma form of SM is in itself the storage form.

PLASMA STATES

The plasma form is another unique feature of SM among peptide hormones. Unlike other peptide hormones that circulate freely in plasma, the SM peptides have plasma-binding proteins to which they are specifically bound with a high affinity.[61, 62] In addition to the SM-binding protein and a bound SM peptide, there is probably also a third subunit to make up the 150,000 molecular weight (mol wt) complex, which is the main circulating form of SM. There are also variable amounts of a smaller (50,000 mol wt) SM complex and some free-binding protein.[40, 63] There is very little or no free-circulating SM peptide. Whether the complex forms of SM are active or whether there is a small amount of free SM, perhaps generated at the tissue level, that accounts for the activity, remains unclear. What does seem clear is that this unique complex form of SM accounts for the very long (hours-long) half-life in plasma[64] and thus its constancy in plasma. There is also evidence that the complex form serves to decrease the insulin-like actions of the bound form.[65] It is important to realize that while the differences in SM levels usually reflect changes in secretion rate, this may not be necessarily so. Changes in binding protein and saturation could in theory affect SM levels profoundly, just as is the case with thyroxine.

CONTROL

Plasma SM levels appear to a large extent to be under GH control. The earliest observations with bioassays for "sulfation factor" were about the GH dependency of the factor, and the bioassays achieved a brief role in clinical medicine as tools for diagnosis of acromegaly and hypopituitarism before the radioimmune assay for hGH became widespread. When the radioreceptor assays for SM-C, SM-A, and NSILA-S (IGF) were first validated, it became clear that the bioassay data could be essentially duplicated in a general way with most of the RRAs. The SM-C and A placental membrane radioreceptor assays show that hypopituitary patients as a group have SM levels one third of normal levels and that acromegalic patients have values roughly three times the norm. These values are very similar to bioassay results using rat, porcine, or chick cartilage tissue. The NSILA RRA using rat liver membranes and the IGF RRA using plasma-binding protein show hypopituitary patients to be lower than normal, but show little or no increase in acromegalic plasma. On the basis of information garnered using more specific RIAs it is now possible to say that this discrepancy is due to the fact that the SM-A and C placental membranes RRAs preferentially detect IGF-I/SM-C, while the other RRAs detect IGF-II in preference to IGF-I. IGF-I/SM-C appears to be the most GH-dependent SM peptide and accounts for nearly all the elevation seen in acromegaly. On the other hand, both IGF-I/SM-C and IGF-II are low in hypopituitarism and rise with GH therapy. As more experience is gained with the more specific assays, we will be able to talk more accurately about the control of the SM peptides. It is clear that GH plays a role in the control of both the IGF-I/SM-C and IGF-II SM peptides. Why an excess of GH does not result in an elevation of IGF-II is totally unclear at this point. However, this fact does dictate the choice of assays if one is interested in detecting elevations of SM. Only assays specific for or favoring IGF-I/SM-C would be useful in these clinical circumstances.

As is the case with many other hormones, GH and SM appear to be involved in a reciprocal feedback loop. Thus, while GH has a positive effect on SM secretion, SM has a negative feedback effect on GH secretion. Early clinical evidence for this reciprocal effect came from observations of situations in which SM was low and GH high, such as Laron type dwarfism[66] and malnutrition.[67] More direct evidence has been obtained by in vitro studies of the hypothalamus and pituitary using SM-C.[68] SM-C causes a release of somatostatin from the hypothalamus, which would inhibit hGH secretion from the pituitary. SM-C also has a delayed direct inhibition of GH release from pituitary cell cultures. Thus low SM levels would promote GH secretion, and high SM levels would inhibit GH secretions.

In addition to GH, other factors have been thought to play a role in the control of SM. Prolactin is very similar to GH in structure, and has been said to increase SM levels in rats.[69] However, the studies in man[44, 70] do not show any relationship between elevated prolactin levels and SM. Insulin appears to be synergistic with GH in promoting SM increase in a rat model.[71] Whether this is simply a reflection of the general anabolic effect of insulin or demonstrates a physiologic role for insulin is unclear. Thyroxine also has been shown to play a role in SM secretion in animal models.[73] Probably the biggest factor determining SM levels other than GH levels is nutrition. Severe malnutrition in human beings[67] is associated with very low SM levels despite generally elevated GH values. These human data are backed by experiments in rats that show a rapid drop in SM levels with fasting.[73] On the other side of the coin, overnutrition (obesity) in human beings[74] has been associated with relatively high levels of SM despite low GH levels. Our present ideas about the SM-GH system are summarized in Figure 4.

Another factor that affects SM levels is age. Newborn cord plasmas have low levels of SM by several different assays.[75, 76] The levels of SM then rise slowly throughout childhood,[43] reaching a peak in adolescence.[77] Preliminary data suggest that the levels of SM then fall after the fifth decade of life; these are supported by observations in aging rats.[78] The mechanism of these age-related changes and what physiologic significance they have are unclear. This does emphasize though that levels of SM cannot be viewed in isolation. One approach to the problem of age variability has been to normalize the SM level by an age-related regression equation.[74] A more common solution is to compare to age-matched controls before deciding whether a value is "normal" or not in a given assay.

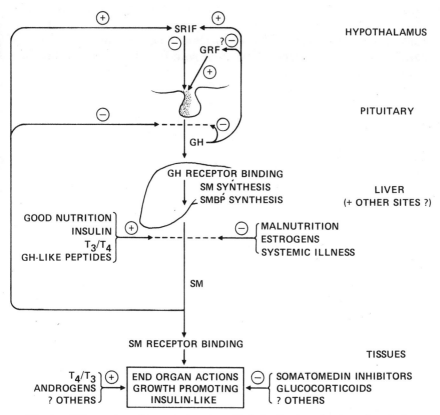

Fig 4.—GH-somatomedin control system. Both feedback and external control systems are represented.

CELLULAR ACTIONS

Like other peptide hormones, the initial event of SM action at the cellular level appears to be binding to specific receptor sites on the surface of cells. The receptor sites for somatomedin are widely distributed in the tissues of the body,[79] including mononuclear blood cells.[80] The binding constant of the reaction is high, estimated to be 2×10^9 by our recent data.[81] Both SM-C and IGF-II appear to share the same receptor site in all tissues studied. The affinity favors SM-C in all tissues except liver. In addition, insulin and proinsulin can cross-react but do so about 1,000-fold less well on a molar basis. The receptor-ligand reaction was originally thought to be a simple reversible bimolecular reaction. However, as in other peptide hormones, there is now reason to think that under physiologic conditions this view is oversimplified. A portion of the hormone enters the cell. Whether this process plays a role in triggering action is a subject of further study.

One thing about the intracellular trigger of SM appears clear: it does not require an increase of cAMP. In fact, in several tissues[82, 83] the cAMP levels seem to drop with SM stimulation, a drop reflected by data obtained with insulin. One possibility is that phosphorylation and activation of one or a few membrane proteins is linked to receptor binding of SM. In any case a number of cellular processes are turned on, including synthesis of protein, RNA, and DNA. Working with a cultured chick chondrocyte system, Kemp and Hintz[84] recently found that protein synthesis is rapidly increased and appears to be the rate-limiting step that SM stimulates on the way to producing sulfated mucopolysaccharides, the mature product of cartilage. Froesch et al.[31] have shown that pure IGF-I is sufficient to stimulate the process, but that T_3 modulates it. The situation with respect to cell division appears to be even more complex. In embryonic chick fibroblasts it appears that pure IGF-I is all that is necessary to stimulate DNA synthesis. However, mouse $3T_3$ cells[85] and human fibroblasts[86] need other factors in addition to SM for normal DNA synthesis and cell division. It appears that many cell lines need an "initiation factor" before SM can work as a "progression factor" to carry a cell through a division. The picture that appears to be emerging is that SM is only a part of the overlapping broader system of growth factors and growth-controlling substances. SM happens to be one growth factor that is under higher hormonal control (GH) and is frequently rate-limiting in a clinical setting. However, it is by no means the only physiologic growth-controlling peptide. The interrelationships of all the growth factors will take many years to dissect.

An area that must be investigated with regard to SM is whether it is sufficient in itself to cause whole body growth. The treatment of GH deficiency with GH causes an increase of SM, and SM has many in vitro actions that are necessary for growth. But can one replace GH with SM and restore normalcy? A number of attempts have been made at giving SM in vivo. It has been relatively easy to show insulin-like effects of

SM peptides given in vivo.[87, 88] In larger scale experiments some changes in sulfation were shown, but the growth response was borderline.[89] An increase in mitotic index in hypox frog lens epithelium has been demonstrated with in vivo treatment[90] but no total body growth. Van Buul-Offers and Vanden Brande[91] showed somatic growth in congenitally hypopituitary mice, although the effects of GH treatment were not totally reproduced. All of these experiments can be criticized on one basis or another. The amounts of SM used were low and sometimes of dubious purity due to the difficulties in obtaining large amounts of pure SM. In addition, all the experiments were done by injecting the small peptide rather than the whole SM complex. The half-life of the peptide is very short compared to the complex, and it is also possible that the complex has other roles in the delivery of SM to the periphery. Thus the ideal in vivo experiment has yet to be done. However, it is also possible that even under ideal circumstances SM will not truly replace GH, and that GH has other actions, both direct and indirect, that are necessary for growth. Only when (and if) large supplies of pure recombinant-DNA synthesized SM peptides are available will it be possible to attack these interesting questions effectively.

CLINICAL CORRELATES

Although the knowledge of these SM hormones has come far in the last two decades, it is clear that new discoveries will (and should) continue to change our viewpoint in the next decade. What can the pediatrician regard as "truth" of clinical importance now, and in what direction will clinical knowledge in the field carry us in the near future? First, as a clinical test SM-C is likely to prove useful in the workup of disorders of children. GH deficiency is associated with low somatomedin levels in essentially all patients. Since there is almost no diurnal variation of SM, a single sample collected and handled properly can serve as a good screening test for GH deficiency, and replace several blood samples for GH obtained after a nonphysiologic stimulus. Although the commercial price for an SM-C RIA is presently rather high, it is still cost effective. If the value is normal, GH deficiency is essentially ruled out of further consideration. If the value is low, several other possi-

TABLE 2.—CAUSES OF LOW SOMATOMEDIN LEVELS

GH deficiency
GH resistance syndrome (Laron's dwarfism and variants)
Ineffective GH syndrome
Newborn and < 3 yrs.
Old age
Malnutrition
Maternal deprivation syndrome
Cirrhosis and hepatic failure
Severe acute illness
Renal failure*
Cushing's disease/syndrome*

*In bioassay only.

bilities must be considered. The causes of low SM levels are listed in Table 2. Malnutrition and maternal deprivation syndrome will both have low SM values. Since these may also be difficult to diagnose for other reasons, these possibilities must be kept in mind. GH-provocative testing will then give normal or high results in malnutrition, but often mimic GH deficiency in maternal deprivation. There is no substitute for a careful history, good psychosocial assessment, and a high index of suspicion. Another cause of low SM that should be kept in mind is that children under three will normally have values in a range that would be considered abnormally low in older children, so that good age-related standards are a necessity. Values in renal failure and Cushing's syndrome may be low if the SM is done by bioassay.

Even with the avoidance of these pitfalls there is a group of children with poor growth who have low SM values, yet who are normal according to the GH-provocative tests. Work by Rudman et al.[92] and Kowarski et al.[93] suggests that these patients may benefit from GH treatment even though not technically GH deficient. These patients may represent a defect in GH or GH metabolism and might be said to have an ineffective hGH syndrome. Much work is needed but ultimately the most useful aspect of getting an SM level on a short child may be to aid in deciding who will respond to GH, irrespective of the GH values. This decision is likely to become an increasingly important one as large supplies of hGH synthesized by recombinant DNA technology become available in the future.

At the other end of the spectrum, it seems likely that SM

determinations will be of use in diagnosing cases of over-growth. Its use in the diagnosis and follow-up of acromegaly is already well established.[94, 95] The pediatric correlate of acro-megaly, pituitary gigantism, is also associated with high SM levels. In both of these situations it appears that the elevation is almost totally due to SM-C/IGF-I with normal or nearly nor-mal levels of IGF-II. Thus an assay (such as the SM-C RIA) that measures this component of total SM is most likely to be of use in these cases. Relatively high values of SM-C can be seen in normal teenagers, obese persons, and persons with renal failure and hypercortisolism. The causes of high SM lev-els are listed in Table 3. In addition, if plasma is not handled and stored correctly the whole plasma SM-C RIA can give falsely elevated levels.[96] This phenomenon appears to be due to a rearrangement of the 150,000 mol wt complex into a smaller 50,000 mol wt form more accessible to antibody.[97] This phenom-enon is not seen with acid-treated or acid-chromatographed plasma. A single elevated SM value cannot be taken as diag-nostic of GH excess but must be viewed in relation to all the other information available on the patient. There are even pa-tients with growth failure who have been reported to have ele-vated SM levels.[98] In theory these patients have a block in SM action, but more of these patients need careful study before any conclusions can be drawn.

There are other areas of pediatrics in which the measure-ment of SM may be useful. It may be a useful monitor of ther-apy in malnutrition and maternal deprivation syndrome, since in both of these situations the SM values are low and rise with successful treatment. It may also be a useful measurement in patients with GH deficiency who are failing to respond to treat-ment. Some cases of hypoglycemia may be due to the secretion

TABLE 3.—Causes of High Somatomedin
Levels

Acromegaly
Pituitary gigantism
Adolescence
Obesity
SM resistance syndrome
Renal failure*
Cushing's disease/syndrome*

*In radioligand assays.

of SM peptides.[39] Of the known SM peptides, IGF-II is the most insulin-like and only specific measurements of IGF-II in patients with undiagnosed hypoglycemia will tell how commonly SM is involved. Finally, there is some evidence that some tumor cells make their own growth factors, including SM-like substances.[99] The measurement of SM might detect these tumors and lead to more rational therapy of them through blocking SM receptor sites.

In our present state of knowledge there is no indication for therapy with SM, nor is it possible to give SM in adequate quantities. In theory, Laron type dwarfs might respond to SM treatment since the metabolic block in these patients appears to be between GH and the release of SM. Only future work with recombinant DNA synthesis of SM and animal testing will put us in a position to answer this question.

Conclusions

The SMs are a group of peptides under the control of GH and other hormonal and nonhormonal factors. These hormones all have in vitro insulin-like and growth-promoting actions, and it is proposed that they play a major role in GH actions. At least two distinct SMs, SM-C/IGF-I and IGF-II, circulate in human plasma, and there may well be others. Biologically related SM peptides are found in the plasma of many animal species. The SM peptides that have been structured so far show strong homology to proinsulin and presumably they share a common ancestral hormone. The assay methods vary in complexity, specificity, and reliability, but determinations of SM-C/IGF-I are now widely available. The measurement of SM-C plays an increasingly important role in the workup of growth abnormalities in childhood, and may develop other clinical indications as experience is gained. Whether SM peptides are *the* major mediators of GH actions remains to be established. However, it is clear that these peptides occupy a crucial niche between classical hormones and tissue factors, and that their study may lead us to new discoveries about growth, aging, and abnormalities of growth control such as neoplasia.

REFERENCES

1. Ellis S., Huble J., Simpson M.E.: Influence of hypophysectomy and growth hormone on cartilage sulfate metabolism. *Proc. Soc. Exp. Biol. Med.* 84:603, 1953.

2. Salmon W.D. Jr., Daughaday W.N.: A hormonally controlled serum factor which stimulates sulfate incorporation by cartilage in vitro. *J. Lab. Clin. Med.* 49:825, 1957.
3. Daughaday W.H., Hall K., Raben M.S., et al.: Somatomedin: Proposed designation for sulfation factor. *Nature* 235:197, 1972.
4. Hall R., Uthne K.: Some biological properties of purified sulfation factor from human plasma. *Acta Med. Scand.* 190:137, 1971.
5. Van Wyk J.J., Underwood L.E., Hintz R.L., et al.: The somatomedins: A family of insulin-like hormones under growth hormone control. *Recent Prog. Hormone Res.* 30:259, 1974.
6. Uthne K.: Human somatomedins: Purification and some studies on their biological actions. *Acta Endocrinol. [Suppl.] (Copenh.)* 175:1, 1973.
7. Liberti J.P.: Purification of bovine somatomedin. *Biochem. Biophys. Res. Commun.* 67:1226, 1975.
8. Chochina R.H., Mariz I.K., Daughaday W.H.: Isolation of a somatomedin from the plasma of rats bearing growth-hormone-secreting tumors. *Endocrinology* 100:549, 1977.
9. Posner B.I., Guzda H.J., Corval M.T., et al.: Partial purification, characterization and assay of a slightly acid insulin-like peptide (ILAs) from human plasma. *J. Clin. Endocrinol. Metab.* 47:1240, 1978.
10. Bala R.M., Bhaumick B.: Purification of a basis somatomedin from human plasma Cohn fraction IV-1, with physiochemical and radioimmunoassay similarity to somatomedin C and insulin-like growth factor. *Can. J. Biochem.* 57:1289, 1979.
11. Growen J., Kanninga C.E., Willebrands A.F., et al.: Evidence for the presence of insulin in serum: A method for the approximate determination of the insulin content of blood. *J. Clin. Invest.* 31:97, 1952.
12. Martin D.B., Renold A.E., Dagenais Y.M.: An assay for insulin-like activity using rat adipose tissue. *Lancet* 2:76, 1958.
13. Yalow R.S., Berson S.A.: Immunoassay of endogenous plasma insulin in men. *J. Clin. Invest.* 39:1157, 1960.
14. Froesch E.R., Bürgi H., Ramseier E.B., et al.: Antibody-suppressible and nonsuppressible insulin-like activities in serum and their physiologic significance. *J. Clin. Invest.* 42:1816, 1963.
15. Bürgi H., Müller W.A., Humbel R.E., et al.: Nonsuppressible insulin-like activity of human serum I: Physicochemical properties, extraction and partial purification. *Biochim. Biophys. Acta* 121:349, 1966.
16. Dulak N.C., Temin H.M.: A partially purified polypeptide fraction from rat liver cell conditioned medium with multiplication-stimulating activity for embryo fibroblasts. *J. Cell. Physiol.* 81:153, 1973.
17. Moses A.C., Nissley S.P., Rechler M.M., et al.: The purification and characterization of MSA from media condition by a rat liver cell line, in Giordano G., et al. (eds): *Somatomedins and Growth*. London: Academic Press, 1979, vol 23, pp 45–59.
18. Rinderknecht E., Humbel R.E.: The amino acid sequence of human insulin-like growth factor I and its structural homology with proinsulin. *J. Biol. Chem.* 253:2769, 1978.
19. Rinderknecht E., Humbel R.E.: Primary structure of human insulin-like growth factor II. *FEBS Lett.* 89:283, 1978.
20. Blundell T.L., Bedarkar S., Rinderknecht E., et al.: Insulin-like growth factor: A model for tertiary structure accounting for immunoreactivity and receptor binding. *Proc. Natl. Acad. Sci. U.S.A.* 75:180, 1978.
21. Van Wyk J.J., Suoboda M.E., Underwood L.E.: Evidence from radioligand assays that SM-C and IGF-I are similar to each other. *J. Clin. Endocrinol. Metab.* 50:206, 1980.
22. Hintz R.L., Liu F., Marshall L.B., et al.: Interaction of somatomedin-C with an

314   RAYMOND L. HINTZ

antibody directed against the synthetic C-peptide region of insulin-like growth factor I. *J. Clin. Endocrinol. Metab.* 50:405, 1980.
23. Hintz R.L., Liu F., Rinderknecht E.: Somatomedin-C shares the carboxy-terminal antigenic determinants with insulin-like growth factor I. *J. Clin. Endocrinol. Metab.* 51:672, 1980.
24. Svoboda M.E., Van Wyk J.J., Klapper D.G., et al.: Purification of Somatomedin-C from human plasma: Chemical and biological properties, partial sequence analysis, and relationship to other somatomedins. *Biochemistry* 19:790, 1980.
25. Sievertsson H., Fryklund L., Uthne K., et al.: Isolation and chemistry of human somatomedins A and B. *Adv. Metab. Disord.* 8:47, 1975.
26. Zapf J., Rinderknecht E., Humbel R.E., et al.: Non-suppressible insulin-like activity from human serum: Recent accomplishments and their physiologic implications. *Metabolism* 27:1803, 1978.
27. Ginsberg B.H., Kahn C.R., Roth J., et al.: Identification and high yield purification of insulin-like growth factors from human plasma by use of endogenous binding proteins. *J. Clin. Endocrinol. Metab.* 48:43, 1979.
28. Moses A.C., Nissley S.P., Short P.A., et al.: Purification and characterization of multiplication-stimulating activity. *Eur. J. Biochem.* 103:387, 1980.
29. Hall K.: Quantitative determination of the sulfation factor activity in human serum. *Acta Endocrinol.* 63:338, 1970.
30. Van den Brande J.L., DuCaju M.U.L.: An improved technique for measuring somatomedin activity in vitro. *Acta Endocrinol.* 75:233, 1974.
31. Froesch E.R., Zapf J., Audhya T.K. et al.: Nonsuppressible insulin-like activity and thyroid hormones: major pituitary-dependent sulfation factors for chick embryo cartilage. *Proc. Natl. Acad. Sci. U.S.A.* 73:2904, 1976.
32. Salmon W.D. Jr.: Interaction of somatomedin and a peptide inhibitor in serum of hypophysectomized and starved pituitary intact rat. *Adv. Metab. Res.* 8:183, 1975.
33. Phillips L.S., Young H.S.: Nutrition and somatomedin II: Serum somatomedin activity and cartilage growth activity in streptozotocin diabetic rats. *Diabetes* 25:516, 1976.
34. Hintz R.L., Siskind R., Amatayakul K., et al.: Plasma somatomedin and growth hormone values in children with protein calorie malnutrition. *J. Pediatr.* 92:153, 1978.
35. Phillips L.S., Belosky D.C., Reichard L.A.: Nutrition and somatomedin V.: Action and measurement of somatomedin inhibitor in serum. *Endocrinology* 104:1513, 1979.
36. Marshall R.N., Underwood L.E., Voina S.J., et al.: Characterization of the insulin and somatomedin-C receptors in human placental membranes. *J. Clin. Endocrinol. Metab.* 39:283, 1974.
37. Meggesi K., Kahn C.R., Roth J., et al.: Insulin and nonsuppressible insulin-like activity: Evidence for separate plasma membrane receptor sites. *Biochem. Biophys. Res. Commun.* 57:307, 1974.
38. Kemp S.F., Rosenfeld R.G., Liu F., et al.: Acute somatomedin response to growth hormone: Radioreceptor assay vs. radioimmunoassay. *J. Clin. Endocrinol.* 52:616, 1981.
39. Hall K., Takano K., Fryklund L.: Radioreceptor assay for somatomedin A. *J. Clin. Endocrinol. Metab.* 39:973, 1974.
40. Rosenfeld R.G., Hintz R.L.: Induction of homologous receptor loss: A sensitive assay for human growth hormone (hGH) in acromegalic, newborn and stimulated plasma. *J. Clin. Endocrinol. Metab.* 50:62, 1980.
41. Kahn C.R.: The riddle of tumor hypoglycemia revisited. *J. Clin. Endocrinol. Metab.* 9:335, 1980.
42. Borsi L., Liu F., Hintz R.: Somatomedin and somatomedin binding protein in newborns. American Pediatric Society-Society for Pediatric Research, 1980.

43. Zapf J., Kaufmann U., Eigennamm J.E., et al.: Determination of nonsuppressible insulin-like activity in human serum by a sensitive binding assay. *Clin. Chem.* 23:677, 1977.
44. Schalch D.S., Heinrich U.E., Koch J.G., et al.: Nonsuppressible insulin-like activity: I. Development of a new competitive protein binding assay. *J. Clin. Endocrinol. Metab.* 46:669, 1978.
45. Furlanetto R.W., Underwood L.E., Van Wyk J.J., et al.: Estimation of somatomedin C levels in normals and patients with pituitary disease by RIA. *J. Clin. Invest.* 60:648, 1977.
46. Zapf J., Morel B., Walter H., et al.: Serum levels of insulin-like growth factor and its carrier protein in various metabolic disorders. *Acta Endocrinol.* 95:505, 1980.
47. Hall K., Brandt J., Enberg G., et al.: Immunoreactive somatomedin A in human serum. *J. Clin. Endocrinol. Metab.* 48:271, 1979.
48. Bala R.M., Bhaumick B.: Radioimmunoassay of basic somatomedin: Equilibrium method without chromatography of serum. *Clin. Res.* 26:839A, 1978.
49. Kemp S.F., Rosenfeld R.G., Liu F., et al.: Acute somatomedin response to growth hormone: Radioreceptor assay vs. radioimmunoassay. Submitted for publication.
50. Hintz R.L., Liu F.: Insulin-like growth factor-II radioimmunoassay based on an antiserum against the synthetic C-peptide segment. Submitted to annual meeting of American Federation for Clinical Research of Western Section, 1981.
51. Daughaday W.H., Trevedi B., Mariz I.K.: Elevated insulin-like growth factor II in non-islet tumor induced hypoglycemia detected by a new specific radioreceptor assay. *Diabetes* 29(suppl. 2):A19, 1980.
52. McConaghey P., Sledge C.B.: Production of "sulfation factor" by the perfused liver. *Nature* 225:1249, 1970.
53. Phillips L.S., Herington A.C., Karl I.G., et al.: Comparison of SM activity inperfusates of normal and hypophysectomized rat livers with and without added growth hormone. *Endocrinology* 98:1214, 1976.
54. Hintz R.L., Clemmons D.R., Van Wyk J.J.: Growth hormone induced somatomedin-like activity from liver. American Pediatric Society-Society for Pediatric Research, 1972.
55. Uthne K., Uthne T.: Influence of liver resection and regeneration on SM activity in sera from normal and hypox rats. *Acta Endocrinol.* 71:255, 1972.
56. Rechler M.M., Eisen H.J., Higa O.Z., et al.: Characterization of a somatomedin (IGF) synthesized by fetal rat liver organ cultures. *J. Biol. Chem.* 254:7942, 1979.
57. McConaghey P., Dehnel J.: Preliminary studies of "sulfation factor" production by rat kidney. *J. Endocrinol.* 52:587, 1972.
58. D'Ercole A.J., Applewhite G.T., Underwood L.E.: Evidence that somatomedin is synthesized by multiple tissues in the fetus. *Dev. Biol.* 75:315, 1980.
59. Atkison P.R., Weidman E.R., Bhaumick B., et al.: Release of somatomedin-like activity by cultured WI-38 human fibroblasts. *Endocrinology* 106:2006, 1980.
60. Todaro G.J., De Larco J.E., Marquant H., et al.: Polypeptide growth factors produced by tumor cells: A possible growth advantage for the producer cells, in Sato G.H., et al. (eds): *Hormones and Cell Culture*. Cold Springs Harbor Laboratory, 1979, pp 113–127.
61. Hintz R.L., Liu F.: Demonstration of specific plasma protein binding sites for somatomedin. *J. Clin. Endocrinol. Metab.* 45:988, 1977.
62. Zapf J., Waldvogel M., Froesch E.R.: Binding of NSILA to human serum: Evidence for a carrier protein. *Arch. Biochem. Biophys.* 168:638, 1975.
63. Furlanetto R.W.: The somatomedin C binding protein: Evidence for a heterologous subunit structure. *J. Clin Endocrinol. Metab.* 51:12, 1980.
64. Kaufmann U., Zapf J., Torretti B., et al.: Demonstration of a specific serum carrier protein of nonsuppressible insulin-like activity in vivo. *J. Clin. Endocrinol. Metab.* 44:160, 1977.

65. Horner J.M., Hintz R.L.: A comparative study of the 125-I-SM-A and 125-I-SM-C radioreceptor assays for somatomedin peptide content in whole and acid-chromatographed plasma, in Giordano G., et al. (eds): *Somatomedins and Growth.* New York: Academic Press, 1979, pp 177–184.
66. Laron Z.: Syndrome of familial dwarfism and high plasma immunoreactive growth hormone. *Isr. J. Med. Sci.* 10:1247, 1974.
67. Hintz R.L., Suskind R., Amatayakul K., et al.: Somatomedin and growth hormone in children with protein calorie malnutrition. *J. Pediatr.* 92:153, 1978.
68. Berelowitz M., Szabo M., Frohman L.A., et al.: Somatomedin-C mediates growth hormone negative feedback by effects on both the hypothalamus and the pituitary. *Science* 212:1279, 1981.
69. Bala R.M., Bohnet H.G., Carter J.N., et al.: Efffects of prolactin on serum somatomedin activity in hypophysectomized rats. *Clin. Res.* 24:655A, 1976.
70. Spencer E.M.: Lack of response of serum somatomedin to hyperprolactinemia in humans. *J. Clin. Endocrinol. Metab.* 50:182, 1980.
71. Daughaday W.H., Phillips L.S., Mueller M.D.: The effects of insulin and growth hormone on the release of somatomedin by the isolated rat liver. *Endocrinology* 98:1214, 1976.
72. Schalch D.S., Heinrich U.E., Draznin B., et al.: Role of the liver in regulating somatomedin activity: Hormonal effects on the synthesis and release of insulin-like growth factor and its carrier protein by the isolated perfused rat liver. *Endocrinology* 104:1143, 1979.
73. Phillips L.S. and Young, H.S.: Nutrition and somatomedin I. Effect of fasting and refeeding on serum somatomedin activity and cartilage growth activity in rats. *Endocrinology* 99:304, 1976.
74. Vanden Brande J.L., Du Caju M.U.L.: Plasma somatomedin activity in children with growth disturbances, in Raita S. (ed): *Advances in Human Growth Hormone Research.* Washington, D.C.: U.S. Government Printing Office, 1974.
75. Hintz R.L., Seeds J.M., Johnsonbaugh R.E.: Somatomedin and growth hormone in the newborn. *Am. J. Dis. Child.* 131:1249, 1977.
76. Tato L., Du Caju M.U.L., Prevot C., et al.: Early variations of plasma somatomedin activity in the newborn. *J. Clin. Endocrinol. Metab.* 40:534, 1975.
77. Bala M., et al.: Serum immunoreactive somatomedin levels in normal adults, pregnant women at term, children at various ages and children with constitutional delay in growth. *J. Clin. Endocrinol. Metab.* 52:508, 1981.
78. Florini J.R., Roberts S.B.: Effect of rat age on blood levels of somatomedin-like growth factors. *J. Gerontol.* 35:23, 1980.
79. D'Ercole A.J., Underwood L.E., Van Wyk J.J., et al.: Specificity, topography and ontogeny of the somatomedin C receptor in mammalian tissues, in Pecile A., et al. (eds): *Growth Hormone and Related Peptides.* New York: Elsevier North-Holland, 1976.
80. Thorsson A.V., Hintz R.L.: Specific ^{125}I-somatomedin receptor on circulating human mononuclear cells. *Biochem. Biophys. Res. Commun.* 74:1566, 1977.
81. Rosenfeld R., Thorsson A.V., Hintz R.L.: Increased somatomedin receptor sites in newborn circulating mononuclear cells. *J. Clin. Endocrinol. Metab.* 48:456, 1979.
82. Tell G.P., Cuatrecasas P., Hintz R.L., et al.: Somatomedin: Inhibition of adenylate cyclase activity in subcellular membranes of various tissues. *Science* 180:312, 1973.
83. Bourret L.A., Goetinick P.F., Hintz R.: Cyclic 3', 5'-AMP changes in chondrocytes of the proteoglycan-deficient chick embryonic mutant nanomelia. *FEBS Lett.* 108:353, 1979.
84. Kemp S.F., Hintz R.L.: The action of somatomedin on glycosaminoglycan synthesis by cultured chick chondrocytes. *Endocrinology* 106:744, 1980.

85. Stiles C.D., Capone G.T., Scher C.D. et al.: Dual control of cell growth by somato-medins and platelet-derived growth factor. *Proc. Natl. Acad. Sci. U.S.A.* 76:1279, 1979.
86. Plet A., Berwald-Netter Y.: The relative contribution of somatomedin to the serum-starved growth of human fibroblasts. *Biochem. Biophys. Res. Commun.* 94:794, 1980.
87. Oelz O., Jakob A., Froesch E.R.: Non-suppressible insulin-like activity of human serum V.: Hypoglycemia and preferential metabolic stimulation of muscle by NSILA-S. *Eur. J. Clin. Invest.* 1:48, 1970.
88. Underwood L.E., Hintz R.L., Voina S.J., et al.: Somatomedin, the growth hormone-dependent sulfation factor is antilipolytic. *J. Clin. Endocrinol.* 35:194, 1972.
89. Uthne K.: Preliminary studies of somatomedin in vitro and in vivo in rats. *Adv. Metab. Disord.* 8:115, 1975.
90. Rothstein H., Van Wyk J.J., Hayden J.H., et al.: Somatomedin C.: Restoration in vivo of cycle traverse in Go/6, blocked cells of hypophysectomized animals. *Science* 208:410, 1980.
91. Van Buul-Offers S., Vanden Brande, J.L.: Effect of growth hormone and peptide fractions containing somatomedin on growth and cartilage metabolism of small dwarf mice. *Acta Endocrinol.* 92:242, 1979.
92. Rudman D., Kutner M.H., Goldsmith M.A., et al.: Further observations on four subgroups of normal variant short stature. *J. Clin Endocrinol. Metab.* 51:1378, 1980.
93. Kowarski A.A., Schneider J., Ben-Galin E.: Growth failure with normal serum RIA-GH and low somatomedin activity. *J. Clin. Endocrinol. Metab.* 47:461, 1978.
94. Clemons D.R., Van Wyk J.J., Ridgway E.C., et al.: Evaluation of acromegaly by radioimmunoassay of somatomedin-C. *N. Engl. J. Med.* 301:1138, 1979.
95. Wiedemann E., Uthne K., Tang R.G., et al.: Serum somatomedin activity by rat cartilage bioassay and human placental membrane radioreceptor assay in acromegaly and Cushing's disease, in Giordano G., et al. (eds): *Somatomedins and Growth.* New York: Academic Press, 1975, pp 289–294.
96. Blethen S.L., Van Wyk J.J., Underwood L.E., et al.: Somatomedin-C is generated in serum by a temperature time pH and divalent action dependent process. 61st Annual Endocrine Society, 1979, p 220.
97. Daughaday W.H., Mariz I.K., Blethen S.L.: Inhibition of access of bound somato-medin to membrane receptor and immunobinding sites. *J. Clin. Endocrinol. Metab.* 51:781, 1980.
98. Lanes R., Plotnick L.P., Spencer E.M., et al.: Dwarfism associated with normal serum growth hormone and increased bioassayable, receptor assayable and immu-noassayable somatomedin. *J. Clin. Endocrinol. Metab.* 50:485, 1980.
99. DeLarco J.E., Todaro G.J.: A human fibrosarcoma cell line producing multiplica-tion stimulating activity-related peptides. *Nature* 272:356, 1978.

Enteric Alimentation in Specialized Gastrointestinal Problems: An Alternative to Total Parenteral Nutrition

ALAN M. LAKE, M.D.,
RONALD E. KLEINMAN, M.D.,
AND
W. ALLAN WALKER, M.D.

The Gastroenterology and Nutrition Units, Johns Hopkins Hospital, Baltimore, Maryland; Massachusetts General Hospital, Boston, Massachusetts; Department of Pediatrics, Johns Hopkins University School of Medicine; and Harvard Medical School

Introduction

OVER THE PAST THREE DECADES, many infant formulas have been introduced as alternatives to human milk in the nutriture of the human infant. While none has all of the qualities of human milk, most have been demonstrated to be sufficient as the sole source of nutrients in normal infants during the first year of life. In the past few years there have been excellent reviews of normal infant nutrition[1] and of the nutritional problems in premature infants.[2]

It is our intention here to focus on the nutritional management of infants with digestive and/or absorptive limitations who require specialized infant formulas or specialized feeding techniques. Although the nutritional requirements of some of these infants will be recognized and met early, thereby maxi-

0065-3101/81/0028-0319-0339-$03.75

mizing their potential for growth, most present as a "failure to thrive"; that is, they do not gain weight or grow at a normal rate after having been fed a variety of formulas. Indeed, it has been our observation that parents make an average of three formula changes prior to consulting their pediatrician and as many as five changes before the advice of a hospital-based subspecialist is sought. Emphasis here will be on the assessment and individualized management of this latter group of infants who from birth to the first year of life present with retarded growth.

Presentation as a failure to thrive implies, simplistically, that nutrient intake or absorption has not met requirements. In the normal infant who weighs less than 10 kg, approximately 50–60 kcal/kg of body weight must be provided daily for basal metabolism. An additional 15–20 kcal/kg of body weight per day are required for stool losses and activity. In infancy, these so-called maintenance requirements vary from an average of 80 kcal/kg of body weight per day in normal infants to nearly 120 kcal/kg of body weight per day in infants recovering from malnutrition. An additional 4–7 kcal/kg of body weight per day must be provided for each gram of daily weight gain, even in the absence of increased metabolic demands. The daily energy intake required for growth in infancy may vary from 100 kcal/kg of body weight per day in normal infants to over 200 kcal/kg of body weight per day with imposed digestive or absorptive limitations.

Failure to achieve adequate energy intake may develop for any number of reasons, some of which are listed in Table 1. Reduced nutrient intake may be the primary manifestation of an abnormal mother-child bond. In addition to multiple social or economic factors, reduced intake can be the result of neurologic or anatomical abnormalities in suck or swallow. Increased losses from the gastrointestinal tract may occur with recurrent emesis or protracted diarrhea. Because the young infant derives most of its nutrients from fluids, fluid restriction can be a major cause of caloric deprivation, especially in infants with heart disease, renal failure, or chronic lung disease such as bronchopulmonary dysplasia. Digestion may be significantly impaired as a function of prematurity, reduced brush border enzyme activity, pancreatic insufficiency, or cholestatic hepatobiliary disease. The absorption of nutrients is primarily dependent on small intestinal surface area, which may be re-

TABLE 1.—FACTORS LIMITING ENERGY
AVAILABILITY FOR GROWTH IN INFANCY

FACTOR	EXAMPLE
Caloric deprivation	Neglect, impaired suck/swallow
Fluid restriction	Cardiopulmonary failure
Impaired digestion	Pancreatic insufficiency
Impaired absorption (reduced surface area)	Celiac disease, malnutrition
Increased metabolism	Chronic inflammation
Impaired utilization	Storage diseases

duced by surgical resection, prolonged malnutrition, or chronic mucosal inflammation, as encountered in enteropathies induced by gluten, milk, or soy protein, in immunodeficiency states, or in bacterial overgrowth. Energy requirements are also increased by metabolism altered by chronic inflammation, cardiopulmonary disease, or storage diseases of glycogen or lipid.

Enteral Feeding Alternatives

What alternatives are available to populations that may require specialized infant feedings? Table 2 is an overview of some of the presently marketed infant formulas. This table is representative rather than all-encompassing, for more than 30 formulas are marketed. Each formula is listed by brand name, followed by the content of protein, carbohydrate, and fat expressed as quantity, form, and percentage of total calories. In the final two columns, we list the osmolality and estimated solute load. All formulas are presented as prepared in standard concentrations of 0.67 calorie/ml or 20 kilocalories/oz, except for Similac LBW and Enfamil Premature, which are 0.80 kilocalorie/ml or 24 kilocalories/oz.

Compositions of Formulas

PROTEIN

While commercially prepared formulas often attempt to mimic the protein composition of human milk, casein is the standard to which alternative protein sources are compared, al-

322 ALAN M. LAKE, RONALD E. KLEINMAN, & W. ALLAN WALKER

TABLE 2.—ORAL FEEDING

FORMULA	GM/dL	PROTEIN TYPE	CAL (%)	GM/dL	CARBOHYDRATE TYPE
Breast milk	1.2	Human	6	6.8	Lactose
Cow's milk	3.3	Bovine	21	4.9	Lactose
Similac/Enfamil	1.8	Skim	9	7.0	Lactose
S.M.A./PM60/40	1.5	Whey/casein	9	7.2	Lactose
Similac LBW	2.2	Whey/casein	11	8.5	Lactose Glucose polymer
Enfamil Premature	2.4	Skim whey	12	8.9	Lactose Glucose polymer
Isomil	2.0	Soy	12	6.8	Sucrose Corn syrup
Prosobee	2.5	Soy	15	6.8	Corn syrup
Goat's milk	3.2	Goat	19	4.6	Lactose
MBF (Meatbase)	2.9	Beef	20	4.2	Sucrose Tapioca
Probana	3.9	Milk Casein hydrol	24	7.3	Dextrose Banana lactose
Nutramigen	2.2	Casein hydrol	13	8.7	Sucrose Tapioca
Portagen	2.3	Sodium caseinate	14	7.6	Sucrose Dextrose malt.
Pregestimil	1.9	Casein hydrol Amino acids	13	9.1	Glucose polymer Tapioca
Carbohydrate-free	1.8	Soy	12	6.4	Must be added

though casein is an imperfect reference standard.[3] Modification of casein-based formulas to make them more like human milk includes enrichment with whey proteins such that the ratio of whey to casein is 60:40, in contrast to cow's milk, which is 18:82. Formulas constituted in this way include SMA, PM 60/40, and Enfamil Premature. Other protein sources, such as vegetable protein, must be supplemented with amino acids to make them nutritionally adequate.

ALTERNATIVES IN INFANCY

CAL (%)	GM/dL	FAT TYPE	CAL (%)	OSMOLALITY mOSM/KgHOH	RENAL SOLUTE mOSM/dl
38	4.0	Human	56	300	7.5
29	3.7	Butter	50	288	23.0
41	3.7	Soy, corn Coconut	50	290	11.0
43	3.6	Vegetable oleo	48	295	13.6
42	4.5	Soy, coconut Medium chain triglyceride (50%)	47	290	15.0
44	4.1	Corn, coconut Medium chain triglyceride (40%)	44	300	22.0
40	3.6	Corn, soy Coconut	48	230	13.0
40	3.4	Soy	45	258	15.0
28	4.0	Animal	53	340	27.0
29	3.3	Animal Sesame	51	147	19.0
47	2.0	Corn	29	592	25.0
52	2.6	Corn	35	443	13.0
44	3.3	Corn MCT (88%)	42	236	15.0
52	2.7	Corn MCT (40%)	35	338	13.0
40	3.5	Soy	48	480 (Dextrose) 250 (Glucose poly.)	13.0

In infancy, recommended protein intake is expressed as percentage of total calories or as gm/kg of body weight, due, as cited above, to the tremendous variation in energy requirements for growth. With high-quality protein, protein intake should ideally be 8% of total calories.[5] Higher levels do not further improve growth. While human milk, with but 6% of its calories as protein, is undeniably adequate for growth in normal infants, its adequacy in premature and malnourished infants remains under investigation. In neonates, protein toxicity has been documented with intakes exceeding 4 gm/kg of body weight per day. Acute manifestations of toxicity include CNS irritability, acidosis, and increased serum urea nitrogen.

Soy protein is a protein of lower quality due to its reduced content of essential amino acids, especially methionine. The marketed soy formulas are thus methionine-enriched. While soy protein formulas are adequate for normal infant nutrition[4] they are not recommended for use in premature infants or infants with cystic fibrosis. A major indication for prolonged use of soy protein formulas is for infants raised by families who adhere to vegetarian diets.

The casein hydrolysates are routinely amino-acid supplemented due to loss of essential amino acids in hydrolysis. Recent studies have confirmed that protein absorption occurs more rapidly in the form of dipeptides and oligopeptides rather than as individual amino acids.[6] The use of amino acid formulas in infancy has thus essentially ceased in favor of casein hydrolysates.

CARBOHYDRATE

The major carbohydrates in infant formulas have been disaccharides with lactose in the milk-based formulas and sucrose in the soy-based formulas. In an effort to reduce reliance on the more fragile brush border lactase and sucrase, manufacturers have turned to an alternative carbohydrate source, starch. This is primarily provided as tapioca, corn syrup solids, or the hydrolysis product of cornstarch referred to as dextrins or glucose polymers. Digestion of starch requires amylase (pancreatic or mucosal gluco-D-amylase) and maltase, a brush border disaccharidase. The only complete formulas that are free of lactose and sucrose are Prosobee and Pregestimil. CHO-free is marketed without carbohydrate with careful instructions on the can for supplementation with dextrose or alternatives. The use of honey is no longer recommended due to recent reports of contamination with botulism spores.[7]

FAT

The lipid content of infant formulas is generally a mixture of saturated and polyunsaturated long-chain fats (LCT). All of the standard formulas have been vitamin E-enriched due to the polyunsaturated fat content. Infants with reduced lipolytic capacity may benefit from the use of medium-chain triglycerides (MCT), which have less than 12 carbon atoms. Medium-chain triglycerides do not require micellar solubilization for absorption and following absorption are transported via the portal vein rather than lymphatics. MCT-containing formulas are thus recommended for infants whose LCT absorption is restricted by prematurity, operative jejunal or ileal resection, mucosal inflammation, lymphangiectasia, pancreatic insufficiency, or cholestatic liver disease. None of the formulas provides fat exclusively as MCT, because the requirements for linoleic acid, an essential fatty acid that has 18 carbon atoms, would not be met.

OSMOLALITY AND RENAL SOLUTE LOAD

The osmolality of the formula may be a critical factor in gastric emptying and intestinal transit, though the latter is usually of consequence only with intrajejunal feedings or the short bowel syndrome. In normal infants, impairment of gastric emptying does not appear to develop until osmolality exceeds 450 milliosmol (mOsm)/kg H_2O.[8] At standard concentration, only Probana and CHO-free prepared with dextrose exceed this.

Renal solute load is rarely a factor in infants with normal renal function. When formulas are concentrated, however, the reduction in free water may become significant.

ELECTROLYTES AND MINERALS

Sodium potassium, chloride, calcium, phosphorus, and iron contents of the formulas are presented in Table 3. The values are those present when the formula is prepared at standard 20 or 24 calories/oz as noted previously. This table is presented for reference rather than extensive discussion. Routine iron supplementation is now recommended in infancy,[9] though the requirements may alternatively be met with cereals or supplements.

TABLE 3.—ELECTROLYTE AND MINERAL COMPOSITION
OF SELECTED INFANT FORMULAS

FORMULA	Na	K	MEQ/L Cl	Ca	Phos	MG/L Fe
Human milk	7	13	11	17	9	1.0
Cow's milk	24	35	29	60	54	0.5
Similac/Enfamil	12	19	15	26	23	1.4 or 12
SMA	7	14	10	22	16	12.7
PM 60/40	7	15	7	20	12	2.6
Similac LBW	16	26	24	36	33	3.0
Enfamil Premature	14	23	19	48	28	1.2
Isomil	13	18	15	35	29	12.0
Prosobee	18	19	12	40	31	12.7
Goat's milk	15	46	32	61	54	1.0
MBF	8	10	7	50	39	15.0
Probana	27	31	21	58	53	1.4
Nutramigen	14	17	13	32	28	12.0
Portagen	14	22	16	32	28	12.0
Pregestimil	14	18	16	32	28	12.0
Carbohydrate-free	16	23	15	42	25	8.5

Specific Formulations for Infants

MILK-BASED FORMULAS

The nutritional, immunologic, and psychological virtues of human breast milk have been repeatedly extolled.[10] We do, however, encounter limitations to the exclusive use of breast milk in infants with severe lactase deficiency, short bowel syndrome, hepatobiliary disease, and volume restriction secondary to congestive heart failure. Similac, Enfamil, SMA, PM 60/40, and related milk protein-based formulas share these limitations for infants with impaired digestive and absorptive capacity, for they contain lactose and long-chain fat. The advantage of milk-based formulas is their low cost and ready availability.

In an effort to meet some of the unique needs of premature infants, Similac LBW and Enfamil Premature have been introduced. They have more protein (11% to 12% of calories), vitamin D, and phosphorus than breast milk. Because premature infants have reduced lactase, approximately 50% of carbohydrate calories are derived from glucose polymer. Although lactose "intolerance" may appear in neonates as osmotic diarrhea and/or acidosis, it appears that some lactose is essential for the development of normal colonic flora[11] and for maximal calcium uptake.[12] In light of the premature infant's well-documented reduction in jejunal micelle concentration, both formulas provide over 40% of lipid calories as MCT. The widespread use of these formulas has been restricted by frequent constipation and scattered reports of lactobezoar formation.[13]

SOY-BASED FORMULAS

The soy-based formulas were introduced for use in infants who are "milk intolerant." When such intolerance is secondary to isolated reductions in lactase, soy formulas are well tolerated. Soy formulas are extensively used in "allergic" children, but recent studies suggest that soy protein is highly antigenic.[14] The major indication for soy formula is therefore the infant recovering from acute enteritis with acquired lactase deficiency or for infants on vegetarian diets. Casein hydrolysate formulas are also lactose-free but are too expensive for routine use.

GOAT'S MILK

Goat's milk has also been heavily used in "cow's-milk-sensitive" infants. Its value in diarrheal disease is limited because its carbohydrate is lactose. Goat's milk is high in essential fatty acids and also has a higher MCT content than cow's milk. Although its availability is restricted, it is an acceptable substitute for cow's milk with several precautions. Its high protein content precludes its exclusive use in early infancy due to acidosis. Routine folic acid supplementation of goat's milk is mandatory.

MEAT-BASED

Meat-based formula (MBF) is yet another lactose-free, milk-protein-free alternative for infant feeding. Nutritional adequacy for healthy infants has been demonstrated. Experience in infants requiring nutritional rehabilitation is too limited to recommend routine application.

PROBANA

Probana is a high-protein, low-fat formula with milk solids, casein hydrolysate, banana powder, lactose, and long-chain fat. It is marketed as a high-protein formula for infants with malabsorption whose diet is otherwise protein-restricted (e.g., celiac disease). There are no clear-cut indications for its use.

NUTRAMIGEN

Nutramigen is the suitable formula for infants with milk or soy protein sensitivity with or without lactose intolerance. Protein is provided as casein hydrolysate. Because sucrose provides 72% of carbohydrate calories and all of its fat is long chain, its use in severe malabsorption is restricted.

PORTAGEN

Portagen is the only formula providing the majority of fat as MCT on the market today. It is therefore the formula of choice in infants with severe steatorrhea, as in pancreatic insufficiency, cholestatic liver disease, or severe malnutrition. Some sucrase activity is necessary, as sucrose provides 25% of its carbohydrate calories. Until further studies are done, caseinate should not be considered hypoallergenic.

PREGESTIMIL

Pregestimil was reformulated in 1978 from an amino acid, dextrose, MCT preparation of excessive osmolality to its present form. A major appeal is that it is free of lactose and sucrose. Protein is provided as casein hydrolysate supplemented with cystine, tyrosine, and tryptophan. MCT provides 40% of the lipid. It is therefore a suitable formula for infants recovering from severe diarrhea with attendant reductions in small bowel surface area and brush border enzymes.

CARBOHYDRATE-FREE FORMULA

A carbohydrate-free soy protein, soy oil formula, was temporarily withdrawn from the market in late 1979 due to a reduction in chloride concentration. Following reformulation, it was rereleased early in 1980. Its present electrolyte content is noted in Table 3. If carbohydrate is not added to the formula, this is a ketogenic diet. In infants recovering from diarrheal disease, we provide carbohydrate as glucose polymer. Honey, as noted above, is no longer recommended in the first year of life.

Estimation of the Infant's Nutritional Status and Absorptive Capacity

Having reviewed the available alternatives, we turn now to the individualized assessment of the infant's nutritional capacity. The limiting factors to be considered in each patient are summarized in Table 4.

The methods for detailed investigation of nutritional status have been fully outlined elsewhere.[15] However, certain aspects can be reemphasized here. A careful medical history, including a detailed dietary history, may elucidate the causes and duration of the malnutrition and indicate which deficiencies to anticipate. The physical examination should include several anthropometric values, which are helpful in determining both duration and type of malnutrition. Since weight change is an index of recent malnutrition, whereas a decrease in linear growth rate usually develops over longer periods of time, indices such as weight for height, height for age, skinfold thickness, and midarm muscle circumference will give important information on the chronicity of the deprivation. Of the biochemical markers of nutritional status, the serum albumin concentration is a standard reference, though measurement of proteins with shorter half-lives, such as transferrin[16] or retinol-binding protein,[17] are more sensitive indicators of acute protein malnutrition. The majority of malnourished infants in the United States

TABLE 4.—DETERMINANTS OF PATIENT'S
ABSORPTIVE CAPACITY

Severity of malnutrition
Intestinal surface area
Volume tolerance
Osmotic tolerance
Protein tolerance
Carbohydrate tolerance
Fat (long-chain) tolerance

present with mild manifestations of marasmus, such as reduced weight for height, skinfold thickness reduced less than 85% of the ideal, and serum albumin concentrations maintained above 3 gm/dl. For more extensive discussions of marasmus or kwashiorkor, the reader is referred to an excellent review.[18] Nutritional surveys of hospitalized patients have revealed a significant number of infants and children with moderate to severe protein-energy malnutrition.[19]

A major nutritional consequence of prolonged malnutrition in infancy is a reduction in intestinal villus height, which in turn reduces absorptive surface area. Such reduction in surface area is also encountered following enteric inflammation and is most pronounced immediately following bowel resection. As a rough index of upper small bowel surface area, we use the D-xylose absorption test. Assuming that neither gastric emptying nor renal function is impaired, the one-hour blood level is a function of mucosal surface area. Following administration of 5 gm of D-xylose, a serum level at one hour that exceeds 25 mg/ 100 ml is normal in infancy.[20]

Volume tolerance is determined by age, cardiac status, renal function, and fluid losses. In normal infants a peak intake of approximately 180 ml/kg of body weight per day is noted at four months of age.[21] In infants with congestive heart failure, chronic pulmonary disease, or renal failure, the volume and rate limits inhibit caloric intake.

The importance of the osmotic load of a formula is probably overplayed. It is primarily of significance in delaying gastric emptying in sick infants and in decreasing intestinal transit time in infants with surgically shortened bowels. Gastric emptying is a complex process influenced in part by volume, duodenal osmoreceptors, and enteric hormonal responses to feeding.[22] With continuous intragastric drip feedings, an increase in osmolality seems to interfere less with gastric emptying than a calorically equivalent increase in volume. With jejunal feedings, on the other hand, increases in volume may be tolerated better than increases in osmolality. The capacity of a high osmotic load to directly induce small-bowel mucosal damage remains controversial.[23]

Studies on protein utilization in chronically malnourished children suggest that hydrolysates are rarely necessary for recovery.[24] In infants recovering from enteric inflammation, a role for less antigenic hydrolysates has been suggested.[25] As noted previously, soy protein formulas are not ideally suited for nutritional rehabilitation. In infants with confirmed protein sensitivity, severe pancreatic insufficiency, or enterokinase deficiency, hydrolyzed casein is indicated.

Patients with inborn errors of protein metabolism will require much more highly specialized diets. Such diets require supervision by trained nutritionists. Mead Johnson and Company markets formulas designed for infants with phenylketonuria (LOFENALAC), maple syrup urine disease (MSUD Diet Powder), tyrosinemia (Product 3200AB), and homocystinuria (Product 3200K), as well as a formula (Product 80056), which is a protein-free base to which appropriate amino acids may be added. Wyeth Laboratories markets a low-protein formula designed for infants with leucine-sensitive hypoglycemia (S-14). Further information about these diets should be obtained from the manufacturers prior to their use.

Carbohydrate absorption can be assessed by a variety of clinical and laboratory techniques. A less invasive alternative to standard carbohydrate tolerance tests involves measurement of breath H_2 instead of serum glucose concentration following an oral carbohydrate load.[27] When carbohydrate is not absorbed by the small bowel, it can be fermented by colonic bacteria, one product of which is hydrogen gas. The quantity of hydrogen produced is related to the amount of carbohydrate that is not absorbed. The hydrogen is excreted primarily in the breath, which can be analyzed by means of the gas chromatograph. The malabsorbed carbohydrate that undergoes bacterial fermentation may not be totally lost as an energy source, for the bacterial fermentation also produces volatile fatty acids, which can be absorbed by the colon.

Disaccharide intolerance due to reductions in brush border disaccharidases may be noted following any condition that reduces small bowel surface area. As a rule, reductions in lactase will be more severe and prolonged than reductions in sucrase. These acquired reductions in disaccharidase activity should be considered transient in infancy, as even in blacks and orientals the acquired forms of lactase deficiency are rarely permanent until school age. Monosaccharide intolerance has also been reported following severe enteritis.[28] As noted previously, Pregestimil and Prosobee are the only lactose-free and sucrose-free complete formulas on the market. Two formulas requiring carbohydrate supplements are available: CHO-free, from Syntex, and Product 3232A, from Mead Johnson and Company.

Lipid malabsorption, primarily of long-chain fat, will most often be seen in infants with pancreatic insufficiency or cholestasis. Quantitation of the severity of steatorrhea is best obtained with a 72-hour stool fecal fat obtained while on a diet with at least 40% of total calories as long-chain fat. Formulas that contain medium-chain triglycerides as a source of lipid calories include Similac LBW, Enfamil Premature, Portagen, and Pregestimil and may be useful in reversing the steatorrhea in the clinical situation mentioned.

General Management Principles

Working within the constraints cited above, one tries to deliver the appropriate formula in such a fashion as to maximize caloric intake. Unfortunately, simply offering the "ideal" formula is commonly not sufficient to meet the increased caloric demands of these infants. Techniques to meet these "hypercaloric" needs—a reduction of metabolic demands, an increase in the volume of feedings, and an increase in the energy density of feedings—are required.

The first step is to reduce the infant's metabolic demands. The infant with cardiopulmonary disease must have aggressive medical therapy. As a rule, all infants less than six months of age with severely impaired growth are placed in an incubator to reduce caloric demand.

The second step is to determine the enteric as well as cardiopulmonary volume limit for the patient. All solid food is discontinued, as the caloric density of solids rarely approaches that achievable with formulas alone. In the severely compromised infant, we proceed directly to continuous infusion feedings. Formula is delivered by small flexible feeding catheter into the stomach and regulated by infusion pump or intravenous drip chamber. Due to concern for possible aspiration with intragastric infusions, a feeding that will last no longer than two hours should be in the chamber or syringe at any time. Aspirates are checked without prior cessation of the infusion. While normal data on gastric aspirates in infancy are lacking, an aspirate in excess of the previous hour's feeding is considered significant. The advantage of continuous infusion feeding is that it appears to reduce the influence of both volume and osmolality of gastric emptying. A theoretical advantage is the associated reduction in bolus substrate load to the mucosal and intraluminal enzyme systems, thus enhancing efficiency. The advantages of delivering nutrients directly into the stomach are obvious in infants with impaired suck and swallow or excessively rapid respiratory rate. Intraduodenal infusion is rarely undertaken due to the increased risks.

The third step is taken once the infant's volume limit has been reached. Additional nutrients have to be delivered by increasing the density of the formula. Increasing the concentration of the formula has the advantage of maintaining the distribution of calories derived from protein, carbohydrate, and fat. The reduction in free water means that osmolality and renal solute load will increase. Fomon has suggested that urine osmolality be monitored closely and not be allowed to exceed 400 mOsm/L in infancy.[29] The electrolyte and mineral loads will also increase and the sodium load alone may militate against formula concentration in patients with heart disease.

Our technique to increase calorie density is to concentrate the formula initially in a stepwise fashion to 1 kcal/ml. If this is not possible due to the sodium, solute, or protein load, or if further calorie increases are necessary, we supplement the formula with carbohydrate and fat, diluting the protein intake to no less than 8% of total calories. Fat (9 calories/gm) and carbohydrate (4 calories/gm) are usually added in equal caloric concentrations. Unless lipolysis is severely impaired, fat is added as long-chain corn oil to minimize the increase in osmolality. Carbohydrate is usually supplemented as glucose polymer. Supplementation of protein is rarely indicated.

In an effort to illustrate more precisely the principles and alternatives cited above, an approach to the nutritional management of infants with lactose intolerance, protein "sensitivity," intractable diarrhea, the short bowel syndrome, and severe congestive heart failure is discussed below.

LACTOSE INTOLERANCE

Lactose intolerance is a symptom, not a diagnosis. Low intestinal lactase in infancy is usually a self-limited process induced by an acute infectious enteritis or ischemic episode. When low intestinal lactase is secondary to chronic intestinal inflammation, intestinal surface area will also be reduced and chronic growth impairment will be noted. In previously ill children, we proceed directly to Portagen, Pregestimil, or Carbohydrate-Free. Lactose is reintroduced into the diet gradually after a minimum of two to four weeks.

PROTEIN "SENSITIVITY"

In early infancy, sensitivity to both milk and soy proteins present as acute enterocolitis, usually manifested as blood-tinged diarrhea. Formula protein "allergies" no doubt also exist in this age group, but confirmation remains very difficult. We recommend initiation of casein hydrolysate formulas such as Nutramigen or Pregestimil. Goat's milk and MBF remain alternatives in previously healthy infants. We do not reintroduce the potential offending protein until at least nine months of age.

INTRACTABLE DIARRHEA

Intractable diarrhea is defined as frequent, loose stools for longer than four weeks with severe reduction in rate of weight gain. Estimation of absorptive capacity will generally confirm moderate malnutrition with associated reductions in mucosal surface area and brush border enzyme activity. Steatorrhea will be modest and an inflammatory infiltrate may be present. The cause often remains unknown.[30]

Emphasis in the first 48 hours is on correction of fluid, electrolyte, and acid/base imbalance. Enteric feedings are then initiated with either Portagen or Pregestimil. Initial feedings are usually by continuous gastric infusion to control volume and caloric load. On the first day, the infant receives no more than 40 kcal/kg of body weight with continued intravenous (IV) hydration as appropriate for fluid and electrolyte needs. While the formula may be diluted slightly to facilitate hydration, we discourage "quarter-strength" ad-lib feeding where overzealous volume intake and caloric load may induce an overload diarrhea.

If the feedings at 40 kcal/kg of body weight per day are tolerated, increases are made in increments of 10 kcal/kg of body weight per day. If intakes of 75 kcal/kg of body weight per day are not achieved in seven days, peripheral venous alimentation, if not previously initiated, is indicated. Caloric increments are initially made by increasing volume, with energy density held at 0.67 kcal/ml (20 calories/ounce). Once volume limits are reached, generally at 180–200 ml/kg of body weight per day, the energy density is increased, as previously discussed, in 1–2 kcal/ounce increments. If the formula is Portagen, we add LCT up to the amount of MCT already present in the formula. Carbohydrate is generally added as glucose polymer. Weight gain usually occurs at 120–150 kcal/kg of body weight per day; however, energy intakes of up to 200 kcal/kg of body weight per day may be required for weight gain.[31] If diarrhea ensues, we first reduce the volume of feedings by one third, continue parenteral supplementation, and allow a couple of days for stabilization before gradually increasing calories again.

When the desired energy intake is achieved and steady weight gain resumes, we begin to wean the infant slowly to bolus feedings. Any systematic technique will generally suffice, though we begin by infusing four hours of formula over three hours progressing to nipple feedings on an every three-hour to four-hour regimen. Solid feedings are not resumed until at least four weeks of sustained growth are achieved so as to maintain control over caloric intake. Lactose restriction is continued for at least eight weeks. If diarrhea recurs on liberalization of the diet, a malabsorption workup, often including a small bowel biopsy procedure, is appropriate to determine etiology. The concurrent use of parenteral nutrition, antibiotics, bile acid binding resin, etc., has been discussed elsewhere.[30–32]

SHORT BOWEL SYNDROME

Infants with this syndrome, who have less than 50 cm of residual small bowel, present at the extreme of absorptive limitation.[33] The principles of management are similar to those outlined above for intractable diarrhea. While these infants will universally require an extended course of IV alimentation, studies have confirmed the need for enteric nutrition to maximize mucosal hypertrophy and regeneration.[34] Compared to other patients with diarrhea, infants with short bowel are more sensitive to volume and osmolality.

Intragastric feedings by tube or gastrostomy are begun as

soon as viability of the residual bowel is confirmed. As the residual bowel has usually been ischemic, severe villus atrophy is assumed. The initial feedings are thus with Pregestimil or Portagen. On day 1, the formula is prepared as .3 kcal/ml and delivered at 10 kcal/kg of body weight per day. A formula regimen based on Carbohydrate-Free has also been suggested.[35] Calorie increases are made very slowly and it is usually at least one month before 50% of calories can be delivered enterically. Lactose and solids are generally withheld for at least three months.

CONGENITAL HEART DISEASE

Impaired growth is a frequent complication of congestive heart failure in infancy.[36] Growth failure may be both an indication as well as a relative contraindication to surgery. Recent studies have confirmed that there is no specific absorption defect in heart failure in infancy, which further substantiates the hypothesis that the growth failure reflects inadequate energy intake relative to needs, most often due to volume restrictions. Krieger[37] has demonstrated that intakes can be boosted by up to 60 kcal/kg of body weight per day over normal requirements and lead to improved nitrogen retention and weight gain without cardiac decompensation.

Tolerance of volume will be the initial limiting factor in nutritional management. Superimposed malnutrition may also lead to moderate reductions in intestinal surface area. If lactose is tolerated and intervention is early, both PM 60/40 and SMA can be concentrated to 1 kcal/ml with sodium content still below 11 mEq/L (see Table 3). Because volume control is nearly always necessary, we commonly request that breast-feeding mothers initially express the milk and then bottle-feed it to determine volume limits. If desired, the energy density of expressed breast milk can be increased, including supplementation with protein.

If lactose-free feedings are necessary, we use Pregestimil or Portagen. Because they contain 14 mEq/L of sodium and 13% of calories from protein at 0.67 kcal/ml, we prepare the formula as 0.5 kcal/ml and then supplement with fat and carbohydrate to return the caloric density to 0.67 kcal/ml or more. Protein is thus kept at 8% to 10% of total calories, with sodium reduced to 8 to 10 mEq/L. As the electrolyte, mineral, and vitamin contents are also reduced by one third, reassessment of each infant's need will be necessary when volume is severely restricted.

Infants with severe growth failure and congestive failure are placed in incubators, and feedings are again initiated by continuous drip intragastric infusion. We advance the volume steadily to determine each infant's threshhold for failure. Energy density is then slowly increased with close monitoring of sodium, protein, and solute load. Energy densities exceeding 1.5 kcal/ml may be required.

Economic Factors

The cost of the specialized infant formulas should not be a major factor in choosing the most appropriate one, but it is a significant factor in outpatient compliance. As a result, efforts are made to wean the infant to a lower priced and generally more available formula as soon as possible. All too often an infant is readmitted because of family economic priorities. Most will have been switched back to whole milk too quickly, while others present with acute metabolic complications secondary to dilution of the more expensive formula. The relative costs of the formulas are listed in Table 5.

TABLE 5.—COMPARISON OF FORMULA COSTS

FORMULA	AVAILABLE IN	APPROXIMATE COST PER QUART ($)
Similac/Enfamil Premature	RTU,* concentrated liquid, powder	1.07
SMA	RTU, concentrated liquid, powder	1.06
PM 60/40	Powder	1.77
Isomil	RTU, concentrated liquid	1.13
Prosobee	RTU, concentrated liquid	1.13
Probana	Powder	4.03
Nutramigen	Powder	3.26
Portagen	Powder	2.73
Pregestimil	Powder	3.77
Carbohydrate-Free	Concentrated liquid	1.30

*RTU = ready to use.

Summary

This review has focused on the enteric nutritional management of infants with abnormalities of volume tolerance, digestion, and/or absorption. The necessity of individually assessing the patient's needs vis-à-vis the alternatives cannot be overemphasized. In some patients, enteral feedings are precluded and IV alimentation is the only alternative. For a discussion of IV nutrition options we refer the physician to an excellent review.[38] We also wish to emphasize that in a review of this nature we cannot discuss the relative virtues of closely related formulas. We therefore encourage the physician to obtain product handbooks from the manufacturers.

REFERENCES

1. Fomon S.J., Filer L.J., Anderson T.A., et al.: Recommendations for feeding normal infants. *Pediatrics* 63:52, 1979.
2. Committee on Nutrition, American Academy of Pediatrics: Nutritional needs of low-birth-weight infants. *Pediatrics* 60:519, 1980.
3. Committee on Nutrition, American Academy of Pediatrics: Commentary of breast feeding and infant formulas including proposed standards for formulas. *Pediatrics* 57:278, 1976.
4. Fomon S.J., Thomas L.N., Filer J.L., et al.: Requirements for protein and essential amino acids in early infancy: Studies with a soy-isolate formula. *Acta Paediatr. Scand.* 62:33, 1973.
5. MacLean W.G., Graham G.G.: The effect of level of protein intake in isoenergetic diets on energy utilization. *Am. J. Clin. Nutr.* 32:1381, 1979.
6. Mathews D.M., Adibi S.A.: Peptide absorption. *Gastroenterology* 71:151, 1976.
7. Arnon S.S., Midura T.F., Damus K., et al.: Honey and other environmental risk factors for infant botulism. *J. Pediatr.* 94:331, 1979.
8. Hunt J.N., Pathak J.D.: The osomotic effects of some simple molecules and ions on gastric emptying. *J. Physiol.* 154:254, 1960.
9. Committee on Nutrition, American Academy of Pediatrics: Iron supplementation for infants. *Pediatrics* 58:765, 1976.
10. Committee on Nutrition, American Academy of Pediatrics: Breast feeding. *Pediatrics* 62:591, 1978.
11. Barbero G.J., Runge G., Fischer D., et al.: Investigations on the bacterial flora, pH, and sugar content on the intestinal tract of infants. *J. Pediatr.* 40:152, 1952.
12. Duncan D.H.: The physiological effects of lactose. *Nutr. Abst. Rev.* 25:309, 1955.
13. Eaenberg A., Shaw R.D., Yousefzadeh D.: Lactobezoar in the low-birth-weight infant. *Pediatrics* 63:692, 1979.
14. Eastham E.J., Lichauco T., Grady M.I., et al.: Antigenicity of infant formulas: Role of immature intestine on protein permeability. *J. Pediatr.* 93:561, 1978.
15. McLaren D.S., Pillet P.H., Read W.C.: A simple scoring system for classifying the severe forms of protein-calorie malnutrition of early childhood. *Lancet* 1:533, 1967.
16. Smith M.F., Moldawer L.L., Bistrian B.R.: Transferrin as a measure of the efficiency of parenteral and enteral nutrition. *J. Parent. Enter. Nutr.* 1:9A, 1977.
17. Smith F.R., Suskind R., Thanangkul O., et al.: Plasma vit. A retinol binding protein and prealbumin concentration in protein calorie malnutrition. *Am. J. Clin. Nutr.* 29:1089, 1976.

18. MacLean W.C., Romana G.L., Massa E., et al.: Nutritional management of chronic diarrhea and malnutrition: Primary reliance on oral feeding. *J. Pediatr.* 97:316, 1980.
19. Merritt R.J., Suskind R.M.: Nutritional survey of hospitalized pediatric patients. *Am. J. Clin. Nutr.* 32:1320, 1977.
20. Buts J.P., Morin C.L., Roy C.C., et al.: One hour blood xylose tests: A reliable index of small bowel function. *J. Pediatr.* 90:729, 1978.
21. Fomon S.J., Thomas L.N., Filer L.J., et al.: Food consumption and growth of normal infants fed milk-based formulas. *Acta Pediatr. Scand.* 233:1971.
22. Cavell B.: Gastric emptying in infants. *Acta Pediatr. Scand.* 60:370, 1971.
23. Wheeler P.G., Menzies J.S., Creamer B.: The effect of hyperosmolar stimuli and coeliac disease on the permeability of the human gastrointestinal tract. *Clin. Sci. Mol. Med.* 54:495, 1978.
24. Viteri F.E., Flores J.M., Alvarado J., et al.: Intestinal malabsorption in malnourished children before and during recovery. *Am. J. Dig. Dis.* 18:201, 1973.
25. Walker W.A., Isselbacher K.J.: Uptake and transport of macromolecules by the intestine: Possible role in clinical disorders. *Gastroenterology* 67:531, 1974.
26. Newcomer A.K., McGill D.B., Thomas P.J., et al.: Prospective comparison of indirect methods of detecting lactose deficiency. *N. Engl. J. Med.* 298:1232, 1975.
27. Klish W.J., Udall J.N., Rodriguez J.T., et al.: Intestinal surface area in infants with acquired monosaccharide intolerance. *J. Pediatr.* 92:566, 1978.
28. Fomon S.J.: *Infant Nutrition,* ed 2. Philadelphia: W.B. Saunders Co., 1974, p 260.
29. Sunshine P., Sinatra F.R., Mitchell C.H.: Intractable diarrhea of infancy. *Clin. Gastroenterol.* 6:445, 1977.
30. Greene H.L., McCabe D.R., Merenstein G.B.: Protracted diarrhea in infancy. *J. Pediatr.* 87:5, 695, 1975.
31. Lloyd-Still J.D., Shwachman H., Filler R.M.: Protracted diarrhea of infancy treated by intravenous alimentation. *Am. J. Dis. Child.* 125:358, 1973.
32. Wilmore D.W.: Factors correlating with a successful outcome following extensive intestinal resection in newborn infants. *J. Pediatr.* 80:88, 1972.
33. Feldman E.J., Dowling R.H., McNaughton J., et al: Effects of oral venous intravenous nutrition on intestinal adaption after small bowel resection in the dog. *Gastroenterol.* 70:712, 1976.
34. Tepas J.J., Maclean W.C., Kolbach S., et al.: Total management of short gut secondary to midget volvulus without prolonged total parenteral alimentation. *J. Pediatr. Surg.* 13:622, 1978.
35. Mehrizi A., Drash A.: Growth disturbances in congenital heart disease. *J. Pediatr.* 61:418, 1962.
36. Sondheimer J.M., Hamilton J.R.: Intestinal function in infants with severe congenital heart disease. *J. Pediatr.* 92:572, 1978.
37. Krieger I.: Growth failure and congenital heart disease. *Am. J. Dis. Child.* 120:497, 1970.
38. Heird W.C., Winters R.W.: Total parenteral nutrition. *J. Pediatr.* 86:2, 1975.

Lymphadenopathy in Children

ANTRANIK A. BEDROS, M.D.

AND

JULIE P. MANN, M.D.

Loma Linda University School of Medicine
Department of Pediatrics
Loma Linda, California

Introduction

ENLARGED LYMPH NODES are a common finding in children. Most of the time these enlarged nodes represent normal age-related physiologic changes or transient responses to benign local or generalized infections originating from the upper respiratory tract or skin. However, since lymph node enlargement may herald more serious problems such as neoplasm, histiocytosis, or autoimmune disease, it is necessary to be able to distinguish benign lymph node enlargement and enlargement due to life-threatening conditions. The term lymphadenopathy is defined literally as disease of lymph nodes, but it will be used here interchangeably with lymph node enlargement. In this chapter we cover the mechanism of lymph node enlargement and causes of lymphadenopathy and propose a simple approach to reach an etiologic diagnosis in the child with lymphadenopathy.

General Considerations

Lymph nodes are discrete ovoid structures varying in size from a few mm to one to two cm in length, and are widely distributed throughout the body. Anatomically, lymph nodes

0065-3101/81/0028-0341-$03.75

342   ANTRANIK A. BEDROS AND JULIE P. MANN

are divided into the occipital, preauricular, submaxillary and submental, cervical, supraclavicular, mediastinal, axillary, epitrochlear, inguinal, iliac, popliteal, abdominal, and pelvic regions. Each node is divided into a cortical part, with its secondary germinal follicles, and a medullary part. These are both supported by a reticular stroma. The entire structure is surrounded by a fibrous capsule pierced in different directions by afferent lymphatics. All lymphatics are lined by reticuloendothelial cells. Lymph empties into the subcapsular sinuses, filters through the lymphoid tissue, and exits through the hilus of the lymph node into the efferent lymphatic.[1]

Germinal follicles of the cortical portion of the lymph node contain lymphocytes, lymphoblasts, histiocytes, and rare reticulum stem cells. Normally the lymphocytes and lymphoblasts outnumber the histiocytes, but their relative proportions change in different disease states. The subcapsular zones contain lymphocytes; the medullae of the nodes are composed of adult lymphocytes, reticular cells, fibroblasts, and plasma cells.

Both B and T lymphocytes enter the node through peripheral sinuses by exiting into the cortex via postcapillary venules. For undetermined reasons, B cells find their way to the follicles and T cells "home" to the deep cortical areas. The medullary cords contain mostly B cells, including many plasma cells, and it is there that antibody formation occurs.[2]

The "normal" lymph node is usually represented as a static structure. In reality, lymph nodes are among the most labile structures in the body. At birth a considerable amount of lymphoid tissue is present even though lymph nodes are not normally palpable in the neonate.[3] As a result of environmental antigenic stimulation, this intrinsic lymphoid tissue steadily grows until puberty, when it undergoes a relative reduction and progressive atrophy throughout life.[4] Therefore, most children have palpable lymph nodes. These are commonly the cervical, axillary, and inguinal nodes. In contrast, the posterior auricular, supraclavicular, epitrochlear, popliteal, mediastinal, and abdominal nodes are always abnormal when demonstrated either by palpation or radiographic examination.

Lymph node enlargement results from either proliferation of intrinsic lymph node structures or from invasion by extrinsic cells. Proliferation of intrinsic lymph node structures may include the germinal follicles, interfollicular areas, or subcapsular sinuses, and lymphocytes, lymphoblasts, or histiocytes. Lymphocyte or lymphoblast proliferation usually occurs in response to antigenic stimulation. Due to their specific surface receptors, lymphocytes recognize foreign antigens and react by either hyperplasia and differentiation into larger secretory cells, which in turn recruit "bystander" lymphocytes into undergoing a similar process, or by proliferation with repeated cell divisions. This results in a greatly increased number of lymph node lymphocytes and consequent detectable lymph node enlargement. This enlargement is transient if the antigen is removed and lymphocyte activation ceases. If, however, the antigen persists, as in the case of intracellular parasites capable of prolonged survival, the lymph node may be chronically enlarged. Lymphoid hyperplasia as seen in hyperthyroidism and lymphomas is unrelated to antigenic stimulation. Histiocytic accumulation is seen in histiocytosis, some lipid storage diseases, and some forms of Hodgkin's disease.

Generally, bacterial infections are associated with follicular lymphoid reactions, and viral infections are associated with interfollicular lymphoid proliferation. But this is not always so. In certain chronic viral infections such as infectious mononucleosis, the germinal folliculi may appear small and widely separated or even absent due to interfollicular lymphoid proliferation, which is predominately lymphocytic but associated with plasma cells and histiocytes. Cell proliferation in the sinusoidal lining is a constant finding in nodes that drain the extremities, especially the legs. Lymph nodes that drain areas of chronic dermatitis with heavy deposits of lipid and melanin pigment show a striking proliferation of phagocytic sinusoidal cells.

Extrinsic invasion and consequent enlargement occurs with polymorphonuclear leukocytes in infectious lymphadenitis or with malignant cells in leukemias or metastatic tumors such as neuroblastoma or rhabdomyosarcoma.[1, 5-7]

Generalized Lymphadenopathy

Generalized lymphadenopathy is defined as enlargement of more than two noncontiguous lymph node regions. Hepatosplenomegaly may be present. Causes of generalized lymphadenopathy include infections, autoimmune diseases, neoplasms, histiocytoses, storage diseases, benign hyperplasia, drug reaction, and miscellaneous causes (Table 1).

TABLE 1.—ETIOLOGIES OF GENERALIZED
LYMPHADENOPATHY

Infections
  Bacterial
  Viral
  Fungal
  Spirochetal
Autoimmune diseases
  Juvenile rheumatoid arthritis
  Systemic lupus erythematosus
  Serum sickness
Neoplasms
  Primary to the lymph node
    Hodgkin's disease
    Non-Hodgkin's lymphoma
    Angioimmunoblastic lymphadenopathy
  Metastatic to the lymph node
    Acute lymphocytic leukemia
    Acute myelogenous leukemia
    Neuroblastoma
Histiocytosis
  Disseminated histiocytosis (Letterer-Siwe disease)
  Histiocytic medullary reticulosis (malignant histiocytosis)
  Familial erythrophagocytic lymphohistiocytosis
  Sex-linked reticulohistiocytosis with hypergammaglobulinemia
  Familial histiocytosis associated with eosinophilia and
    primary immunodeficiency
Storage diseases
  Niemann-Pick disease
  Gaucher's disease
Drug reaction
  Phenytoin
  Mephenytoin
  Pyrimethamine
  Antileprosy medication
  Antithyroid medication
  Phenylbutazone
  Allopurinol
  Isoniazid
Miscellaneous causes
  Chronic pseudolymphomatous lymphadenopathy
  Primary dysgammaglobulinemia with lymphadenopathy
  Beryllium exposure
  Hyperthyroidism

INFECTION

Infection causes lymph nodes to enlarge from either intrinsic
reactions with antibody formation and hyperplasia, or from direct infection of the node with invasion by organisms and polymorphonuclear cells. Lymph node enlargement from infection

may be accompanied by signs of acute inflammation with heat, reddening of overlying skin, and tenderness. The nodes may remain discrete or may become matted together with resulting necrosis, rupture, and sinus formation. Localized infections cause lymphadenopathy limited to the regional nodes that drain the area of infection. Generalized lymphadenopathy, however, results from systemic infections such as bacterial seeding of the bloodstream from infective endocarditis or staphylococcal abscess.

Generalized exanthems may be associated with generalized lymphadenopathy. Rubella has, as a prominent feature, enlarged, tender lymph nodes that develop four to ten days before the onset of the characteristic rash. Posterior auricular, suboccipital, and posterior cervical nodes are most commonly involved. Adenopathy is at its height during the rash, persists during the following week, and may on occasion last for several months afterward.

Rubeola produces hyperplasia of all lymphoid tissue, including the lymph nodes, tonsils, adenoids, Peyer's patches, thymus, and spleen. Generalized lymphadenopathy is common, but the nodes at the angle of the jaw and in the posterior cervical region are especially prominent. Mesenteric lymphadenopathy may result in abdominal pain, and changes in the mucosa of the appendix may obliterate the lumen and mimic symptoms of acute appendicitis. These lymphoid changes tend to subside with the disappearance of Koplik's spots.

Infectious mononucleosis, caused by the Epstein-Barr virus (EBV), has tender, enlarged cervical lymph nodes as a hallmark of the disease. But generalized lymphadenopathy occurs, with axillary, epitrochlear, inguinal, mediastinal and mesenteric adenopathy being the most common. Cytomegalovirus also produces a mononucleosis-like picture with generalized lymphadenopathy and hepatosplenomegaly. Other exanthematous diseases like scarlet fever, varicella, and adenovirus infections may also produce a mild generalized lymphadenopathy.

Coccidioidomycosis (valley fever) is usually a respiratory disease acquired by inhalation of airborne spores and produces prominent hilar adenopathy. However, disseminated disease with generalized lymphadenopathy, meningitis, bony lesions, and abscesses does occur. This is more common in children than in adults, although the disease does follow a more benign course in the five-to-twelve-year-old age group. Histoplasmosis is another fungal disease that produces respiratory symptoms and hilar adenopathy. It may be disseminated among infants and immunosuppressed patients. Generalized lymphadenopathy, hepatosplenomegaly, fever, endocarditis, pericarditis, or meningitis may develop.

Syphilitic nodes appear within a few weeks to six months after exposure to syphilis. They seldom become massively enlarged but may remain palpable for months after other signs of secondary syphilis have disappeared. In primary syphilis the nodes involved are those in the neighborhood of the chancre, while generalized lymphadenopathy is seen in secondary syphilis. Cervical nodes (Winterbottom's sign), occipital, and epitrochlear nodes are commonly involved. Histopathology of the lymph node shows a follicular hyperplasia with extension into the medulla that sometimes resembles follicular lymphoma.[8, 9]

AUTOIMMUNE DISEASE

Forty-three percent of children with juvenile rheumatoid arthritis [10] of systemic onset have generalized lymphadenopathy. Splenomegaly may be found but hepatomegaly is less common. The lymphadenopathy may be present with other systemic symptoms before joint involvement is apparent and will disappear as the acute inflammatory phase of the disease wanes. Active systemic lupus erythematosus has lymphadenopathy in 70% of patients; this is generalized in 34%.[11, 12] Hepatosplenomegaly is also common. Serum sickness,[13] a hypersensitivity reaction characterized by urticaria, edema, fever, and polyarthralgia, is also associated with generalized lymphadenopathy. The exanthem and generalized lymphadenopathy regress at the same time.

NEOPLASM

Lymphadenopathy due to neoplasm may be either primary to the lymph node, originating from nodal structure, or secondary due to invasion by metastatic malignant cells. Primary involvement of lymph nodes is seen in Hodgkin's disease. Here it presents as a painless swelling of one or more groups of superficial lymph nodes. Cervical adenopathy is present in 80–90%

of patients. Mediastinal adenopathy, seen in 70% of patients, may be suggested by a persistent nonproductive cough and can be demonstrated by chest radiograph. Inguinal adenopathy and extranodal primary sites are both uncommon and occur in less than 1% of patients. Systemic symptoms of intermittent fever (Pel-Ebstein), anorexia, nausea, weight loss, and pruritus may be present in 30% of children, but these are more likely seen in advanced stages of the disease.[14] On physical examination the involved nodes are discrete and firm, even though they may reach considerable size. They do not break down and suppurate, nor do they become fixed to either the skin or deeper structures as in inflammatory reactions. Histologically, the involved lymph nodes show either partial or total obliteration of normal architecture by lymphocytes, histiocytes, eosinophils, and plasma cells. The diagnostic feature is the presence of Reed-Sternberg cells, which are large, pleomorphic, multinucleated cells with prominent nucleoli. The histologic subclassification of Hodgkin's disease is based on the variations in the cellular composition of the infiltrate and the degree of lymphocytic or histiocytic involvement.[15]

Non-Hodgkin's lymphoma designates a heterogenous group of lymphoid malignancies. They are more common than Hodgkin's disease, especially in younger children, and show a male predominance. About 80% of lymphoma arises from lymphatic tissue and 20% originates from such extralymphatic sites as skin, breast, orbit, parotid, ovary, and bone. In contrast to Hodgkin's disease, localization of lymphoma is unusual, for there is both early hematogenous dissemination and lymphatic spread. The presenting symptoms depend on the site of primary tumor and the extent of local and distant disease. Peripheral lymph nodes, commonly the cervical but also axillary, inguinal, epitrochlear, or preauricular, are involved. Enlargement is rapid, often within one to two weeks, and unaccompanied by systemic symptoms. At first the nodes are nontender, firm, and discrete but may later become confluent. The abdomen is the second most frequently involved site and the tumor may occur retroperitoneally or anywhere along the gastrointestinal tract. These children present with abdominal pain, vomiting, and diarrhea. Lymphoma is the most common anatomical lesion causing intussusception in children over six years of age. Mediastinal involvement may present with persistent cough and dyspnea accompanied by clinical signs of superior vena cava obstruction.[15, 16]

Angioimmunoblastic lymphadenopathy or immunoblastic lymphadenopathy is a recently reported, hyperimmune, prelymphomatous condition of unknown etiology that is a rare cause of generalized lymphadenopathy in children.[17-19] It is characterized by mildly enlarged, minimally tender, generalized lymphadenopathy, hepatosplenomegaly, pleuropulmonary infiltration, and systemic symptoms of fever, malaise, polyarthralgia, skin rash, and weight loss. Histologically, the entire node is involved, with proliferation of capillaries, immunoblasts, and plasma cells. Depletion of lymphocytes and interstitial infiltration with acidophilic material may be seen. The course is chronic and unpredictable, with exacerbation and occasional spontaneous remission. Death results from infection, renal or cardiovascular failure, or malignant transformation into immunoblastic sarcoma.

Invasion by extrinsic malignant cells may also be a source of lymphadenopathy. Generalized lymphadenopathy has been reported in 70% of children with acute lymphocytic leukemia and 31% of children with acute myelogenous leukemia.[20, 21] But hepatosplenomegaly, anemia, and thrombocytopenia with accompanying purpura or hemorrhage is frequently the presenting sign. Bone marrow examination is usually diagnostic.

A cervical or supraclavicular mass may be the first physical abnormality detected in neuroblastoma.[15] The tumor arises from neural crest tissue and presents as an abdominal mass in half of the patients. However, because of rapid spread by local invasion or hematogenous or lymphatic metastasis, 70% of children will have metastatic disease at the time of diagnosis. Other nodal groups are less commonly involved than cervical nodes but generalized lymphadenopathy may occur. Diagnosis is made by proper radiographic studies and detection of elevated urine catecholamines.

HISTIOCYTOSES

The histiocytic disorders are a group of diseases that have as their main feature infiltration of tissues by histiocytic cells with varying degrees of differentiation.[22] They may present as either a local, multifocal, or disseminated syndrome. In the disseminated form, Letterer-Siwe disease, generalized lymphade-nopathy and massive hepatosplenomegaly are seen in addition to seborrheic rash, pulmonary infiltrations, marrow failure, and bony lesions.

Histiocytic medullary reticulosis (malignant histiocytosis) is a rapidly fatal disease of young adults. It is characterized by generalized lymphadenopathy, hepatosplenomegaly, fever, ane-mia, thrombocytopenia, and meningitis. Widespread histiocytic infiltration of many organs is found at autopsy. Familial eryth-rophagocytic lymphohistiocytosis is another malignant form of histiocytosis in which generalized lymphadenopathy is in-volved. It is inherited as an autosomal recessive trait. Bone marrow examination is diagnostic; numerous histiocytes show erythrophagocytosis.[23]

Other less commonly seen histiocytoses that may have gen-eralized lymphadenopathy as a part of the disease complex are sex-linked reticulohistiocytosis with hypergammaglobulinemia and familial histiocytosis associated with eosinophilia and pri-mary immunodeficiency.[22, 23]

Storage Disease

In Niemann-Pick and Gaucher's diseases, lipid-laden histio-cytes accumulate in lymph nodes, liver, or spleen, resulting in detectable enlargement. Diagnosis is made by either bone mar-row examination or lymph node biopsy.[24]

Drug Reaction

Lymphadenopathy associated with phenytoin (DPH) and other anticonvulsant drug administration has been well docu-mented. The lymphadenopathy may either be generalized or lo-calized to one (usually the cervical)[31] area, and appears one to two weeks after DPH therapy has begun. A severe, pruritic, maculopapular rash[32] with fever, hepatosplenomegaly, jaun-dice, anemia, leukopenia, and plasmacytosis in the bone mar-row and peripheral blood may appear at the same time or fol-lowing the lymphadenopathy. When DPH is discontinued, symptoms will spontaneously regress over three to four weeks. However, there have been a few reported cases of subsequent development of lymphoma and Hodgkin's disease after DPH

administration.[33, 34] Mephenytoin,[35] pyrimethamine,[36] antileprosy and antithyroid drugs, phenylbutazone, allopurinol, and
isoniazid have all been reported to cause generalized lymphadenopathy.[35, 37]

MISCELLANEOUS

Chronic pseudolymphomatous lymphadenopathy, or chronic
benign lymphadenopathy, in childhood has been described in a
small group of children between one month and 13 years of age
who exhibit generalized lymphadenopathy, splenomegaly and,
less often, hepatomegaly.[30, 38] These children have diffuse hypergammaglobulinemia (usually immunoglobulin G (IgG) and
A (IgA)), thrombocytopenia, lymphocytosis, and autoimmune
hemolytic anemia with a positive Coombs test. Anterior cervical, supraclavicular, and axillary nodes are most frequently involved, but femoral, abdominal, inguinal, and epitrochlear
nodes may also be enlarged. Histologically, the nodes show
nonspecific hyperplasia, primarily of the B cell area. Nodal size
varies from one to ten cm, enlarges with bouts of hemolysis,
and decreases with infections. The disease follows a chronic
course and responds to immunosuppressive drugs.[39] The cause
of this disease is unknown.

Primary dysgammaglobulinemia with a decrease in IgG and
IgA and an increase in IgM has been reported in a 19-month-
old child. This patient also developed fever, macular rash,
lymphadenopathy, and hepatosplenomegaly. Histologically, the
node exhibited nonspecific hyperplasia of the reticuloendothelial areas and small lymphoid follicles.[40]

Other miscellaneous causes of generalized lymphadenopathy
are the granulomatous changes associated with beryllium exposure[41] and the nonspecific lymphoid hyperplasia associated
with hyperthyroidism.[3]

Regional Lymphadenopathy (Table 2)

OCCIPITAL NODES

Occipital nodes are located at the back of the head close to
the edge of trapezium. They drain the posterior scalp. They are
palpable in 5% of normal children and are frequently enlarged

when generalized lymphadenopathy is present. When enlargement is restricted to the occipital nodes, rubella or septic absorption from inflammatory conditions like pediculosis capitis, tinea capitis, or seborrheic dermatitis are common causes.

PREAURICULAR NODES

Preauricular nodes, which are not normally palpable, drain the lateral portion of the eyelids, conjunctivae, skin of the cheek, and temporal region of the scalp. The oculoglandular syndrome, or keratoconjunctivitis, consists of severe conjunctivitis, corneal ulceration, and eyelid edema associated with ipsilateral preauricular or anterior cervical lymphadenopathy, and is caused by a variety of organisms. Trachoma, the obligate intracellular member of the *Chlamydia* family, is the most common cause of this syndrome. It is found worldwide and is endemic in the Middle East and North Africa and among North American Indians living on reservations. Chlamydia is also responsible for a neonatal inclusion conjunctivitis that appears one to two weeks after birth. The presence of preauricular adenopathy may separate chlamydial from gonococcal ophthalmitis, which it closely resembles. Adenovirus infections, characterized by sore throat, follicular conjunctivitis, low-grade fever, and enlarged preauricular and/or posterior cervical nodes, are responsible for "swimming pool epidemics" of the childhood oculoglandular syndrome.[42] Type VIII adenovirus is another etiology of epidemic keratoconjunctivitis associated with intense follicular conjunctivitis, punctate keratitis, low-grade fever, and preauricular adenopathy.[43] Tularemia, listeriosis, tuberculosis, syphilis, cat-scratch fever, herpes simplex, and sporotrichosis have also been described as causes of the oculoglandular syndrome. Swollen preauricular nodes can sometimes be confused with branchial cleft cysts or parotid gland inflammation.[3]

SUBMAXILLARY AND SUBMENTAL NODES

Submaxillary and submental nodes lie under the body of the mandible or between the anterior bellies of the musculus digastricus; drain the teeth, gums, tongue, and buccal mucosa; and are commonly enlarged when those structures are infected.

TABLE 2.—ETIOLOGIES OF REGIONAL
LYMPHADENOPATHY

Occipital nodes
  Septic absorption
    Pediculosis capitis
    Tinea capitis
    Seborrheic dermatitis
  Viral
    Rubella
Preauricular nodes
  Oculoglandular syndrome
    Trachoma and other chlamydia
    Adenovirus
    Tularemia
    Listerosis
    Tuberculosis
    Syphilis
    Sporotrichosis
    Cat-scratch fever
    Herpes simplex
Submaxillary and submental nodes
  Septic absorption from local infection
  Secondary syphilis
  Cat-scratch fever
  Staphylococcus aureus
  Mycoplasma hominis
Cervical nodes
  Infection and infestation
    Viral
      Upper respiratory tract infection
      Infectious mononucleosis (Ebstein-Barr virus)
      Heterophile negative mononucleoses
        Cytomegalovirus
        Toxoplasmosis
        Leptospirosis
        Brucellosis
        Tularemia
    Bacterial
      S. aureus
      Brucellosis
      Group A β-hemolytic streptococcus
      Haemophilus influenzae type B
      Diphtheria
      Tuberculosis
      Atypical tuberculosis
      Leprosy
      Tularemia
    Fungal
      Histoplasmosis
      Candida albicans
      Sporotrichosis
    Parasitic
      Toxoplasmosis

    Hypoderma bovis larva
    Leptospirosis
    Miscellaneous
      Sarcoidosis
      Cat-scratch fever
  Neoplasm
    Hodgkin's disease
    Non-Hodgkin's lymphoma
    Neuroblastoma
    Rhabdomyosarcoma
    Leukemia
  Histiocytosis
    Sinus histiocytosis with massive lymphadenopathy (SHML)
    Histiocytosis X
  Miscellaneous causes
    Mucocutaneous lymph node syndrome (Kawasaki's disease)
    Postvaccination lymphadenopathy
Supraclavicular nodes
  Left supraclavicular node
    Intra-abdominal lesions
  Right supraclavicular node
    Thoracic lesions
Mediastinal nodes
  Bacterial
    Tuberculosis
    Atypical tuberculosis
  Fungal
    Coccidioidomycosis
    Histoplasmosis
    Pneumoconiosis
  Neoplasm
    Lymphoma
  Miscellaneous
    Cystic fibrosis
    Sarcoidosis
    Benign giant lymph node hyperplasia
Axillary nodes
  Septic absorption from local infection or inflammation
  Neoplasm
    Non-Hodgkin's lymphoma
    Malignant histiocytosis
  Miscellaneous
    Rat-bite fever
    Baccillus Calmette-Guérin (BCG) vaccine
    Cat scratch disease
    Sporotrichosis
Epitrochlear nodes
  Septic absorption from local infection or inflammation
  Syphilis
  Cat-scratch fever
  Tularemia
  Sporotrichosis
Inguinal nodes
  Septic absorption

TABLE 2.—*Continued*

Lymphogranuloma venereum and chancroid
Plague and anthrax
Malignant histiocytosis, lymphoma
Scleroderma
Rickettsial infection
Iliac nodes
  Bacterial infection
Popliteal nodes
  Septic absorption
Abdominal and pelvic nodes
  Septic absorption
  Acute nonspecific mesenteric adenitis
  Lymphoma

Nonspecific pharyngitis, diphtheria, scarlet fever, coxsackievirus, secondary syphilis, or herpetic gingivostomatitis may cause this lymphadenopathy. Dental caries or abscesses are associated with an acute unilateral enlargement, as is cat-scratch fever. If the node is unilateral and chronically swollen, especially if it develops gradual adherence to the skin or enlargement of nodes further down the neck with a lilac-red discoloration of the skin, tuberculosis must be considered. *Staphylococcus aureus* has been shown to cause rare cases of neonatal submandibular adenitis, and one patient with submandibular adenitis from *Mycoplasma hominis* has been reported.[44]

CERVICAL NODES

Cervical node enlargement is probably the most frequently encountered childhood lymphadenopathy.[45] These nodes include the superior deep, superficial, and inferior deep cervicals. The superior deep cervicals are located below the angle of the mandible and drain the tongue. The superficial cervicals include the anterior group, which lie along the anterior jugular vein, and the posterior group, which are found in the posterior triangle along the course of the external jugular vein. These drain the external ear and parotid gland. The inferior deep cervicals, including the scalene and supraclavicular nodes, are located in the lower neck. They receive lymphatic drainage from the superficial tissues of the head and neck and also from deeper structures such as the larynx, trachea, and thyroid gland. The scalene and supraclavicular nodes also receive drainage from the entire head and neck, the arms, the superficial thorax, lungs, mediastinum, and abdomen.

Etiologies of cervical lymphadenopathy include infection and infestation, neoplasm, histiocytoses, and miscellaneous causes. Nonlymphoid cervical masses may also mimic cervical lymphadenopathy.

INFECTION AND INFESTATION—Viral upper respiratory tract infections are by far the most common cause of cervical lymphadenopathy. These nodes are soft, minimally tender, and not associated with evidence of redness or warmth of the overlying skin.[46]

Infectious mononucleosis, which is caused by EBV infection, presents with fever, malaise, and tonsillitis following an upper respiratory tract infection. Tender and enlarged cervical lymph nodes are the hallmark of infectious mononucleosis, the anterior and posterior cervical chains being those most commonly involved. The lymph nodes are enlarged singly or in groups, vary from five to 25 mm in diameter, and are firm, discrete, and tender on palpation. The diagnosis in children and adolescents can be confirmed by a positive heterophile reaction. Children and infants, however, may be heterophile negative, and determination of antibody response to EBV antigens may be necessary to confirm the diagnosis in them.[47]

Heterophile negative mononucleoses are caused by other infectious agents and can clinically be similar to EBV-caused infectious mononucleosis. This group includes cytomegalovirus (CMV) infection, toxoplasmosis, leptospirosis, brucellosis, and tularemia.

A CMV infection can cause cervical adenopathy, fever, tonsillitis, and atypical lymphocytosis. But CMV infection is more frequently associated with the administration of blood products and organ transplantation. This postperfusion syndrome results in fever and atypical lymphocytosis without tonsillitis or adenopathy.[48]

Toxoplasmosis is not a rare disease. Approximately 35% of the United States population is infested with the *Toxoplasma gondii* parasite, which is responsible for 10% of heterophile negative mononucleosis in children and adults.[49] Household cats and undercooked meat are the most common sources of infestation. Asymptomatic lymphadenopathy is the most common manifestation of the disease. Clinically, toxoplasmosis may result in generalized lymphadenopathy involving superficial nodes or the deep mediastinal, mesenteric, or peritoneal chains. The cervical region is involved in 82% of patients. The nodes are slightly tender, nonadherent to each other, unilateral or bilateral, and variable in size. Enlargement may persist for months. A diffuse maculopapular, nonpruritic rash that spares the palms, soles, and scalp may be present for three to four days. Splenomegaly and pharyngitis are uncommon, but myocarditis and meningitis may be part of the syndrome. IgM fluorescent antibody titers to toxoplasmosis rise very early in the course of the disease and reflect active infection. Clinically, the condition is mild but should be treated in order to prevent reactivation in later life.[49-51]

Leptospirosis should be suspected in a mononucleosis-like illness with both cervical lymphadenopathy and central nervous system involvement. Diagnosis is made by agglutination titers; blood or urine cultures will occasionally reveal leptospiral organisms.[52]

Brucellosis is transmitted to man from contact with infected domestic animals or by the ingestion of milk or milk products containing viable *Brucella* organisms. Patients present with a mononucleosis-like syndrome of myalgia, weakness, chills, headache, and arthralgia. Many acutely ill patients have small, nontender cervical and axillary lymph nodes. Cervical adenopathy occurs in 50% of patients, splenomegaly in 50% of bacteremic patients and moderate hepatomegaly in 25%. Both organs are occasionally tender. Diagnosis is made either by positive blood culture or by an elevated agglutination titer for brucellas.[53]

Tularemia may assume many forms depending on the mode of infection. It may be transmitted by tick bite, handling of infected animals, ingestion of contaminated meat or water, or inhalation of bacteria. The ulceroglandular form accounts for four fifths of all cases. The skin may be insignificantly ulcerated at the point of entry, but the regional nodes draining the site of the lesion are tender and enlarged and may suppurate. Generalized lymphadenopathy may be present. An oculoglandular syndrome accounts for less than 1% of cases. Pain, photophobia, intense congestion, and lacrimation is present and the cervical and preauricular lymph nodes are enlarged and frequently suppurative. A diagnosis of tularemia should be suspected in the patient with suppurative lymphadenitis who fails to respond to routine antibiotics, especially if there is a history of recent insect bite. Diagnosis is made either serologically, using the agglutination test, or by immunofluorescent studies of infected tissues.[54, 55]

Bacterial infections of the upper respiratory tract, impetigo, severe acne of the head and neck, or dental abscesses may result in acute cervical lymphadenitis. Clinically, the nodes are enlarged and tender and may become fluctuant with erythema of the overlying skin. Group A β-hemolytic streptococcus is a common etiology of cervical lymphadenitis in children but the incidence of S. aureus is increasing.[43, 56] Suppurative adenitis is unusual in infants less than four months of age but several cases have been reported due to S. aureus.[57-60] Haemophilus influenzae type B,[61] Candida albicans,[62] and histoplasmosis[63] are less common etiologies of cervical lymphadenitis. Diphtheria presents with bilateral cervical adenitis, which occasionally gives the child a "bull neck" appearance.[3]

Mycobacteria causes between 1% and 6% of all cases of serious cervical lymphadenitis in children. When Mycobacterium tuberculosis is the responsible organism, pulmonary or systemic disease is apparent. Cervical nodes are involved bilaterally and are initially discrete, mobile, and tender but as the infection progresses they become fixed, matted, and suppurative. The incidence of pulmonary tuberculosis has decreased significantly over the last 25 years with efficient public health control. The incidence of mycobacterial cervical lymphadenitis, however, has not dropped proportionately. It is now recognized that the majority of these infections are due to atypical mycobacteria or mycobacteria other than tuberculosis (MOTT).[64] M. avium, M. intracellulare, and M. fortuitum[65] have been reported as etiologic agents. A node at the angle of the mandible is frequently involved. This node is initially freely movable but becomes attached to the overlying skin, which then looks hyperemic or like parchment. A chest radiograph is usually negative. Skin testing with Double Mantoux or PPD will help differentiate mycobacterial adenitis from pyogenic bacterial adenitis.[64] In addition, repetitive skin testing with PPD over a three- to five-month period is also useful in differentiating adenitis caused by MOTT from that due to M. tuberculosis. Chil-

358

dren with atypical mycobacterial lymphadenitis will have a decreasing tuberculin response to repeated testing with PPD, while children with tuberculous adenitis will show a stable response.[66] A history of recent exposure to tuberculosis is frequently elicited and evidence of extralymphatic tuberculosis is also helpful in differentiating typical from atypical mycobacterial infections. Since response to drug therapy in atypical infections is disappointing and dissemination of the disease is rare, total surgical excision of the involved node is the definitive treatment. Antituberculous drugs should be used only when surgery is impossible or complete excision cannot be performed.[67-70]

Sarcoidosis should be considered in black children who present with bilaterally enlarged, discrete, rubbery cervical lymphadenopathy. Generalized lymphadenopathy in 23–37% of patients[71] and keratitis, iritis, skin lesions, bone cysts and spotty decalcifications may also be associated with it. Chest radiograph shows enlarged hilar nodes, peribronchial fibrosis, midlung field streakiness, or diffuse mottling simulating hilar tuberculosis. Over 80% of children will also have involvement of the scalene nodes. Noncaseous granuloma will be noted on pathologic study of the biopsied node.[72-73]

Cat-scratch fever develops four to 30 days after contact with an infected kitten, dog, or monkey. Preauricular nodes may enlarge secondary to conjunctivitis, but cervical nodes are more frequently involved. Occasionally unusual nodes will be affected in the drainage area of the lesion and present under the edge of the pectoral or trapezius muscle, beneath the sternocleidomastoid in the midline of the neck, or in epitrochlear nodes. Infected nodes are grossly enlarged and tender and are associated with fever, headache, and malaise. Generalized adenopathy does not occur and the white blood cell count remains normal.[74] Diagnosis can be made by demonstrating a delayed reaction to cat-scratch antigens, but the safety of this agent has been questioned.[75]

Leprosy[76] and invasion of cervical lymph nodes with gadfly larvae[77] are rare etiologies of cervical lymphadenopathy.

NEOPLASM.—Approximately 27% of malignant childhood tumors present in the head and neck region and, excluding the orbit and brain, cervical lymph nodes are the most common site of involvement.[72] Etiology of malignant cervical nodes varies according to the age of the child. During the first six years of life, neuroblastoma and leukemia are the most common causes, followed by non-Hodgkin's lymphoma and rhabdomyosarcoma. In contrast, Hodgkin's disease followed by non-Hodgkin's lymphoma is the most common etiology over age six. Although non-Hodgkin's lymphoma is twice as common as Hodgkin's disease, a child with a malignant neck mass has an equal chance of having either disease. This is because 80–90% of children with Hodgkin's disease but only 40% of children with non-Hodgkin's lymphoma have a neck mass.[78]

Rhabdomyosarcoma is the most common solid tumor of the head and neck in children aged one to six years,[78–80] and usually arises in the nasopharynx or the ear. Children may present early in the course of the disease with chronic adenoiditis or serous otitis media as a result of eustachian tube obstruction. However, enlarging cervical adenopathy and chronic serosanguineous nasal discharge should raise a suspicion of neoplasm. Weight loss and involvement of the fifth, sixth, and seventh cranial nerves due to basilar skull invasion are late signs.

HISTIOCYTOSIS.—Sinus histiocytosis with massive lymphadenopathy (SHML) is a benign form of histiocytosis.[81, 82] More than 130 patients ranging from one year to 51 years of age have reportedly had it.[83] However, 62% of such patients present in the first ten years of life and 80% present before age twenty. Males are affected twice as often as females. Clinically, patients present with massive, painless lymph node enlargement, usually in the cervical area (95%), but in 78% of patients other nodes are affected as well. Symptoms of fever (56%), weight loss (18%), arthralgia, myalgia, and weakness are seen. Anemia (78%), leukocytosis (38%) with neutrophilia (45%), a high sedimentation rate, and diffuse hypergammaglobulinemia with marked IgG elevation may be found on laboratory investigation. On physical examination about 25% of patients will have extranodal manifestations of the disease with histiocytic infiltration of the eyelids, upper respiratory tract, skin, salivary glands, and testes. Proptosis with palpable orbital tumors in the absence of obvious lymphadenopathy has been reported in a few children.[84] Osteolytic or osteoblastic bone lesions are rare, and hepatosplenomegaly does not occur. There have been a few reported patients with cranial nerve impairment secondary to involvement of the epidural space. Treatment with cytotoxic agents resulted in a dramatic decrease in nodal size and disappearance of neurological symptoms.[85] Children with SHML are often initially suspected of having lymphoma, but lymph node biopsy is diagnostic. Histologically, the nodes show dilatation of the sinuses, with benign-appearing macrophages that contain phagocytosed lymphocytes. Clinically, SHML runs a protracted course with spontaneous remission and exacerbations. The response to steroids and chemotherapy is questionable, but in some patients irradiation reduces the size of the nodes. Follow-up of 65 patients showed that in 20 the disease disappeared in six months to ten years from diagnosis, but that in 40 others the disease persisted for six months to 21 years after diagnosis. The etiology of SHML is unknown; EBV and leptospirosis have been suspected.

The localized form of histiocytosis X may also present with cervical lymphadenopathy.

MISCELLANEOUS CAUSES.—The mucocutaneous lymph node syndrome (Kawasaki's disease) is a rare childhood disease of unknown etiology that causes nonsuppurative cervical lymphadenopathy.[86] Infants and children under nine years of age are primarily affected and present with a diffuse polymorphous exanthem, hyperemia of the palms, soles, lips, and tongue, conjunctivitis, fever, and cervical node enlargement. Nonpurulent, often unilateral, cervical lymph node enlargement (1.5 cm. or more in diameter) is noted commonly at the first presentation or thereafter. Cervical lymphadenopathy can be of such marked degree that retropharyngeal or peritonsillar abscess may be suspected. The mass diminishes in size usually at the time of defervescence. Generalized lymphadenopathy does not occur. Histological abnormalities in cervical lymph node biopsy specimens are nonspecific. Approximately 1–2% of children will develop coronary artery aneurysms and may die of myocardial infarction. There is no specific therapy for this syndrome and treatment is symptomatic.

Painless cervical node enlargement mimicking lymphoma has been reported three to four days after deltoid administration of DPT vaccine and one to three weeks after smallpox vaccine.[87] Lymphadenopathy has also been reported following immunization with live attenuated measles virus,[88] Salk vaccine, or typhoid fever vaccination.[33]

Nonlymphoid cervical masses.—Nonlymphoid masses may be discovered in a child's neck and must be differentiated from cervical lymphadenopathy.[46] Cervical ribs are firm, immovable, and readily diagnosed by cervical radiographs. Thyroglossal duct cysts are usually located at the level of the hyoid in the midline, may have a fistula, and retract with protrusion of the tongue or move with swallowing. Branchial cleft cysts also retract with swallowing but are located along the anterior border of the sternocleidomastoid muscle and may have a mucus-producing fistula. Cystic hygromas compress, transilluminate, and enlarge with straining. Hemangiomas are similar to cystic hygromas but are smaller and have a bluish tinge. Sternocleidomastoid tumors are transient, hard, spindle-shaped fibromas found in the upper half of the sternocleidomastoid muscle of two- to five-week-old infants. These tumors are associated with faciocranial asymmetry, scoliosis, or thoracic asymmetry and usually disappear by two years of age. Neonatal goiters are midline and move with swallowing. Café au lait spots are helpful in differentiating cervical neurofibromas from enlarged cervical nodes. Dermoid cysts found in the midline feel doughy, cystic, and nontender and do not transilluminate. Teratomas are similar to dermoid cysts. Calcifications or tooth remnants, however, may be noted on radiographs.

SUPRACLAVICULAR NODES

Supraclavicular nodes drain the entire head and neck, the arms, superficial thorax, lungs, mediastinum, and abdomen. The left supraclavicular node is close to the thoracic duct, and is frequently enlarged secondary to intra-abdominal lesions (Troisier's sign), and when present without other cervical lymphadenopathy, suggests an intra-abdominal tumor or inflammation. The right supraclavicular node drains areas of the lung and mediastinum and is often enlarged in thoracic lesions.

MEDIASTINAL NODES

Lymph from the thoracic viscera, including the lungs, heart, thymus, and thoracic esophagus, drains through the mediastinal lymph nodes before entering the thoracic duct or right lymphatic duct. Supraclavicular lymphadenopathy implies mediastinal lymphadenopathy; a variety of physical signs and symptoms should also lead to that suspicion. Signs of bronchial obstruction with cough and wheezing, laryngeal paralysis with hoarseness and inspiratory stridor, paralysis of the left leaf of the diaphragm, dysphagia from esophageal compression, compression of the superior or inferior vena cava with swelling of the neck and face, and swelling of the arm due to subclavian vein compression, may all be found. However, mediastinal node enlargement can only be demonstrated by chest radiograph. Chronic pulmonary diseases cause mediastinal lymphadenopathy, in contrast to acute bacterial or viral infections, which rarely do. Tuberculosis causes unilateral hilar lymphadenopathy in 86% of patients but bilateral enlargement in only 9%. Occasionally, a caseous node may obstruct the right bronchus in early postprimary tuberculosis, or pulmonary atelectasis may result from peritracheal node enlargement. Coccidioidomycosis, histoplasmosis, and sarcoidosis can cause bilateral hilar adenopathy; these nodes are frequently calcified.[3] Childhood lymphomas also result in bilateral hilar adenopathy but are not associated with nodal calcification. Other chronic pulmonary diseases such as cystic fibrosis and pneumoconiosis may cause hilar lymphadenopathy.[89]

Benign giant lymph node hyperplasia (BGLNH), or Castleman-Iversen disease,[25] presents as a large lymphoid tumor up to 20 cm in diameter, most commonly in the hilar areas of the mediastinum. The cervical, axillary, retroperitoneal, mesenteric, and pelvic regions may less frequently be involved, as may soft tissues of the shoulder and broad ligament of the uterus.

Histologically, BGLNH has been divided into the hyaline-vascular (80–90% of patients) and the plasma-cellular (10–20%) types.[25] Clinically, children with the hyaline-vascular type may be totally asymptomatic despite a large tumor or may present as having a space-occupying lesion. Systemic symptoms are rare.[26] In contrast, children with the plasma-cellular type commonly present with a syndrome of fever, polyarthralgia, iron-deficiency anemia,[27, 28] a high sedimentation rate, and hypergammaglobulinemia (usually IgG and IgA).[29, 30] Peripheral lymphadenopathy, hepatosplenomegaly, abnormal liver functions, thrombocytosis, leukocytosis, bone marrow plasmacyto-

sis, growth retardation, peripheral neuropathy, and the nephrotic syndrome have also been reported. These symptoms disappear with removal of the giant node. The etiology of BGLNH
is unknown.

The normal thymus may be quite large in early childhood
and may be mistaken for mediastinal lymphadenopathy, but
its location in the anterior superior mediastinum is apparent
on lateral chest radiograph. Dermoid cysts and teratomas are
also located in the anterior mediastinum but may demonstrate
skeletal elements or teeth on chest radiograph. Ganglioneuro-
mas and neuroblastomas are located in the posterior mediastinum. Bronchial adenomas are located more peripherally than
hilar nodes. Substernal goiters can be associated with palpable
suprasternal goiters, and barium swallow examination will
show the mediastinal shadow rising with swallowing and the
mass will show radioactive iodine uptake. Pericardial cysts are
usually located in the right cardiophrenic angle.[90]

AXILLARY NODES

Axillary nodes drain the hand, arm, chest wall, upper and
lateral abdominal wall, and part of the breast. Septic absorption from local bacterial infection or inflammation, as in rheumatoid arthritis of the upper extremities, is the most common
cause of axillary adenopathy. However, if the axillary nodes
enlarge rapidly without an obvious infective cause, malignancy
must be considered. Non-Hodgkin's lymphoma and malignant
histiocytosis are more likely to present in this manner than is
Hodgkin's disease. Rat-bite fever, with maculopapular rash and
relapsing fever, is associated with large tender axillary nodes
following a bite on the hand.[91] *Bacillus Calmette-Guérin* (BCG)
vaccine in the deltoid can cause axillary node calcification detectable on chest radiograph.[62] Cat-scratch fever may cause
massive axillary lymphadenopathy. Sporotrichosis is characterized by multiple subcutaneous nodules that appear along the
course of lymphatics draining the primary lesion, usually on
the hand or fingers. These nodules and regional (usually axillary or epitrochlear) lymph nodes may become discolored and
drain spontaneously but are not painful, and there are no systemic symptoms.

EPITROCHLEAR NODES

Epitrochlear nodes drain the superficial lymphatics of the middle, ring, and little fingers and the medial aspect of the hand and forearm. Lymphadenopathy of epitrochlear nodes is most often the result of septic absorption from a streptococcal or staphylococcal skin infection. However, rheumatoid arthritis or more deep-seated infections such as cellulitis or arthritis may also cause epitrochlear lymphadenopathy. Cat-scratch fever or tularemia may cause suppurative epitrochlear adenopathy. In secondary syphilis chronically enlarged bilateral epitrochlear nodes can be found and may remain enlarged for life. Epitrochlear nodes are also commonly involved when generalized lymphadenopathy is present.[93]

INGUINAL NODES

Inguinal nodes drain the scrotum and penis in the male, the vulva and vaginal mucosa in the female, the skin of the lower abdomen, perineum, and gluteal region, the lower part of the anal canal, and the lower extremities. One should search for local signs of infection because septic absorption is the most common cause of inguinal lymphadenopathy. Most children with lymphogranuloma venereum acquire the disease by direct transmission from an infected adult. Chronically enlarged and tender inguinal lymph nodes are the most prominent manifestation of the disease and may be the only sign. These nodes often suppurate, become matted together, and form draining sinuses. Rectal and anal strictures are uncommon in children, and systemic symptoms are mild.[94] In chancroid, which is caused by *Hemophilus ducreyi*, lymphadenopathy is frequently suppurative and the organism will be demonstrated on Gram stain of the pus.[95] Bubonic plague is transmitted from wild animals to man and occurs in the western United States. It is a rare disease but 75% of the reported cases occur in patients less than 25 years of age. Onset is variable; patients present with malaise, fever, and pain or tenderness in an area of regional lymph nodes or significant lymph node enlargement (the bubo). The inguinal and axillary regions are most commonly involved, but supraclavicular, epitrochlear, cervical, or popliteal lymphadenopathy may occur. The progress of the disease may be extremely rapid: a patient may appear mildly ill, with fever and adenitis, and progress to a moribund state within hours. Suppurative lymphadenopathy is also seen in anthrax. Fever, rash, and inguinal lymphadenopathy are seen in rickettsial infections following arthropod bites on the lower extremities. A rapidly enlarging inguinal node without other obvious cause, as is seen in axillary nodes, is reason for concern about neoplasm. Malignant histiocytosis has been reported in inguinal nodes. Patients present with fever, lymphadenopathy, weakness, anemia, leukopenia, and thrombocytopenia. Bone marrow aspirate reveals proliferation of abnormal histiocytes showing phagocytosis of red cells, platelets, and white cells. Lymph node biopsy will be diagnostic in 30–50% of patients.[96] Scleroderma, a connective tissue disorder of unknown etiology, involves the skin, gastrointestinal tract, heart, lung, and kidney but has been reported as presenting with inguinal lymphadenopathy.[97] Lymph node biopsy shows noncharacteristic reactive changes and hyperplasia, but microscopic examination of skin and muscle biopsies may be diagnostic.

Inguinal hernias, lipomas, aneurysms, ectopic testes, ectopic spleens, and inguinal endometriosis can also be confused with enlarged inguinal nodes.

ILIAC NODES

Iliac nodes drain the lower abdomen, including the infraumbilical abdominal wall and portions of the genitalia, urethra, and bladder. These can be detected by deep palpation over the inguinal ligament. Acute iliac adenitis, secondary to group A β-hemolytic streptococcus or S. aureus, may follow abdominal trauma, appendicitis, infections of the urinary tract, lower extremities, or occasionally upper respiratory tract. Patients will present with fever, abdominal and/or hip pain, and psoas spasm and will limp, lie in bed with the thigh flexed and abducted, and be unable to extend the leg. No limitation of hip motion except for extension will be demonstrated on examination and this will help differentiate the condition from true hip disease. Acute iliac adenitis can also be differentiated from appendicitis by lack of nausea and vomiting and initial hip or thigh pain rather than abdominal pain.[98]

POPLITEAL NODES

These nodes drain the knee joint and skin on the lateral side of the lower leg and foot, and are not palpable unless quite enlarged. The only cause for popliteal lymphadenopathy is local septic absorption from etiologies similar to those that cause epitrochlear lymphadenopathy.

ABDOMINAL AND PELVIC NODES

These nodes drain the lower extremities and all the pelvic and abdominal organs. Any inflammatory condition of the bowel may lead to their enlargement, especially if there is a break in the mucous membrane, as in patients with ulcerative colitis, dysenteric tuberculosis of the bowel, typhoid fever, or undulant fever. Abdominal and pelvic lymphadenopathy may cause abdominal pain or discomfort, backache, constipation, urinary frequency, hematuria, jaundice, and intestinal obstruction due to intussusception. Nodal enlargement may occasionally be detected by direct abdominal palpation or rectal examination. Any disorder that causes generalized adenopathy will also result in abdominal adenopathy and many of the abovementioned symptoms may follow. This explains the frequent association of abdominal pain and vomiting with streptococcal pharyngitis and abdominal pain in 20% of patients with acute rheumatic fever.[99]

The abdominal masses noted in a patient with tuberculosis are rarely the calcified nodes themselves but rather extensive inflammatory and caseous mattings formed around a node nucleus. These may result in recurrent right lower quadrant pain, nausea, vomiting, and weakness. Unlike appendicitis, there is no fever or leukocytosis, and radiographic studies show local intestinal spasm and reverse peristalsis in addition to calcification of nodes. These nodes, unlike superficial nodes involved in tuberculosis, seldom suppurate.

Nonspecific mesenteric adenitis in children is accepted as being of viral origin. It is relatively common in children and is characterized by recurring right lower quadrant abdominal pain associated with enlarged inflamed mesenteric nodes in the region of the ileocecal valve. Patients may exhibit Brennan's sign when turned on the left side, which is a shift of the point of maximal abdominal tenderness to the left because of the mobility of the mesentery.[99]

About one half of all childhood lymphomas involve abdominal nodes but these are rarely palpable. These nodes, however, can cause ascites due to portal vein compression or edema due to iliac vein compression and will change rapidly in size with infection or chemotherapy.

Management of the Child With Lymphadenopathy

Although lymphadenopathy, whether generalized or localized, is a frequently encountered childhood problem, there is no diagnostic size, appearance, or shape of a lymph node mass that will absolutely distinguish it from insignificant masses. Even neoplasms such as lymphoma or metastatic neuroblastoma begin as small insignificant swellings. Obviously, a careful history and physical examination will indicate the correct diagnosis in many patients. An infant with a large, warm, tender, fluctuant cervical mass must be considered to have staphylococcal cervical adenitis and does not present the diagnostic dilemma of a relatively asymptomatic patient with generalized lymphadenopathy, low-grade fever, and fatigue. However, some arbitrary guidelines—history and physical examination, observation, testing, treatment, and biopsy—can aid in the management of the child with lymphadenopathy.[100]

The history should include the duration of the lymphadenopathy and any associated symptoms or current medications. Complaints of skin lesions, abrasions, or other infections in the region drained by the involved nodes should be elicited, as should a history of cat scratch, insect or rodent bite, or exposure to other ill persons.

Physical examination should include location of the lymphadenopathy—isolated supraclavicular or axillary lymphadenopathy is of much more concern than cervical lymphadenopathy. Lymph node size should be measured and recorded and the character of the node, whether tender, fluctuant, adherent to adjacent structures, or firm, should also be noted. Other pertinent physical findings, such as hepatosplenomegaly or petechiae, are also important.

The physician can elect to observe an enlarged lymph node for a period of weeks, provided that the history and physical

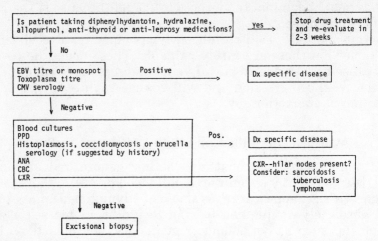

Fig 1.—Basic algorithm for workup of child with generalized lymphadenopathy.

examination do not strongly indicate an infectious or malignant etiology. Measurement of the lymph node and notation of any changes in the character of the involved node or the presence of any new systemic complaints should be recorded at every office visit.

Testing by complete blood count, erythrocyte sedimentation rate, or other specific tests suggested by the history and physical examination, such as chest radiograph, tuberculin and other skin tests, toxoplasmosis or cytomegalovirus antibody titer tests, reaction tests or needle aspiration of a fluctuant node, may be done either at the initial or during follow-up office visits.

Treatment with two to four weeks of appropriate antibiotic therapy is necessary in suspected infectious etiologies to document response. Failure of reduction in nodal size is an indication for further diagnostic workup and consideration for excisional biopsy.

Excisional biopsy with microscopic examination is used to more definitively reach an etiologic diagnosis. A patient becomes a candidate for the procedure if the initial physical examination and history suggests malignancy, laboratory testing is inconclusive and the lymphadenopathy persists or enlarges, or appropriate antibiotic therapy fails to shrink the node.[101, 102]

The algorithm presented in Figures 1–3 is a basic guideline for evaluation of the child with lymphadenopathy.[72, 101, 102] It is

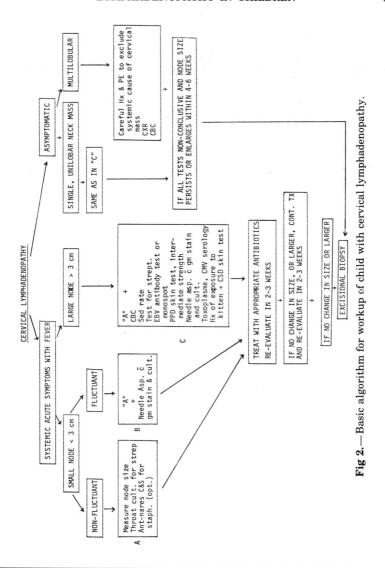

Fig 2.—Basic algorithm for workup of child with cervical lymphadenopathy.

not intended as a comprehensive outline, nor does it include diagnostic tests for rare diseases. It includes only those groups of lymph nodes detectable on physical examination. However, this algorithm will provide a starting point for a stepwise approach to diagnosing the majority of causes for childhood lymphadenopathy.

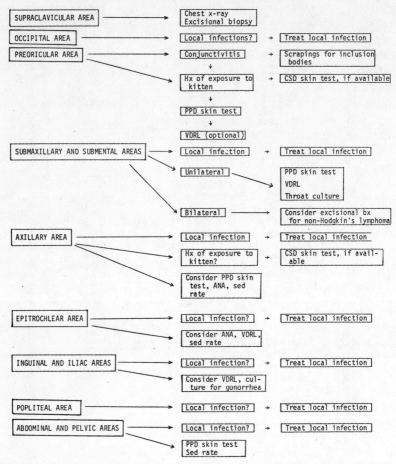

Fig 3.—Basic algorithm for workup of child with localized lymphadenopathy.

Excisional Biopsy

Pediatricians must frequently decide whether and when to biopsy an enlarged lymph node. In most patients, consideration of the child's age, history, associated physical findings, routine hematologic studies, skin tests, and simple radiographic studies are all that are necessary to arrive at a correct diagnosis. If, however, after these initial diagnostic procedures one suspects but cannot otherwise confirm a diagnosis of neoplasm, storage disease, CMV infection, or sarcoidosis, lymph node biopsy for histopathologic examination is indicated. In children with acutely enlarged and inflamed lymph nodes suspected of having lymphadenitis, aspiration rather than biopsy of lymph nodes is indicated because examination and culture of such aspirates can be helpful in choosing an appropriate antibiotic therapy.

When the decision has been made to biopsy an enlarged lymph node, a positive yield in which the clinical diagnosis is confirmed, changed, or excluded can be expected in 40–60% of patients. Lake and Oski,[103] in a series of 75 pediatric patients, found that 55% had nondiagnostic hyperplasia, 21% noncaseating granulomatous lymphadenitis, 7% caseating granulomatous lesions, and 17% lymphoreticular malignant neoplasm.

The three major reasons for diagnosis failure in biopsy of lymph nodes are inadequacy or distortion of the specimen during biopsy, biopsy of the wrong lymph node, or biopsy of the right lymph node early in the course of an illness, when changes may be subtle and nondiagnostic. The largest, firmest palpable node available should be chosen for excisional biopsy, particularly if there are reactive changes between the nodes and surrounding tissues. More than one node should be removed if possible and irradiated areas avoided. Lymph nodes must be meticulously handled during the procedure, and crushing clamps or retractors should not be placed directly on the nodes to avoid injury to the node itself. As a general rule, biopsy of cervical or supraclavicular nodes are preferable to biopsy of inguinal nodes when other considerations are the same. Inguinal nodes are frequently enlarged from chronic infection and their architecture is often distorted. Unless they are grossly enlarged, axillary nodes may be difficult to find during surgery because of the complex anatomy of this area.[104, 105]

Since the interpretation of lymph node biopsy specimens is based primarily on cellular characteristics, the handling of lymph nodes after removal must be carefully considered in order to produce the highest possible positive yield.[106] Margolis et al.[107] have devised a practical protocol for processing specimens of lymph nodes for biopsy. The entire node is bisected under sterile conditions immediately upon removal by a pathologist or surgeon in the operating room. Further studies are then performed, depending on the appearance of the cut surface of the lymph node. These are divided into three main groups:

372 ANTRANIK A. BEDROS AND JULIE P. MANN

GROUP 1.—If there is pus or caseous necrosis, permanent microscopic sections and Gram and acid-fast stains and cultures (aerobic and anaerobic, acid-fast and fungal) are obtained.

GROUP 2.—If there is nodular or diffuse infiltration of the lymph node, a frozen section is immediately obtained. If malignant disease is present, the remainder of the node is submitted for permanent section and lymphocyte markers, and a portion of the sterile specimen is placed in glutaraldehyde for potential electron microscopic studies. If the frozen specimen is negative for tumor, the lymph node is handled in the same manner as in Group 3.

GROUP 3.—If the consistency of the node is normal or homogeneous, permanent sections and additional studies are requested, including bacteriologic smears and cultures (as defined in Group 1), lymph node imprint, and the preservation of a small portion of a node frozen to − 70 C under sterile conditions to obtain immunofluorescent studies and viral or tissue cultures if indicated by permanent section studies. The fixation of the entire specimen in formaldehyde precludes the possibility of carrying out these additional procedures.

With this protocol these investigators obtained a positive yield in 62% of their lymph node biopsy samples.

What happens to children in whom the pathologic report of the lymph node biopsy specimen is nondiagnostic? Of the 37 children described by Kissane and Gephardt, 25% developed severe lymphoreticular disease.[38] Of the 41 patients seen by Lake and Oski, who were initially found to have nondiagnostic reactive hyperplasia, 17% ultimately proved to have a specific pathologic disease.[103] Therefore, should the initial workup and biopsy specimen of the child with lymphadenopathy fail to show a specific diagnosis, close follow-up for persistent or recurrent symptoms is essential, with repeated biopsy when indicated.[108]

Acknowledgment

The authors would like to thank Anna Meyers and Terri Picard for the secretarial assistance.

REFERENCES

1. Anderson W.A.D., Kissane J.M.: *Pathology*. St. Louis: C.V. Mosby Co., 1977, p 1325.
2. Alexander J.W., Good R.A.: *Fundamentals of Clinical Immunology*. Philadelphia: W.B. Saunders Co., 1977, pp 25–26.

3. Zuelzer W.W., Kaplan J.: The child with lymphadenopathy. *Semin Hematol.* 12(3):323, 1975.
4. Emery J.C., Dinsdale F.: The postnatal development of lymphoreticular aggregates and lymph nodes in infants' lungs. *J.Clin. Pathol.* 26:529, 1973.
5. Brunson J.G., Gall E.A.: *Concepts of Disease.* New York: Macmillan Publishing Co., 1971, pp 914–916.
6. Dehner L.P.: *Pediatric Surgical Pathology.* St. Louis: C.V. Mosby Co., 1975, pp 643–665.
7. Robbins S.L.: *Pathologic Basis of Disease.* Philadelphia: W.B. Saunders Co., 1974, pp 749–750.
8. Nayeem S.A., Bernhardt B.: Syphilitic lymphadenopathy. *J.A.M.A.* 239(6):495, 1978.
9. Turner D.R., Wright D.J.M.: Lymphadenopathy in early syphilis. *J.Pathol.* 110:305, 1973.
10. Calabro J.J., Holgerson W.B., Conpal G.M., et al.: Juvenile rheumatoid arthritis: A general review and report on 100 patients observed for 15 years. *Semin. Arthritis Rheum.* 5:257, 1976.
11. Cruickshank B.: The basic pattern of tissue damage and pathology of systemic lupus erythematosis, in Dubois E.L. (ed): *Lupus Erythematosis,* ed 2. Los Angeles: University of Southern California Press, 1974, pp 12–71.
12. Fox R.A., Rosahn P.D.: The lymph nodes in disseminated lupus erythematosus. *Am. J. Pathol.* 19:73, 1943.
13. Kojis F.G.: Serum sickness and anaphylaxis *Am. J. Dis. Child.* 64:133, 1942.
14. Jenkin R.D.T., Brown T.C., Peters M.V., et al.: Hodgkin's disease in children: A retrospective analysis: 1958–73. *Cancer* 35:979, 1975.
15. Altman A.J., Schwartz A.D.: *Malignant Diseases of Infancy, Childhood and Adolescence.* Philadelphia: W.B. Saunders Co., 1978, pp 234–303.
16. Sutow W.W., Vietti T.J., Fernbach D.J.: *Clinical Pediatric Oncology.* St. Louis: C.V. Mosby Co., 1977, pp 408–463.
17. Frizzera G., Moran E.M., Rappaport N.: Angioimmunoblastic lymphadenopathy diagnosis and clinical course. *Am. J. Med.* 59:803, 1975.
18. Lukes R.J., Tindle B.H.: Immunoblastic lymphadenopathy: A hyperimmune entity resembling Hodgkin's disease. *N. Engl. J. Med.* 292:1, 1975.
19. Howarth C.B., Bird C.C.: Immunoblastic sarcoma arising in child with immunoblastic lymphadenopathy. *Lancet* 2:747, 1976.
20. Lascari A.D.: *Leukemia in Childhood.* Springfield, Ill.: Charles C. Thomas, Publisher, 1973, p 37.
21. Freedman M.H., Finkelstein J.Z., Hammond G.C., et al.: The effect of chemotherapy on acute myelogenous leukemia in children. *J. Pediatr.* 78:526, 1971.
22. Newton W.A., Hamoudi A.B.: *Histiocytosis: A Histologic Classification with Clinical Correlation, Perspective in Pediatric Pathology.* Chicago: Year Book Medical Publishers, Inc., 1973, vol 1, pp 251–281.
23. Leikin S.: *The Histiocytoses: Clinical Management of Cancer in Children.* Acton, Mass.: Science Group Inc., 1975, pp 203–221.
24. Debuch H., Wiedemann H.R.: Lymph node excision as a simple diagnostic aid in rare lipidoses. *Eur. J. Pediatr.* 129:99, 1978.
25. Keller A.R., Hochholzer L., Castleman B.: Hyaline-vascular and plasma-cell types of giant lymph node hyperplasia of the mediastinum and other locations. *Cancer* 29:670, 1972.
26. Miller J.S., Miller J.J.: Benign giant lymph node hyperplasia presenting as fever of unknown origin. *J. Pediatr.* 87(2):237, 1975.
27. Geary C.G., Fox H.: Giant lymph node hyperplasia of the mediastinum and refractory anaemia. *J. Clin. Pathol.* 31:757, 1978.
28. Neerhout R.C., Larson W., Mansur P.: Mesenteric lymphoid hamartoma associated with chronic hypoferremia, anemia, growth failure and hyperglobulinaemia. *N. Engl. J. Med.* 280:922, 1969.

29. Mutz I., Stögmann W.: Immunodeficiency with lymphoid hyperplasia. *Eur. J. Pediatr.* 124:207, 1977.
30. Rieger C.H.L., Lustig J.F., Justman R.A., et al.: Immunologic function of patients with chronic benign lymphadenopathy. *Eur. J. Pediatr.* 124:51, 1976.
31. Greene D.A.: Localized cervical lymphadenopathy induced by diphenylhydantoin sodium. *Arch. Otolaryngol.* 10:446, 1975.
32. Holland P., Mauer A.M.: Diphenlhydantoin-induced hypersensitivity reaction. *J. Pediatr.* 66:322, 1965.
33. Dorfman R.F., Warnke R.: Lymphadenopathy simulating the malignant lymphomas. *Hum. Pathol.* 5:519, 1974.
34. Hyman G.A., Sommers S.C.: The development of Hodgkin's disease and lymphoma during anticonvulsant therapy. *Blood* 28:416, 1966.
35. Snead C., Siegel N., Hayslett J.: Generalized lymphadenopathy and nephrotic syndrome as a manifestation of mephenytoin (Mesantoin) toxicity. *Pediatrics* 57(1):98, 1976.
36. Costello J.M., Becroft D.M.: Drug reaction simulating malignant lymphoma: A case due to pyrimethamine. *N.Z. Med. J.* 86(599):430, 1977.
37. Hart F.D.: *French's Index of Differential Diagnoses,* ed 10. Baltimore: Williams & Wilkins, 1973, pp 473–477.
38. Kissane J.M., Gephardt G.N.: Lymphadenopathy in childhood: Long-term follow-up in patients with nondiagnostic lymph node biopsies. *Hum. Pathol.* 5(4):431, 1974.
39. Canale V.C., Smith C.H.: Chronic lymphadenopathy simulating malignant lymphoma. *J. Pediatr.* 70(6):891, 1967.
40. Stiehm E.R., Fudenberg H.H.: Clinical and immunologic features of dysgammaglobulinemia type I: Report of a case diagnosed in the first year of life. *Am. J. Med.* 40:805, 1966.
41. Constantinidis K.: Acute and chronic berylliosis disease. *Br. J. Clin. Pract.* 32(5):127, 1978.
42. Ryan R., O'Rourke J.F., Iser G.: Conjunctivitis in adenoidalpharyngeal-conjunctival virus infection. *Arch. Ophthalmol.* 54:211, 1955.
43. Barton L.L., Feigin R.D.: Childhood cervical lymphadenitis: A reappraisal. *J. Pediatr.* 84:846, 1974.
44. Powell D.A., Miller K., Clyde W.A.: Submandibular adenitis in a newborn caused by mycoplasma hominus. *Pediatrics* 63(5)798, 1979.
45. Schmitt B.D.: Cervical adenopathy in children. *Postgrad. Med.* 60(3):251, 1976.
46. Jones P.G.: Swellings in the neck in childhood. *Med. J. Aust.* 1:212, 1963.
47. Shurin S.: Infectious mononucleosis. *Pediatr. Clin. North Am.* 26(2)315, 1979.
48. Starr S.E.: Cytomegalovirus. *Pediatr. Clin. North Am.* 26(2):283, 1979.
49. Rafaty F.M.: Cervical adenopathy secondary to toxoplasmosis. *Arch. Otolaryngol.* 103:547, 1977.
50. Beverly J.K.A., Beattie C.P.: Glandular toxoplasmosis: A survey of 30 cases. *Lancet* 2:379, 1958.
51. Thomaidis T., Anastassea-Vlachou K., Mandalenaki-Lambrou C., et al.: Chronic lymphoglandular enlargement and toxoplasmosis in children. *Arch. Dis. Chil.* 52:403, 1977.
52. Taber L.H., Feigin R.D.: Leptospirosis. *Pediatr. Clin. North Am.* 26(2):400, 1979.
53. Bagnarello A.G.: Mononucleosis-like picture: Brucella suis infection. *Pa. Med.* 79:58, 1976.
54. Pollen R.C., Stuart B.M.: Tularemia: Analysis of 225 cases. *J.A.M.A.* 129:495, 1945.
55. Speert D.P., Britt W.J., Kaplan E.L.: Tick-borne tularemia presenting as ulcerative lymphadenitis. *Clin. Pediatr.* 18(4):239, 1979.
56. Dajani A.S., Garcia R.E., Wolinsky E.: Etiology of cervical lymphadenitis in children. *N. Engl. J. Med.* 268:24, 1963.

57. Ayliffe G.A.J., et al.: Staphylococcal infection in cervical glands of infants. *Lancet* 2:479, 1972.
58. Wald E.R., Sivasubramanian K.: Cervical adenitis in infancy: Report of four cases due to staphylococci. *Clin. Pediatr.* 15(12):1168, 1976.
59. Dewar J., et al.: Staphylococcal infection in cervical glands of infants. *Lancet* 2:712, 1972.
60. Hieber J.P., Davis A.T.: Staphylococcal cervical adenitis in young infants. *Pediatrics* 57(3):424, 1976.
61. Fishaut J.M., Mokrohisky ST: Cervical lymphadenitis caused by *Haemophilus influenzae* type B. *Am. J. Dis. Child.* 131:925, 1977.
62. Khoo B.H., Cho C.T., Smith S.D., Cervical lymphadenitis due to *Candida albicans* infection. *J. Pediatr.* 86(5):812, 1975.
63. Ginsburg C.M.: An unusual cause of cervical lymphadenitis. *Laryngoscope* 87(7):1180, 1977.
64. MacKellar A.: Diagnosis and management of atypical mycobacterial lymphadenitis in children. *J. Pediatr. Surg.* 11(1):85, 1976.
65. Rivron M.J., Hughes E.A., Sibert J.R., et al.: Cervical lymphadenitis in childhood due to mycobacterial of the Fortuitum Group. *Arch. Dis. Child.* 54:312, 1979.
66. Schuit K.E., Powell D.A.: Mycobacterial lymphadenitis in childhood. *Am. J. Dis. Child.* 132:675, 1978.
67. Altman R.P., Margileth A.M.: Cervical lymphadenopathy from atypical mycobacteria: Diagnosis and surgical treatment. *J. Pediatr. Surg.* 10(3):419, 1975.
68. Black B.G., Chapman J.S.: Cervical adenitis in children due to human and unclassified mycobacteria. *Pediatrics* 33:887, 1964.
69. Brock R.C., Cann R.J., Dickinson R.J.: Tuberculosis mediastinal lymphadenitis in childhood: Secondary effects on the lungs. *Guys Hosp. Rep.* 87:295, 1937.
70. Schaad U.B., Votteler T.P., McCracken G.H., et al.: Management of atypical mycobacterial lymphadenitis in childhood: A review based on 380 cases. *J. Pediatr.* 95(3):356, 1979.
71. Siltzbach L.E., James D.G., Neville E., et al.: Course and prognosis of sarcoidosis around the world. *Am. J. Med.* 57:847, 1974.
72. May M.: Neck masses in children: Diagnosis and treatment. *Ear Nose Throat J.* 57:136, 1978.
73. Snapper I.: The bedside diagnosis of cervical lymphadenopathies. *Med. Clin. North Am.* 51:627, 1962.
74. Carithers H.A., Carithers C.M., Edwards R.O. Jr.: Cat-scratch disease: Its natural history. *J.A.M.A.* 207:312, 1969.
75. Carithers H.A.: Cat-scratch skin test antigen: Purification by heating. *Pediatrics* 60(6):928, 1977.
76. Noussitov F.M., et al.: *Leprosy in Children.* Geneva: Geneva World Health Organization, 1976.
77. Donner L., Chalupsky J.: Unusual form of lymphadenopathy. *Vnitr. Lek.* 23(7):702, 1977.
78. Jaffe B., Jaffe N.: Head and neck tumors in children. *Pediatrics* 51:731, 1973.
79. Sessions D.G., Ragab A.H., Vietti T.J., et al.: Embryonal rhabdomyosarcoma of the head and neck region in children. *Laryngoscope* 83:890, 1973.
80. Healy G.B., Jaffe N., Cassidy J.R.: Rhabdomyosarcoma of the head and neck: Diagnosis and management. *Head Neck Surg.* 1:334, 1979.
81. Brostrom K., Baandrup U.: Sinus histiocytosis with massive lymphadenopathy. *Acta Pediatr. Scand.* 66:257, 1977.
82. Rosai J., Dorfman R.F.: Sinus histiocytosis with massive lymphadenopathy. *Arch. Pathol.* 87:63, 1969.
83. Pruzanski W.: Lymphadenopathy associated with dysgammaglobulinemia. *Semin. Hemat.* 17(1):44, 1980.

84. Friendly D.S., Font R.L., Rao N.A.: Orbital involvement in "sinus" histiocytosis. *Arch. Ophthalmol.* 95:2006, 1977.
85. Haas R.J., Helmig M.S., Prechtel K.: Sinus histiocytosis with massive lymphadenopathy and paraparesis: Remission with chemotherapy. *Cancer* 42:77, 1978.
86. Yanagihara R., Todd J.K.: Acute febrile mucocutaneous lymph node syndrome. *Am. J. Dis. Child.* 134:603, 1980.
87. Hartsock R.J.: Postvaccinial lymphadenitis. *Cancer* 21:632, 1968.
88. Dorfman R.F., Herweg J.C.: Live, attentuated measles virus vaccine: Inguinal lymphadenopathy complicating administration. *J.A.M.A.* 198:320, 1966.
89. Hodgsdon C.H., Olson A.M., Good C.A.: Bilateral hilar adenopathy: Its significance and management. *Ann. Intern. Med.* 43:83, 1955.
90. Felson B.: *Chest Roentgenology.* Philadelphia: W.B. Saunders Co., 1973, p 419.
91. Watkins C.G.: Rat-bite fever. *J. Pediatr.* 28:429, 1961.
92. Stein S.C., Sokoloff M.J.: Calcification of regional lymph nodes following BCG vaccination. *Am Rev. Tuber. Pul. Dis.* 73:239, 1956.
93. Currarino G.: Acute epitrochlear lymphadenitis. *Pediatr. Radiol.* 6(3):160, 1977.
94. Favre M., Hellerström S.: The epidemiology, etiology and prophylaxis of lymphogranuloma inguinale. *Acta Derm. Venereol.* (suppl 30) (Stockh) 34:1, 1954.
95. Hadley A.T.: Chanchroid. *Am. Fam. Phys.* 20(6):83, 1979.
96. Nielsen J., Barlow J.F.: Thirteen-year-old boy with fever and inguinal lymphadenophy. Vermillion, S. Dakota: University of South Dakota Clinicopathological Conference, 1978, pp 29–32.
97. Tangsrud S.E., Skyberg D., Larsen T.E.: Scleroderma with massive regional lymphadenopathy. *Acta Ped. Scand.* 68:627, 1979.
98. Carson M.J., Hartman S.: Acute iliac lymphadenitis. *J. Pediatr.* 29:183, 1946.
99. Wilensky A.O.: General abdominal lymphadenopathy with special reference to nonspecific mesenteric adenitis. *Arch. Surg.* 42:71, 1941.
100. Green M.: Pediatric diagnosis, ed 3. Philadelphia: W.B. Saunders Co., 1980, pp 521–527.
101. Greenfield S., Jordan M.C.: The clinical investigation of lymphadenopathy in primary care practice. *J.A.M.A.* 240(13):1388, 1978.
102. Novack A.H.: Lumps and bumps in the neck. *Pediatr. Digest* 21(10):15, 1979.
103. Lake A.M., Oski F.A.: Peripheral lymphadenopathy in childhood: Ten-year experience with excisional biopsy. *Am. J.Dis. Child.* 132:357, 1978.
104. Wintrobe M.M., et al.: *Clinical Hematology,* ed 7. Philadelphia: Lea & Febiger, 1975, pp 1259–1262.
105. Wintrobe M.M., et al.: *Harrison's Principles of Internal Medicine,* ed 8. New York: McGraw-Hill Book Co., 1977, pp 301–303.
106. Banks P.M., Long J.C., Howard C.A.: Preparation of lymph node biopsy specimens. *Hum. Pathol.* 10(6):617, 1979.
107. Margolis I.B., Matteucci D., Organ C.H.: To improve the yield of biopsy of the lymph nodes. *Surg. Gynecol. Obstet.* 147:376, 1978.
108. Carithers H.A.: Lymphadenopathy: A diagnostic enigma. *Am. J. Dis. Child.* 132:353, 1978.

Current Trends in the Treatment of Self-Injurious Behavior

NIRBHAY N. SINGH, PH.D.

Department of Psychology
University of Canterbury
Christchurch, New Zealand

Introduction

ALTHOUGH THE PROBLEM OF SELF-INJURIOUS BEHAVIOR in children has been reported in the pediatric literature since before the turn of the century,[34, 54, 78, 88] its treatment history is of a more recent vintage.[12, 21, 95, 174, 194, 232] As a pathologic condition, self-injurious behavior is usually associated with schizophrenic and mentally retarded children, although some forms of this behavior are often observed in normal infants and young children.[80, 97, 247] It has been suggested, for example, that head banging, picking, scratching, and hair pulling are usually mild and transient developmental phenomena in normal pediatric populations.[47, 247]

Several terms, including self-destructive, self-punitive, autoplectic, masochistic, autoaggressive, and self-mutilative behavior, have been used to describe such behavior. However, the most widely accepted term for this problem is self-injurious behavior (SIB). SIB refers to any self-inflicted repetitive action that leads to lacerations, bruising, or abrasions of the patient's own body. These behaviors are clinically significant because they are "excessive, unusual, bizarre, and without any immediately apparent desirable consequences."[21]

Self-injurious behavior may take one of several forms, including headbanging, eye-gouging, biting, scratching, self-

377

0065-3101/81/0028-0377-0440-$03.75

pinching and punching, and rectal digging. Recurrent vomiting and/or rumination,[221] self-induced seizures through either hyperventilation[60] or photic stimulation,[259] breath-holding,[218] and hyperventilation[223] have also been regarded by some investigators as self-injurious behaviors.[68] This chapter, however, will not consider such behaviors, since they have either been recently reviewed elsewhere (e.g., rumination[221]) or are reported so rarely that there is not enough evidence to draw conclusions about them.

The purpose of this chapter is twofold: first, to report on the current trends in the treatment of self-injurious behavior in children; and second, to provide a critical evaluation of the various therapeutic methods and research procedures used in the treatment of SIB. A more general aim is to provide a relatively brief but accurate summary of the rapidly growing behavioral literature on SIB for pediatricians and other professionals who are engaged in the treatment of childhood behavior disorders. A brief overview of the various theoretical approaches that attempt to explain the etiology of SIB is provided. In general, only those theories based on a behavioral-psychological orientation appear to provide specific, testable hypotheses about the maintaining variables of SIB. Thus, the bulk of the current therapeutic literature is behavioral. Although the coverage here is not to be taken as exhaustive, an effort has been made to include most of the published clinical and experimental literature from the last decade.

Prevalence

Several studies have surveyed the prevalence of SIB in various populations. These are presented in Table 1. Prevalence data are available for normal infants and young children (Group I), institutionalized mentally retarded children (Group II), and others, namely schizophrenic, abused, and neglected children and psychiatric patients (Group III).

The reported prevalence of SIB varies, depending on which population has been studied. The data presented for Group 1 studies (see Table 1) show that the reported prevalence of SIB in "normal" pediatric populations varied from 3.3% to about 20%; five of the seven studies reported figures only for head-banging. Although definitive statements cannot be made at this point because of insufficient data, a few tentative conclusions can be offered. Current literature indicates that SIB in normal infants, mainly of the headbanging variety, first appears at about eight or nine months of age and stops usually before the age of four years. This behavior is usually preceded by the appearance of other rhythmic habits or stereotyped movements, the most common form being bodyrocking.[51, 118, 196] There appears to be a significant difference between the sexes in terms of prevalence, with a 3:1 ratio of males to females.[51, 118, 126, 196]

The prevalence of SIB in institutionalized mentally retarded persons varied from 5.3% to 37.1% (see Table 1, Group II) depending on the definition of SIB used, the method used to collect data, the observation period, and the average level of retardation of the surveyed population. The study of SIB is replete with definitional problems, and unfortunately few studies have dealt with this issue. Retrospective data were used in some studies, which subjected them to the obvious limitations of potentially inaccurate recall by the children's primary caretakers. More studies based on direct observation techniques are clearly needed. Other studies presented data based on short-term observations or recall. Such data are of limited value, since it is well established that SIB in mentally retarded children can be quiescent for several weeks or months.

Finally, there is a direct relationship between the level of retardation and the prevalence of SIB. Several studies have found prevalence rates to be higher in the more severely and profoundly retarded.[18, 135, 136, 199, 248] Another factor that should be considered is that the high incidence of SIB in some institutions could result from their admission policy. Children who injure themselves are often given priority because their parents and caretakers are unable to cope with this behavior at home.

Several general findings on the prevalence of SIB in mentally-retarded persons have emerged from the studies presented in Table 1. It appears that there are inverse relationships between intelligence and both prevalence and severity of SIB. The frequency, intensity, and durability of SIB differentiate the mentally retarded from "normal" populations who show such behavior. There is some suggestion in the literature from institutionalized populations that, when compared to chil-

TABLE 1.—REPORTED PREVALENCE OF SELF-INJURIOUS BEHAVIOR

AUTHOR	POPULATION SAMPLE	AGE LEVEL	PREVALENCE (%)	TYPE OF SIB
Group I				
De Lissovoy[51]	374 NC*	19–32 months	15.2	Headbanging
Kravitz and Boehm[117]	340 NC		7	Headbanging
Kravitz et al.[118]	1,168 NI†		3.6	Headbanging
Levy and Patrick[126]	422 NI		3.3	Headbanging
Lourie[127]	130 NI	<3 yr	15–20	Unspecified
Sallustro and Atwell[196]	506 NI and NC	3 mo–6 yr	5.1	Headbanging
Shintoub and Soulairac[209]	300 NI and NC	9–18 mo	11–17	Various forms, including self-biting, pinching, scratching, hitting, hairpulling, and headbanging
		<2 yr	9	
		<5 yr	0	
Group II				
Ballinger[18]	626 IMRP‡		15	Various forms, with self-biting and headbanging being most common
Carraz and Erhardt[39]	140 IMRP		37.1	Various forms
MacKay et al.[135]	850 IMRP	4–63 yr	19	Various forms, with regurgitation, face-slapping, skin-picking, headbanging and self-biting being most common
Maisto et al.[136]	1,300 IMRP	10–70 yr (mean = 33.5)	14	Various forms, with headbanging and self-biting being most common
McCoull[145]	4,808 IMRP		5.3	Various forms
Ressman and Butterworth[183]	Mentally retarded school children		2.1	Biting and chewing arms and hands
Ross[193]	11,000 IMRP		12	Various forms
Schroeder[199]	IMRP		9	Various forms, with headbanging being most common

Author	Sample	Age	%	Forms
Schroeder et al.[204]	1,150 IMRP	5–85 yr	10	Various forms
Singh[215]	368 IMRP	5–34 yr	22.8	Various forms, with headbanging, face-slapping and skin-picking being most common
Smeets[231]	400 IMRP and emotionally disturbed persons	M = 19.9 yr F = 16.3 yr (mean)	8.75	Various forms, with headbanging, pinching, scratching, and face-slapping being most common
Soule and O'Brien[234]	966 IMRP		7.7	Various forms, with self-biting and headbanging being most common
Van Velzen[248]	1,929 IMRP	2–66 yr (mean = 18)	30.3	Various forms, with self-biting, beating the head and headbanging being most common
Whitney[255]	950 IMRP		8.8	Various forms, with self-biting and headbanging being most common
Group III				
Green[83]	70 Schizophrenic children	5–12 yr	40	Various forms
Green[85]	59 Abused Children 29 Neglected children 30 Normal children	8–9 yr (mean)	40.6 17.2 6.7	Various forms
Phillips and Muzaffer[173]	2,816 Psychiatric persons	5–17 yr	4.3	Various forms
Shodell and Reiter[210]	58 Schizophrenic persons		38	Various forms, including headbanging, self-biting, self-pinching, hairpulling, and self-scratching or hitting

*NC = normal children.
†NI = normal infants.
‡ IMRP = institutionalized mentally retarded persons.

dren who do not exhibit SIB, those who do exhibit SIB are younger but have been institutionalized for a longer period of time. However, too little comparative data are available from noninstitutionalized mentally retarded populations to show that these findings apply to the mentally retarded in general.

In terms of other populations, Table 1 (Group III) suggests that the prevalence of SIB may be somewhat higher in schizophrenic children than in other populations. However, insufficient epidemiological data are available to confirm this.

The Problem of Etiology

The diversity of theoretical speculation about the nature and etiology of SIB in pediatric populations has been truly remarkable. Yet most speculations have been based on very small samples of children, without adequate supportive evidence from experimental investigations. For example, the following have been suggested at various times as possible causes for some forms of SIB: otitis media,[53, 176] autoerotism,[44, 71, 123] aggression,[75] motor release,[127, 153] disturbed parent-child relationships,[23, 185] intracranial irritations,[76] prior physical abuse,[84, 205] the eruption of central and lateral incisors,[118] maternal deprivation,[212] and sensory deprivation.[125] All of these theories received only limited acceptance, mainly because they could not be experimentally verified nor could they generate effective treatment strategies for controlling SIB in children.

The psychodynamic theories of SIB have had a somewhat wider currency than most of the early theories. Spitz and Wolf[235] have suggested that infants engage in SIB if they are deprived of maternal care, which they say puts the infant in a state of anaclitic depression and turns his aggressive and libidinal drives inward. In a similar vein, Silverstein et al.[212] have suggested that SIB is a substitute for incomplete maternal stimulation. Others have invoked such explanations as an attempt to establish "body reality," the distinction of self from external reality, the reduction of guilt consequent on SIB, an attempt to establish ego boundaries, and regression of the ego identity.[34, 86, 265]

One problem inherent in psychodynamic theorizing is the difficulty in scientifically verifying many of its propositions. Its reliance on underlying deep-rooted causes as determinants of pathological behavior does not provide an adequate data base that can be used for treatment. The few studies that have attempted to treat SIB within a psychodynamic framework have rarely been successful and, in some cases, have had to resort to other approaches.[230, 238] Furthermore, psychodynamic techniques are not deemed to be appropriate in the treatment of SIB in children, since the majority of children with SIB are either too young or too severely and profoundly retarded to be able to respond to such therapy.[211, 221, 240]

The self-stimulating theory accounts for the development of SIB in terms of "an accommodation by the organism to an environment that consistently fails to provide an optimal or homeostatic level of stimulation."[21] That is, a child engages in SIB to increase the level of sensory stimulation available to him.[45, 119]

Some research evidence suggests that certain forms of stimulation, such as vestibular stimulation, may accelerate the development of infants.[196] For example, it has been shown that vestibular stimulation enhances weight gains[69] and motor responsiveness,[42] reduces arousal,[113, 245] and increases visual alertness[112] in both normal and premature infants.

One prediction of this theory is that self-injury may actually increase sensory input in an unstimulating environment. Several studies dealing with the treatment of SIB in mentally retarded persons are relevant here. For example, it has been shown that stereotyped behaviors, including SIB, decrease when play equipment is provided to institutionalized children.[25, 49, 186] However, as noted by Carr,[37] the generality of these findings is rather limited due to certain methodological problems. Furthermore, other research evidence dealing directly with the frequency of SIB has not supported this hypothesis.[93, 94] With the exception of one study,[111] no adequate empirical test has been made of the self-stimulation hypothesis for SIB.

Another etiological speculation, one based on organicism, relates to the observation that SIB is a marked characteristic in certain individuals who suffer from metabolic, chromosomal, or neurological disorders.[175] For example, SIB has been reported in patients with the Lesch-Nyhan syndrome,[122] de Lange's syndrome,[99] the 49XXXXY syndrome,[114] and the 47XYY syndrome.[169] The assumption has been that SIB can be regarded "as some sort of seizure-like episode, deriving from either structural or chemical defects in the brain."[21] Several types of findings have been garnered in support of this view. It has been suggested, for example, that SIB is associated with cerebral catecholamine activity[120, 159] and with amphetamine intoxication and overdosage of levodopa, which leads to dysfunction of basal ganglia.[114] Others have noted that stimulants such as pemoline and caffeine may produce SIB.[79]

As noted by Carr,[37] an explanation of SIB based purely on the concept of organicity does not account for all the data available. If SIB is caused by a specific biochemical abnormality, it should be possible to correct it pharmacologically. Indeed, there is some empirical support for this view. Mizuno and Yugari[154, 155] reported the suppression of SIB following the administration of 1 to 8 mg/kg of L-5-hydroxytryptophan in an open trial. Unfortunately, these results can only be taken as suggestive of the efficacy of L-5-hydroxytryptophan, since Mizuno and Yguari failed to employ the proper experimental controls (e.g., double-blind, measurement of interobserver reliability) required for such studies.[5, 236] Furthermore, at least one controlled study has shown that while L-5-hydroxytryptophan may produce clinically significant reductions in athetoid movements in the Lesch-Nyhan, it does not reduce SIB.[74] Although further investigations are warranted in this area, current evidence suggests that pharmacological interventions are not totally effective in either the appearance[140] or the control of SIB in patients with the Lesch-Nyhan syndrome.[168]

Other evidence also argues against a purely organic etiology. It has been reported that SIB is not present in all patients with the Lesch-Nyhan syndrome.[40, 167, 206, 207] Other reports have indicated that SIB in the Lesch-Nyhan syndrome can be treated by conditioning techniques.[6, 33, 57] Such conditioning has been reported to be effective in controlling SIB in de Lange's syndrome as well.[208, 227] The demonstrated efficacy of conditioning procedures in the control of a condition, which is thought to be produced as a result of a patient's aberrant physiological processes, is certainly not a prediction of an organic explanation. The evidence currently available does not preclude an organic explanation, nor does it fully confirm it. It is plausible, however, to suggest that certain organic conditions may be responsible for the genesis of SIB, but the behavior itself may be maintained by other variables.

The best documented and most popular account of the etiology of SIB has been explained in terms of instrumental conditioning. Skinnner[228] advanced two hypotheses that account for this type of behavior: the discriminative-stimulus hypothesis and the avoidance hypothesis. Since both of these hypotheses have been considered at length in other reviews,[21, 37, 186] only a brief overview of them will be presented here.

A stimulus whose presence has been associated with reinforcement is referred to as an S^D or discriminative stimulus. According to the S^D hypothesis, SIB in children occasions a social response from the child's parents or primary caretakers. For example, when an infant bangs his head, accidentally or otherwise, his parents give him a lot of attention. When there is a history of such association between headbanging and parental attention, headbanging begins to serve as an S^D for parental attention.

One prediction of the discriminative-stimulus hypothesis would be that increased parental attention may result in a greater frequency of headbanging and that a decrease or withdrawal of parental attention would decrease the frequency of headbanging. If one applies that same reasoning to SIB generally, it can be expected that if social reinforcement maintains SIB in children, its removal would suppress the behavior. Indeed, there is some empirical evidence to support the prediction that social reinforcement is facilitative in the maintenance of SIB and that its withdrawal or removal becomes discriminative for SIB.* Of course, the corollary to this prediction, that social reinforcement, if made contingent on the occurrence of SIB, would increase its frequency, has also received some empirical support.[128, 129]

An individual is said to have made a discrimination when he responds differently in the presence of different stimuli (e.g., situations or persons), and when his responses are differentially controlled by antecedent stimuli his behavior is thought to be under stimulus control. In terms of SIB, several studies have shown that such behavior often occurs under tight environmental control.[38, 77, 200, 203] For example, Bucher and Lovaas[31] and Romanczyk and Goren[190] have shown that the rate of SIB is often correlated with the presence or absence of an adult. According to the discriminative-stimulus hypothesis, the pres-

---

*References 31, 57, 63, 90, 101, 129, 166, 233, 244, 257, 258.

ence of an adult is discriminative for SIB, since only the presence of an adult signals social reinforcement. Thus, higher rates of SIB can be expected in the presence of certain adults if a child has had a history of social reinforcement for SIB in their presence. Other studies have shown that children can come under the stimulus control of certain objects, like a blanket, and exhibit high rates of SIB when these are withdrawn.[48, 171] A related finding of some clinical significance is that release from physical restraint has been found to discriminate for increased rates of SIB in certain children.[48, 62, 246, 260]

The avoidance hypothesis views SIB as being "maintained by the termination or avoidance of an aversive stimulus following the occurrence of a self-injurious act."[37]

Several investigators have reported that some children respond to demand situations by engaging in SIB.* In such patients, the onset of SIB has invariably resulted in the removal or termination of the demand situation. Thus SIB effectively functions as an escape response and is thought to be maintained by negative reinforcement, which is produced by the termination of the aversive situation.

The discriminative-stimulus hypothesis appears to have firm empirical support for its predictions that SIB in children can be decreased or increased by either withdrawing social reinforcement or making it available following the occurrence of SIB, and that it may occur under tight stimulus control. Although the literature supporting the avoidance hypothesis is not extensive, it does appear to account for some of the data that cannot be easily explained by the discriminative-stimulus hypothesis. These hypotheses, however, are not necessarily mutually exclusive and some data on SIB can be explained by invoking either hypothesis (e.g., data on release from restraint studies). Although our understanding of the etiology of SIB is still imperfect, these two hypotheses in concert may well handle most of the treatment data from SIB studies.

Methodological Evaluation

The bulk of the treatment-oriented "research" to be evaluated in the next section actually consists of single-case reports,

---

*References 26, 38, 72, 82, 101, 164, 257.

some of which suffer from a lack of experimental sophistication. It is appropriate, therefore, to examine a number of methodological issues that bear strongly on the scientific merit of any study using behavioral treatment techniques.

Single-subject investigations appear to be the major option in conducting research in this area, given the nature of the problem (its topography, frequency, and intensity) and the nature of the subject sample.[92, 115] One crucial question regarding such research is: To what degree are the results of single-subject studies generalizable beyond the given patient? What is questioned here is not only the internal but also the external validity of results. A study is internally valid when one can assume with a large degree of certainty that manipulation of the independent variable alone was responsible for observed changes in the dependent variable (i.e., SIB). That is, the experimental design is robust enough to rule out rival hypotheses for the observed behavioral change. Internal validity is a necessary condition before the results of any study can allow for generalizations about different subjects, settings, and therapists. The extent to which such generalizations can be made is referred to as external validity.

The minimal criteria used in this chapter to evaluate how methodologically sound are the grounds for belief in the efficacy of the various treatment regimens are design, interobserver agreement (reliability), generalization, and follow-up.

Design

Several time-series designs have been proposed that counter possible threats to internal validity.[36, 81, 115] The simplest of the time-series analyses can be obtained by using the B design, where B refers to the treatment or intervention condition.[30] Here no pretreatment data are obtained and the investigator simply monitors the occurrence of the target behavior over the course of treatment. The frequency of occurrence of the target behavior during pretreatment is referred to as the baseline rate. The B design is methodologically an improvement over the uncontrolled single-case studies in that it involves repeated and objective measurement of the target behavior during the course of treatment. However, as noted elsewhere,[92] this design is still plagued with all the complications (e.g., effects of time and placebo) that typify the case-study methodology.

An improvement over the B design is the AB design, which includes objective measurements of the target behavior(s) taken repeatedly throughout the baseline (A) and intervention (B) phases of the study. Although this design has some utility in clinical settings, it is still open to most of the criticisms levelled against the B design, since it can control only some of the sources of internal invalidity.[188] The ABAB design demonstrates a functional relationship between the target behavior and the treatment regimen by alternating the presentation and removal of the therapy over time. That is, the design requires that the therapeutic program be presented and temporarily withdrawn at some point so as to demonstrate experimental control. This design, which is one of the most frequently used single-subject designs, is also referred to as a reversal or replication design. Although it has two major limitations—irreversibility or complete elimination of target behavior after the initial intervention, and the potentially deleterious effects of reversing the target behavior—it is particularly robust in terms of internal validity.

The multiple-baseline design is frequently used in studies of SIB, since it does not have the problems associated with the ABAB design.[14] Instead of relying on a reversal of intervention, the multiple-baseline design demonstrates experimental control by showing that behavioral change is associated with the intervention at different points in time. Multiple-baseline designs can be of three types, depending on whether the data are collected across individuals, behaviors, or situations. Although this design is thought to be somewhat weaker in terms of internal validity when compared to the ABAB design, its robustness can be strengthened by having several baselines and by ensuring that the baselines are not interdependent.[106]

A variety of time-series designs can be used to determine whether programmed intervention or extraneous events account for the observed behavior change in single-subject research. However, the ABAB and multiple-baseline designs appear to be the most frequently used single-subject experimental designs in applied research.[102] Other designs have been infrequently used in the study of SIB; these will be discussed within the context of the studies that employ them.

INTEROBSERVER AGREEMENT

A second methodological issue governing the adequacy of the therapeutic studies is the reliability of the reported data.* To assess the accuracy and consistency with which an observer records the behavior of a patient, a second observer is usually employed who simultaneously but independently records the same behaviors of the given patient on some occasions. Although no single criterion for an acceptable level of agreement between two such observers has been specified in the literature on applied behavioral therapy, convention dictates that agreement should *not* fall below 80%. The demonstration of an acceptable level of interobserver agreement is crucial, since it sets the upper limit to the validity of inferences derived from the data. Observer drift, reactivity of reliability assessment, complexity of response codes and behavioral observations, observer training and expectancies, and feedback, are among the major considerations in the interpretation of reliability data.[104, 108] To control all of these variables in a single study can be difficult; nevertheless, a systematic attempt needs to be made to provide controls for the major variables.

GENERALIZATION

The observation has repeatedly been made that the effective transfer and maintenance of changes in behavior across time and settings does not automatically occur after the termination of programmed treatment.[14, 137, 138, 239, 250] According to Stokes and Baer,[239] generalization is the "occurrence of relevant behavior under different, nontraining conditions (i.e., across subjects, settings, people, behaviors and/or time) without the scheduling of the same events in those conditions as had been scheduled in the training conditions."

They have discussed nine techniques designed to assess or program generalization that are relevant to clinical treatment: (1) *train and hope,* where some form of training has been instituted and it is hoped that generalization will occur in the absence of systematic programming; (2) *sequential modification,* where the unprogrammed generalization of behavior

---

*References 13, 46, 104, 108, 116, 165.

change is assessed and if it is found to be absent or deficient, generalization is programmed systematically across responses, subjects, settings or therapists in a sequential manner; (3) *introduction of natural maintaining contingencies,* where the patient is "trapped" or introduced to natural contingencies in the environment that maintain the behavior change in the absence of treatment contingencies; (4) *training sufficient exemplars,* where a sufficient number of exemplars (in terms of therapists, responses, and settings) are programmed as part of the treatment to achieve generalization; (5) *train loosely,* where training is carried out on an informal basis with the therapist who has little control over the stimuli and correct responses; (6) *use of indiscriminable contingencies,* where the patient is treated or reinforced under intermittent or varied conditions, including schedule of reinforcement, settings, and time; (7) *programming common stimuli,* where generalization is achieved by ensuring that naturally occuring stimuli are present in both training and transfer situations; (8) *mediated generalization,* where a response is established as part of the new learning that is likely to be used in other problems as well; and (9) *train "to generalize,"* where generalization itself is reinforced as if it were another behavior.

The Stokes and Baer classification can be used to analyze generalization procedures followed in the treatment of SIB in children. Of major importance in the present context is the generalization and maintenance of treatment across settings (e.g., different parts of the ward, and in the clinic, home, and school) and across therapists (e.g., different nurses and ward attendants, parents, siblings, and peers).

FOLLOW-UP

Follow-up refers to the durability or maintenance of therapeutic change once the treatment program has been terminated. The durability of therapeutic change is a function of the stimulus context in which the behavior occurs at the time of follow-up evaluation, the patient's reinforcement history since intervention, and the contingencies in operation during the period following termination of treatment. Follow-up can be usefully seen within the Stokes and Baer framework as the assessment of generalization over time, and as such the procedures enumerated for ensuring generalization can be used to program the durability of therapeutic change. Follow-up data needs to be collected systematically over several sessions (much as one collects baseline and intervention data) and periodically, so that the long-term effectiveness of given therapeutic regimens can be compared.

Treatment of SIB

Quite diverse therapeutic interventions have been used in the treatment of SIB in children. Surgery has often been referred to as a possible "cure" and a few studies attesting to its use are available. For example, transorbital leukotomy[16] and amygdalotomy[109] have been used to treat SIB. The surgical treatment of some forms of self-injurious behavior has had a long history,[221] but evidence in support of this technique is very weak.

As noted elsewhere,[4] psychoactive medication has been used extensively in the treatment of various childhood behavior problems and the treatment of SIB has been no exception. Most psychopharmacological agents have been used, but few have been shown to be effective.[24, 177, 249] In one of the very few well-controlled experiments, Primrose[177] showed that SIB in mentally retarded children could be controlled to some degree by using baclofen, a γ-aminobutyric acid (GABA) analogue. However, this finding needs replication before it can be accepted as a reliable phenomenon. The current view on the use of psychopharmacological agents in the treatment of SIB is that, in the absence of reliable data derived from methodologically sound studies, its use should be regarded only as experimental. In terms of the quality of experimental studies, this area of research remains virtually uninvestigated.

Various mechanical devices have been used to control SIB in children, including air splints,[2, 170] protective helmets[17, 260] and custom-designed seating devices to control SIB in patients with the Lesch-Nyhan syndrome.[124]

Psychotherapeutic approaches used to treat SIB, especially those of the psychodynamic variety, have had relatively little success.[230, 238] The population amenable to this form of therapy has invariably been older children and adults, all of "normal" intelligence. If prevalence studies (see Table 1) are any indication, the type of patients who require treatment for SIB are usually infants and the mentally retarded, most of whom are normally found in institutions. Thus it is not surprising that no experimental or clinical studies in the literature attest to the efficacy of psychotherapy in pediatric populations.

The best results have been achieved through behavioral procedures. These are reviewed below. Most of the techniques used in the behavioral treatment of SIB have involved aversive events. The most common way of using aversive events is through a punishment procedure. In behavioral terms, punishment refers to "the presentation of an aversive event or the removal of a positive event following a response which decreases the frequency of that response."[103] This definition emphasizes the two forms that punishment procedures can take, the presentation of aversive events or the removal of positive events following an undesirable response.

Several aversive events have been used to treat SIB, including electric shock, aromatic ammonia, bitter substances, mist, and a harmless face cover. The two principal variants used to remove positive events are response-cost and time-out from positive reinforcement. Other behavioral techniques reviewed below include extinction (the withholding of reinforcement from a previously reinforced response), overcorrection (a mild punishment technique), and positive reinforcement.

ELECTRIC SHOCK

Tate and Baroff[244] were probably the first to use electric shock to treat children with SIB. Their study, although lacking in experimental sophistication (Table 2), strongly suggested that SIB in children could be controlled by painful aversive stimuli. Tate and Baroff were interested in suppressing a variety of self-injurious behaviors in a nine-year-old, functionally blind psychotic boy. This patient had a five-year history of headbanging and face-slapping that had resulted in the complete detachment of his left retina and partial detachment of the other. Earlier treatment regimens, including psychotherapy and drug therapy, had no significant effect on the frequency of occurrence of these behaviors. Partial suppression of SIB was initially achieved through the withdrawal of physical contact following a self-injurious response. However, it was decided to use response-contingent electric shock because of the possibility that even at reduced rates of SIB the patient was in serious danger of completely destroying the right retina by further headbanging. Baseline data were obtained for 24 minutes prior to the administration of electric shock. Following this, the patient was told that if he continued to hit himself he would be shocked and the shock would be painful. A 130-V battery was used to deliver electric shock for 0.5 second to his lower right leg contingent on each occurrence of SIB. SIB was suppressed in 147 days and remained effective for a six-month period. Other positive changes were noted not only in his behavior but also in the behavior of attendants and nurses toward him. Additional details about this patient are provided in the report by Baroff and Tate.[19] Similar findings have been reported in other studies.[180, 256]

Whaley and Tough[253] used mild electric shock (65 V at 1 mamp) to suppress ear- and head-pounding in a severely retarded six-year-old boy. The patient was shocked for the duration of each response but he was taught an avoidance response—touching toys—which could be used to turn off the shock. Since this response was deemed incompatible with ear- and head-pounding, the patient could avoid being shocked by simply holding on to certain toys. Although only an AB design was used and inadequate data were presented in this report, Whaley and Tough suggested that the electric shock contingency and avoidance response was effective in controlling this patient's SIB.

Lovaas and Simmons[129] reported the treatment of three children who engaged in headhitting and headbanging. Electric shock was made contingent on SIB. This resulted in a dramatic suppression of SIB but the withdrawal of electric shock resulted in an immediate reversal of the therapeutic effects. Lovaas and Simmons found that the response suppression was selective in its effects, across both therapeutic settings and therapists. It was evident that this was a direct function of the presence or absence of shock, which suggests that the effects of this treatment may be limited to the situation in which therapy is carried out and to the therapist who carries out the program. The implication for durable and generalized control of SIB is that the electric shock contingency should be applied by several therapists across several settings.

TABLE 2.—METHODOLOGICAL ANALYSIS OF STUDIES USING PHYSICAL PUNISHMENT PROCEDURES

AUTHOR	SUBJECT DESCRIPTION	TOPOGRAPHY	TREATMENT	DESIGN	INTEROBSERVER AGREEMENT	GENERALIZATION	FOLLOW-UP
Tate and Baroff[244]	9-yr-old blind psychotic boy	headbanging, face-slapping, hitting shoulder with chin, self-kicking	electric shock and positive reinforcement (Experiment 2)	AB	—	—	6-month anecdotal information
Baroff and Tate[19]	9-yr-old blind boy with autistic tendencies	headpunching, headbanging	withdrawal of physical contact, electric shock	AB	—	Yes. Treatment programmed across settings	9-month observational data
Whaley and Tough[253]	6-yr-old boy with Down's syndrome	headbanging, earpounding	electric shock	AB	—	—	—
Lovaas and Simmons[129]	8-yr-old severely retarded boy; 8-yr-old severely retarded girl; 11-yr-old severely retarded boy	headhitting, headbanging	electric shock	ABAB/multiple-baseline across settings	3 observers: 95% agreement (reliability assessed prior to the study)	Yes. Treatment programmed across staff and settings	—
Simmons and Reed[213]	5-yr-old mildly mentally retarded girl	hitting hand on the edge of upper incisor teeth	electric shock	ABAB	—	Yes. Treatment programmed across staff and settings	8-mo observational data
Corte et al.[48]	4 profoundly retarded 17- to 20-yr-old adolescents	face-slapping, face-banging, hairpulling, face-scratching, fingerbiting	electric shock	multiple baseline	4 observers: 88–100% agreement	Yes. Treatment programmed across staff and settings	—
Merbaum[149]	12-yr-old boy variously diagnosed as autistic, schizophrenic, retarded, and brain damaged	face-beating	electric shock, electric shock and positive reinforcement	AB	—	Yes. Treatment programmed across school staff and mother, and settings	1-yr anecdotal information

Study	Subject	Target behavior	Treatment	Design	Reliability	Generalization	Follow-up
Kohlenberg et al.[111]	7-yr-old girl with mild quadriplegia	pinching, face-slapping	electric shock	AB	—	—	—
Callias et al.[35]	4.5-yr-old severely retarded boy	headbanging	electric shock and positive reinforcement	AB	—	Yes. Treatment programmed across staff and settings	3–6 mo anecdotal information
Hall et al.[89]	11-yr-old profoundly retarded male	headbanging, face-beating	electric shock	AB	—	Yes. Treatment programmed across staff	5-mo observational data
Prochaska et al.[178]	9-yr-old profoundly retarded epileptic girl	headbanging	electric shock	AB	2 observers: 100% agreement (reliability informally assessed prior to the study)	Yes. Treatment programmed across settings	7-mo anecdotal information
McPherson and Joachim[147]	9-yr-old moderately retarded boy	headbanging, face-hitting	electric shock and positive reinforcement	AB	—	Yes. Treatment programmed across settings and staff	4-mo anecdotal information
Rechter and Vrablic[180]	a. 15-yr-old profoundly retarded blind girl b. 33-yr-old severely retarded woman	facepounding and headbanging	electric shock	AB	—	—	—
Young and Wincze[261]	21-yr-old profoundly retarded woman	headbanging, headhitting	reinforcement of incompatible behaviors electric shock	multiple-baseline	2 observers: 90–99% agreement	—	—
Wilbur et al.[256]	a. 22-yr-old profoundly retarded man b. 15-yr-old boy with Down's syndrome	head- and face-hitting, self-kicking gouging of cheeks headbanging	electric shock and positive reinforcement electric shock	B B	— —	Yes. Treatment programmed across staff and settings	8-mo observational data

AUTHOR	SUBJECT DESCRIPTION	TOPOGRAPHY	TREATMENT	DESIGN	INTEROBSERVER AGREEMENT	GENERALIZATION	FOLLOW-UP
Muttar et al.[162]	10-yr-old mentally retarded girl with enophthalmos. Medication: Valium 10 mg four times a day	face-punching, eyepoking, kneebanging, headbanging	electric shock	AB	—	Yes. Treatment programmed across ward settings	20-mo observational data
Griffin et al.[87]	15-yr-old severely retarded boy, deaf and blind	head- and arm-hitting, throat-and eye-gouging, fingerbiting, scratching	hair tug, electric shock, physical restraint	ABA	2 observers: 85–100% agreement	Yes. Treatment programmed across various settings	34-mo interview data
McFarlain et al.[146]	25-yr-old profoundly retarded male	headbanging	electric shock	ABAB	2 observers: r = .98 (reliability assessed prior to the study)	Yes. Treatment programmed across ward staff	—
Romanczyk and Goren[190]	6.5-yr-old autistic boy	headbanging, face-slapping, scratching	electric shock, electric shock and DRO, extinction	AB	—	Yes. Treatment programmed across staff and settings	1-yr anecdotal information
Duker[59]	16-yr-old profoundly retarded girl	headbanging, face-hitting	electric shock	multiple-baseline across behaviors with a reversal	2 observers: 89 and 98% agreement (reliability assessed during baseline)	Yes. Treatment programmed across staff	—
Duker[58]	a. 10-yr-old boy with Down's syndrome Medication: 1 tab Polaramine three times a day	scratching	slap on the hand and physical restraint	AB	—	Yes. Treatment programmed across staff	—
	b. 18-yr-old severely retarded girl	headbanging	satiation; satiation	AB AB	2 observers: 93–100%	—	18 weeks' observational

Simmons and Reed[213] reported the case of a 5-year-old mildly retarded girl who repeatedly struck the dorsum of either hand on the sharp edge of her upper incisors as an avoidance response to demand situations. Using an ABAB design, Simmons and Reed showed that the rate of SIB varied systematically as a function of the application and withdrawal of the electric-shock contingency for SIB. The treatment was generalized across ward, school, and home settings; the child's respective attendants were trained in its use. Follow-up observations eight months after the termination of treatment showed the maintenance of treatment gains over time.

Similar findings were reported in a study by Corte et al., who found electric shock to be effective in eliminating the SIB of four profoundly retarded adolescents.[48] These investigators compared the effects of three behavioral treatments and found that punishment with electric shock (150 V at 5 mamp and 300 V at 1 mamp) was more effective than differential reinforcement of non-SIB, which, in turn, was more effective than extinction procedures. However, as noted in other studies,[152, 187] the effects of punishment were found to be specific to the setting in which therapy was carried out.

Several studies using response-contingent electric shock have attempted to explicitly program treatment across settings and staff. For example, Merbaum[149] used the patient's mother in the home and teachers at school as therapists. McPherson and Joachim[14] used the patient's teacher and speech therapist at school and nurses in the ward as therapists.[147] Callias et al.[35] and Hall et al.[89] used a number of therapists and locations for treatment. Prochaska et al.[178] used a portable, remote-controlled device, and Duker[59] used a radio-controlled shocker to apply electric shock contingent on SIB to overcome the problems associated with treatment generalization. Although all but one[59] of these studies suffered from obvious methodological flaws (e.g., AB-type designs, no assessment of observer reliability, and anecdotal reporting of follow-up), they are noteworthy for their attempt to overcome the problems of generalization through programmed treatment.

In addition to the limitations of punishment reviewed above, Young and Wincze[261] demonstrated another. A profoundly retarded girl was punished with 0.5 second of electric shock for engaging in headbanging (head-to-rail of bed) but not for head-

hitting (fist-to-head). The results showed that while headbanging was immediately reduced to near-zero levels, headhitting
remained at the pretreatment rate, suggesting that all types of
SIB need to be punished to achieve generalized suppression of
SIB.

Such a technique has been used in some studies. Muttar et
al. reported the case of a 10-year-old mentally-retarded girl
who engaged in face-punching, eye-poking, knee-banging and
headbanging.[162] All types of SIB were punished with electric
shock (300 V at 2 mamp) for 0.5 second following each response. Although a methodologically weak design was used,
the results showed that the introduction of the electric shock
contingency resulted in a dramatic decrease in SIB. It took
three months to completely eliminate SIB in both home and
ward situations. Observational data collected at 20 months following the termination of formal treatment showed that this
patient had remained free of SIB over this period of time. Griffin et al.[87] initially used hair-tug to control multiple forms of
SIB in a deaf and blind, profoundly retarded boy. Since hair-
tug was only partially successful, electric shock and continuous
restraint contingencies were added to the punishment procedure. This resulted in a complete suppression of all types of SIB
in this patient and follow-up data showed that the behavior
had not recurred in several settings over a 34-month period.

McFarlain et al.[146] trained the ward staff in charge of a profoundly retarded boy to use electric shock and a conditioned
aversive stimulus (a loud "No") contingent on each headbanging response. Headbanging was rapidly decreased with this
contingency. The ward staff generalized the suppression to the
patient's usual ward situation by making a loud verbal "No"
contingent on each instance of SIB. The potency of the conditioned aversive stimulus was maintained by occasionally pairing it with electric shock. It would have been useful to know
for practical reasons the exact nature of this pairing (the report
omitted it), particularly in terms of its frequency, and the durability of the response suppression maintained by a conditioned aversive stimulus.

In a detailed experimental report, Romanczyk and Goren[190]
demonstrated the possibility of completely suppressing SIB in
highly controlled environments but only for short periods of

time. Several procedures, including electric shock, extinction, and the differential reinforcement of other behaviors, were used to treat headbanging, face-slapping, and scratching in a 6.5-year-old autistic boy. Problems were encountered when attempts were made to generalize the control of SIB, which had been achieved in the laboratory to extratherapy settings. Romanczyk and Goren suggested that for a problem behavior such as self-injury, the only acceptable criterion for clinical control is its *complete* suppression rather than only a *reduction* to very low or near-zero levels.

In summary, the current literature suggests that electric shock may be effective in eliminating certain types of SIB in some children. However, this optimistic conclusion must be tempered by the fact that most studies were methodologically deficient, some deficient in several respects. As shown in Table 2, only 7 of 20 studies employed methodologically adequate experimental controls required of evaluative studies. Furthermore, a similar number of studies did not report interobserver reliability data and several studies were inadequate in terms of generalization and follow-up.

In addition to the methodological problems associated with studies in which electric shock is used to punish, there are certain practical problems that must be mentioned. Although electric shock is reputed to be the most effective aversive event[9] and is considered the treatment of choice for chronic SIB,[151] current ethical and legal constraints[32, 141] render it the treatment of last resort, if it can be used at all. Furthermore, the problem of generalization of treatment effects has not been satisfactorily dealt with. Finally, the availability of less intense or painful forms of punishment with a high degree of potency militates against the widespread use of electric shock.

AROMATIC AMMONIA

Noxious odor, in the form of aromatic ammonia, has been used as an aversive stimulus in the treatment of tics,[110] infant breath-holding,[218] running away,[217] hyperventilation,[223] and SIB.[3, 20, 224, 241] Its potency, in terms of its effects on the maladaptive behavior of mentally retarded children, is thought to be second only to that of electric shock. In the usual procedure, a

vial of aromatic ammonia is crushed and held under the patient's nose for either a specified time limit (e.g., three seconds)
or for the duration of a self-injurious act.

In a study of a 20-year-old autistic woman, Tanner and
Zeiler[241] crushed a vial of aromatic ammonia and thrust it under her nose whenever she slapped herself and withdrew it
whenever she stopped. Although there was a rapid and immediate suppression of face-slapping, this reduction was not evident outside of experimental sessions. To facilitate generalization of response suppression, the ward staff was trained in the
use of the treatment procedure, and face-slapping was substantially reduced in all ward settings. Follow-up data showed that
this control was maintained for 3 weeks, a period too short to
provide a meaningful prognosis for the long-term control of SIB
with this procedure.

In another study, Baumeister and Baumeister reported two
cases in which they used aromatic ammonia as the aversive
consequence to eliminate mouthing, hairpulling, and self-slapping responses in two severely retarded girls.[20] Although the
response rate was fairly high in one patient (46 to 55 responses
per minute), only 30 applications of aromatic ammonia were
required to produce complete response suppression within three
days; 35 applications were required to achieve similar results
in the other patient. Observations taken at four months subsequent to the termination of the program showed that complete
response suppression had been maintained. In contrast to the
study by Tanner and Zeiler, Baumeister and Baumeister imple-
mented the program of therapy in the patient's own ward environment with the regular ward staff. This technique facilitated the generalization of treatment gains across ward staff
and settings.

In a methodologically elegant study, Altman et al.[3] reported
the successful treatment of hairpulling and hand-biting in two
mentally retarded children. In contrast to the Tanner and
Zeiler technique, in which aromatic ammonia was presented
for the duration of a SIB act, a three-second inhalation of aromatic ammonia was found to be effective in this study.
Through the use of a multiple baseline design, Altman et al.
showed that SIB was sequentially controlled in clinical, home,
and school settings, as the aversive contingency was introduced

in these settings. In one patient a near-zero rate of hairpulling was maintained for seven weeks; thereafter it gradually increased to about one half of the original rate. In the second patient, follow-up data obtained a year after treatment was discontinued showed that the aversive contingency had produced a complete suppression of hand-biting in the home.

Finally, Singh et al.[224] used a reversal design to show that chronic face-slapping and head-hitting could be controlled in a deaf-blind, profoundly-retarded girl through response-contingent inhalation of aromatic ammonia for three seconds. Although the treatment resulted in near-zero levels, complete suppression of SIB was not achieved. Singh et al. suggested that aromatic ammonia could be used to reduce SIB to very low rates and that a subsequent positive reinforcement technique would completely eliminate it. Empirical verification of this suggestion is needed.

Although general conclusions cannot be drawn on the basis of four studies, several tentative conclusions can be offered. Current research is of a reasonably high calibre and suggests that aromatic ammonia is a particularly potent punisher the use of which needs to be further investigated. Its efficacy needs to be tested against electric shock techniques so that their differential effects can be assessed. It would be useful to know, for example, the differential strengths of these two punishers when one is presented with a patient who has a long history of intractable SIB that has apparently not been amenable to modification. In contrast to electric shock, aromatic ammonia has several features that recommend it as an aversive stimulus. It is small, easily portable, easy to use, inexpensive, and more acceptable than electric shock to staffs of institutions. Because of its size, it can be used in most situations and by most people, thereby ensuring that response suppression will be maintained. However, certain limitations and precautions in its use need to be mentioned. Aromatic ammonia, like other aversive procedures, can be misused by staff and parents alike. Excessive use can, of course, damage nasal mucosa, and direct contact can burn patient's skin. This can be a real problem with particularly strong or large patients who are apt to struggle rather vigorously during the application of aromatic ammonia. Although current studies have not reported any severe side effects, the therapist would be well advised to have medical personnel monitor the course of treatment for potential adverse reactions.

BITTER SUBSTANCES

Bitter substances have been used as aversive stimuli in the treatment of certain types of maladaptive behavior in infants and young children. For example, quinine,[43] lemon juice,[22, 195] and pepper sauce[29, 219] have been used as aversive stimuli to treat rumination. Only lemon juice has been used to treat SIB.

Mayhew and Harris[144] demonstrated the effectiveness of lemon juice (food-grade citric acid) in treating face-punching and headbanging in a profoundly retarded boy. A small amount of lemon juice (pH level 1.5) was squirted into the patient's mouth each time he engaged in a self-injurious act. However, the patient received no more than 55 ml of the solution on a given day. During baseline, the patient made 11 SIB responses per minute in a 15-minute session. Introduction of the lemon juice contingency reduced this immediately to only 0.46 responses per minute. Withdrawal of treatment contingencies reversed therapeutic effects; the rate of response now averaged 1.6 per minute over 23 days. Reintroduction of the treatment contingency again resulted in a rapid decrease in SIB to 0.32 responses per minute. The addition of positive reinforcement for alternative behaviors to the lemon juice contingency produced even further reductions in SIB, which was now maintained at near-zero levels.

While the results of this study are encouraging, insufficient experimental data are available to draw conclusions about the procedure. Indeed, the effects of bitter substances on the usual types of SIB remain virtually uninvestigated. If the results of studies with bitter substances in the treatment of other disorders, such as rumination, are any indication, then we can assume that a similar finding can be expected in the treatment of children with intractable SIB. The clinician needs to be cautioned, however, about its potential complications. These include irritation of both internal and external mouth areas and possible aspiration of lemon juice into the patient's lungs.

FACIAL SCREENING

Facial screening,[134] a mildly aversive stimulus, has been used as a punisher to modify a variety of topographically different forms of maladaptive behaviors in children, including high-frequency out-of-seat behavior,[98] persistent disruptive handclapping[263] and self-injurious behavior.[133, 220, 222, 225, 262] Facial screening requires the patient's face to be covered with a terrycloth bib for a few seconds following a maladaptive response.

Lutzker[133] reported the effects of facial screening on head- and face-slapping in a 20-year-old retarded man. Following each SIB, the therapist verbally reprimanded the patient for engaging in head- or face-slapping, quickly put the bib over his face and head, and held it loosely at the back of his head until the SIB had stopped for three seconds. It was shown through the use of a multiple-baseline design that facial screening was effective in reducing SIB across three settings with a different teacher implementing the treatment in each setting.

Singh[220] evaluated the effectiveness of this procedure in the control of infant thumb-biting in a multiple-baseline study. The infant's parents were trained to apply facial screening for three seconds contingent on each occurrence of thumb-biting. Thumb-biting was eliminated within three weeks and monthly follow-up observations showed that complete suppression had been maintained for a year. This finding is of some importance, since Singh's is the only study that has produced observational data on the long-term suppressive effects of this procedure.

In another study using this technique, Zegiob et al.[262] treated the multiple SIB of a profoundly retarded, brain-damaged boy. They found that the suppressive effects of facial screening generalized to nonconsequated, disruptive, and self-injurious acts. In an attempt to determine the necessary conditions to effect this treatment, these investigators made a partial component analysis of the facial screening procedure. They found that presenting the bib without actually covering the patient's face or restraining his head in the same position as used for facial screening was not effective.

Two recent studies have focused on other parameters of this procedure. In one study, the effects of the absence or presence of visual blocking on SIB were evaluated by means of an alternating treatments design.[225] Visual blocking was found to be necessary in the facial screening procedure. In the other study, an alternating treatments design was used to measure the differential impact of three durations (three seconds, one minute, and three minutes) of facial screening on SIB.[222] It was found that the one-minute duration was the most effective in terms of both immediate response reduction and short-term generalization.

On the basis of evidence from current research, one can tentatively conclude that facial screening appears to be an effective response-reduction technique. Because it is only a mild punisher, it offers a viable alternative to the use of painful response-contingent aversive stimuli, such as electric shock and aromatic ammonia. As shown in Table 3, however, evidence attesting to the efficacy of this technique is based on only five N = 1 studies. Further documentation is required. The procedure is socially acceptable and easy to use and most therapists (parents or hospital staff) can be trained in its use given minimal supervision and training. As with most other aversive techniques, however, the ease with which the procedure can be applied depends on such variables as the frequency of SIB and the physical size and characteristics of the patient. Finally, clinicians should not be deceived by the apparent simplicity of this technique, since any aversive procedure carries with it a potential for abuse, especially in large, understaffed, custodial institutions where patients with SIB are usually to be found.

WATER MIST SPRAY

Water mist spray as an aversive stimulus,[55] or hydropsychotherapy,[172] has been used in an attempt to reduce SIB in children (see Table 3). In the usual procedure, a small amount of water is sprayed on the patient's face following each episode of SIB.

The first use of this procedure was made in 1967 by Peterson and Peterson,[172] who evaluated its effectiveness as a treatment for SIB in a severely retarded boy. The patient's mother reported that she had once reduced her son's tantrums by pouring water on him. Peterson and Peterson[172] used DRO but with little success. Then they evaluated the effects of response-contingent water as a punisher using a reversal design and showed some control over the boy's SIB. Although the frequency of SIB was substantially reduced, complete suppression was not achieved and the mother was taught to use time-out (brief isolation) contingent on each occurrence of self-injurious behavior.

Merwin and Kornegay[150] used water spray mist in the treatment of a variety of self-injurious behaviors in a profoundly retarded girl. Each occurrence of SIB was followed by a verbal reprimand, and water, in the form of a fine mist, was sprayed into the patient's face. In the absence of SIB, the patient was reinforced for engaging in certain fine and gross motor tasks. The results showed that SIB was rapidly decreased with the introduction of this procedure and was maintained at near-zero levels during experimental and generalization periods. Although formal data were not presented, these investigators suggested that as a result of their treatment program there was a positive change in their patient's general emotional and social behavior.

In a study with a profoundly retarded boy, Murphy et al.[160] reduced self-choking with 1 ml of response-contingent water and reinforcement for alternative behaviors. These investigators showed that self-choking was amenable with this procedure, although such effects had dissipated by the time follow-up had been conducted 20 months after treatment. Furthermore, the separate effects of water spray mist and reinforcement of alternative behaviors could not be differentially evaluated in this study.

Dorsey et al.[56] evaluated the effects of water mist spray on the SIB of seven profoundly retarded persons for handbiting, skin tearing and headbanging. As in the other three studies, there was substantial reduction in the frequency of SIB responses across patients as a result of treatment.

These studies suggest that water spray mist may be used as a mild punisher in the suppression of a variety of topographically different forms of SIB. Current research indicates that it can be effective in producing clinically significant reductions in the frequency of SIB, but so far no studies have shown it to be completely effective. We do not know much about the effective parameters of this procedure, and future research may well address itself to this important area of investigation. For example, Merwin and Kornegay[150] have provided some data that

TABLE 3.—METHODOLOGICAL ANALYSIS OF STUDIES USING AROMATIC AMMONIA, BITTER SUBSTANCES, FACIAL SCREENING, AND WATER SPRAY PROCEDURES

AUTHOR	SUBJECT DESCRIPTION	TOPOGRAPHY	TREATMENT	DESIGN	INTEROBSERVER AGREEMENT	GENERALIZATION	FOLLOW-UP
Tanner and Zeiler[241]	20-yr-old autistic woman. Medication: chlorpromazine, 100 mg three times a day (first 6 days of study), chlorpromazine 75 mg twice a day and trifluoperazine hydrochloride 10 mg twice a day.	face-slapping	aromatic ammonia	ABAB	2 observers:93–100% agreement	Yes. Programmed across settings and ward staff	3-week's observational data
Baumeister and Baumeister[20]	4-yr-old severely retarded girl with microcephaly. 7-yr-old severely retarded girl	mouthing, self-slapping of face and legs, hair-pulling	aromatic ammonia	AB	2 observers: 95% agreement	Yes. Treatment programmed across staff and settings	4-mo observational data
Altman et al.[3]	4-yr-old severely retarded girl with a seizure disorder	hairpulling (trichotillomania)	aromatic ammonia and DRO	ABAB multiple baseline/reversal multiple-baseline	several observers: 67–100% agreement	Yes. Treatment programmed across staff and settings.	7 weeks' observational data
	3.7-yr-old moderately retarded boy	handbiting				Yes. Treatment programmed across staff and settings	1-yr observational data

Study	Subject	Behavior	Treatment	Design	Observer agreement	Generalization	Follow-up
Singh et al.[224]	15-yr-old profoundly retarded girl, deaf and blind due to congenital rubella	face-slapping, face-hitting	aromatic ammonia	ABAB	2 observers: 89–96% agreement	Yes. Programmed treatment across settings and ward staff	—
Mayhew and Harris[144]	19-yr-old profoundly retarded man. Medication: Mellaril, 75 mg three times a day, and 25 mg Sinequan, three times a day	face-punching, headbanging	citric acid (lemon juice) citric acid and positive reinforcement	ABABCBC	2 observers: 75–100%	—	—
Lutzker[133]	20-yr-old mentally retarded man with unarrested phenylketonuria	head- and face-slapping	facial screening	multiple-baseline across settings	2 observers: 83–100% agreement	Yes. Treatment programmed across settings and school staff	—
Zegiob et al.[262]	13-yr-old profoundly retarded brain-damaged boy	self-hitting	facial screening	ABAB/multiple baseline across settings	2 observers: 96–100% agreement	Yes. Treatment programmed across settings	—
Singh[220]	11-month-old mildly microcephalic boy	thumb-biting	facial screening	multiple-baseline across settings	2 observers: 100%	Yes. Parents trained as therapists	12-mo observational data
Singh et al.[222]	18-yr-old severely retarded girl	face- and jaw-hitting	facial screening	alternating treatments design	4 observers: 86.4–93.7% agreement	Yes. Treatment programmed across ward staff and settings	—
Singh[225]	19-yr-old profoundly retarded woman with deafness probably due to maternal rubella	face-slapping, headhitting	facial screening	alternating treatments design	2 observers: 91–97% agreement	Yes. Treatment programmed across ward staff, and settings	5 weeks' observational data

TABLE 3.—METHODOLOGICAL ANALYSIS OF STUDIES USING AROMATIC AMMONIA, BITTER SUBSTANCES, FACIAL SCREENING, AND WATER SPRAY PROCEDURES *Continued*

AUTHOR	SUBJECT DESCRIPTION	TOPOGRAPHY	TREATMENT	DESIGN	INTEROBSERVER AGREEMENT	GENERALIZATION	FOLLOW-UP
Peterson and Peterson[172]	3.5-yr-old retarded boy with Hurler's syndrome	headbanging, self-hitting	DRO, water spray, time out	ABCACD	2 observers: 70–89% agreement	—	—
Merwin and Kornegay[150]	29-yr-old profoundly retarded woman	face- and head-hitting, beating chin against shoulder, kicking knee to forehead	water spray mist and positive reinforcement	changing criterion	Unspecified number of observers: 85–100% agreement	Yes. Treatment programmed across settings and ward staff	—
Murphy et al.[160]	24-yr-old profoundly retarded man. Medication: Dilantin, phenobarbital for epilepsy	self-choking	water spray mist and positive reinforcement for alternative behaviors	BAB	several observers: 96–100% agreement	Yes. Treatment programmed across staff and settings	20-mo observational data
Dorsey et al.[56]	7 profoundly retarded nonambulatory persons: 6 females (5- to 37-yr-olds) and 19-yr-old man	handbiting, skin-tearing, headbanging	water mist	ABAB (6 subjects) AB (1 subject)	several observers: 96.5–100% agreement	—	—
	21-yr-old woman, profoundly retarded, with severe quadriplegia due to Edwards' syndrome;	handbiting	verbal reprimand, water mist, and DRO	ABCD and multiple-baseline	2 observers: 86–100% agreement	Yes. Treatment programmed across staff and settings	—
	26-yr-old profoundly retarded woman with severe		verbal reprimand and DRO				

408

suggest that applying water spray mist 15–20 times following each instance of SIB is more effective than a single application. Other variables that need further investigation include the amount of water sprayed per application, the temperature of the water, and the distance from which it is sprayed.

RESPONSE COST

There are two forms of punishment that involve the withdrawal of positive events contingent on the performance of a given event: response cost and time out. Both response cost and time-out have been used to treat SIB in children.

Brawley et al.[28] used response cost to achieve partial suppression of face-slapping in a seven-year-old autistic boy. Food and social reinforcement in the form of adult attention were made contingent on all desirable behaviors of the patient, but an occurrence of face slapping or other inappropriate behavior resulted in the withdrawal of adult attention and food. Lucero et al.[130] compared the effects of contingent withdrawal of social and/or edible reinforcers on the frequency of SIB in three children. Using a Latin-square, Lucero et al. withdrew attention, food, or food plus attention for 15 seconds following each occurrence of headhitting or headbanging. The withdrawal of food and food plus attention were found to be effective in reducing the SIB of all three patients; the withdrawal of attention had minimal effects on frequency of SIB.

Nunes et al.[166] used response-contingent withdrawal of vibratory stimulation to control self-slapping in a 16-year-old boy. The patient had access to vibration from a hand vibrator as long as he did not indulge in SIB. Whenever he slapped himself the vibrator was taken away for 15 seconds. Treatment was scheduled in three settings in a multiple-baseline design; the results showed a dramatic reduction in the patient's rate of SIB across all settings.

Other studies[246] have also used response cost procedures but only as a part of a multicomponent package.

In summary, response cost appears to be a procedure with some merit in need of further investigation. However, the recommendation for this procedure as a treatment for SIB in children should be tempered by the fact that only three studies have demonstrated its efficacy in a controlled manner (Table

TABLE 4.—METHODOLOGICAL ANALYSIS OF STUDIES USING RESPONSE COST, TIME-OUT AND EXTINCTION PROCEDURES

AUTHOR	SUBJECT DESCRIPTION	TOPOGRAPHY	TREATMENT	DESIGN	INTEROBSERVER AGREEMENT	GENERALIZATION	FOLLOW-UP
Brawley et al.[28]	7-yr-old autistic boy	face-slapping	response cost	ABAB	2 observers: 70–98% agreement	Yes. Treatment programmed across staff	3-mo observational data
Lucero et al.[130]	18-yr-old profoundly retarded boy, 17-yr-old profoundly retarded girl, 10-yr-old profoundly retarded girl	headhitting, headbanging	response cost	Latin-square, ABACADA ACADABA ADABACA	3 observers: 60–100% agreement	—	—
Nunes et al.[166] (experiment 1)	16-yr-old severely retarded boy	self-slapping	response cost	multiple-baseline across settings	2 observers: 98–100% agreement	Yes. Treatment programmed across staff and settings	—
Wolf et al.[258]	3.5-yr-old autistic boy	headbanging, face-slapping, hairpulling, face-scratching	timeout	B	—	Yes. Treatment programmed across ward staff and parents, and hospital and home settings	6-mo anecdotal information
Wolf et al.[257]	5-yr-old autistic boy	self-slapping	timeout	AB	—	—	2-mo observational data
Hamilton et al.[90]	17.4-yr-old severely retarded girl	headbanging	timeout	AB	—	—	9 mo
	16.5 yr-old severely retarded girl with hypertelorism	bodyslamming	timeout	B	—	—	2-mo observational data

Reference	Subject	Behavior	Treatment	Design	Reliability	Generalization	Follow-up
Duker[58]	15-yr-old profoundly retarded girl	headbanging, handhitting	time-out, positive reinforcement	AB	—	Yes. Treatment programmed across ward staff wardwide	4-mo observational data
Solnick et al.[233] (experiment 2)	16-yr-old severely retarded boy with Down's syndrome	head- and face-hitting	time-out, enriched and impoverished environment	multiresponse baseline	2 observers: 95–100% agreement	—	—
Lovaas et al.[128]	9-yr-old schizophrenic girl	head- and arm-hanging	extinction	ABAB(?)	—	—	—
Lovaas and Simmons[129]	8-yr-old severely retarded boy; 11-yr-old severely retarded boy	headhitting; headbanging	extinction	B	3 observers: 95% agreement (reliability assessed prior to the study)	—	—
Jones[101]	9-yr-old severely retarded autistic girl	self-hitting (against teeth)	extinction	B	several observers: 95% agreement	monitored across settings	18 weeks' observational data
Myers[163]	12-yr-old mentally retarded boy	biting fingertips and nails	extinction, DRO, response-cost	ABCAD	—	—	—
Duker[57]	8-yr-old profoundly retarded boy with Lesch-Nyhan syndrome	thumb-biting, headbanging	extinction, positive reinforcement	AB	2 observers: 100% agreement	Yes. Treatment programmed across ward staff	—

4). Furthermore, clinicians should be cognizant of the finding that withdrawal of strong positive reinforcers may result not only in the overall decrease of SIB, but may also produce negative side effects such as anger in the patient.[157]

TIME OUT

Time-out from reinforcement (or simply time-out) is a form of punishment in which the patient is isolated or removed from a positively reinforcing situation for a specified period of time after making an undesirable response. For example, a patient may be isolated for a few minutes following an SIB response and during the time-out interval he will not have access to social interaction with staff or other patients, activities, privileges, or other events that he may normally find reinforcing.

Wolf et al.[258] used time-out to control the headbanging, face-slapping, hair-pulling, and face-scratching of an autistic preschooler. The patient was isolated in his bedroom following each tantrum (which included SIB). He had to remain in his room until he was quiet. The time spent in isolation varied from a few minutes to about 45 minutes. Headbanging, face-scratching, and hair-pulling disappeared in about 2.5 months, although face-slapping required another three months of treatment before it was completely eliminated. Treatment was generalized across different settings by training several people (e.g., ward staff and parents) to carry out the time-out procedure with the patient. This patient was followed up two years later by Wolf et al.,[257] who found that he now engaged in self-slapping in the nursery school. A time-out procedure was used again to control this behavior. He was sent to his room for 30 minutes following each episode of self-slapping. It was found that time-out had to be used only three times to completely eliminate his self-slapping at school. This suppression was maintained at zero levels for at least two months.

Hamilton et al.[90] used time-out for SIB in two severely retarded girls. For one patient a 30-minute time-out was made contingent on each instance of headbanging, and for the other a two-hour bed restraint was programmed. Headbanging was rapidly eliminated in three weeks and the treatment effects were maintained at a nine-month follow-up after the termination of treatment. Body-slamming was eliminated in seven months and the treatment effects were maintained at a two-month follow-up.

In another study Duker[58] used a time-out procedure to suppress headbanging in a 15-year-old profoundly retarded girl. The patient was isolated for ten minutes. She was released from time-out if she had stopped headbanging for a two-minute interval. To enhance the effects of time-out, reinforcement was available for incompatible behavior on an intermittent basis. The patient's usual ward attendants and nurses instituted the time-out procedure throughout the day. A near zero level of headbanging and headhitting resulted in about 60 days of therapy.

These studies suggest that time-out may be effective in controlling certain types of SIB in children. However, this can only be considered a tentative conclusion, since all time-out studies had several methodological deficiencies (see Table 4). For example, all four studies discussed above uniformly used a weak experimental design and did not report interobserver reliabilities.

Several issues concerning time-out are pertinent here. First, time-out appears to have the advantage over more aversive techniques in that it can be painless and relatively brief. Studies have shown that time-outs only a few minutes long are effective in suppressing maladaptive behavior[27] and that longer durations do not necessarily augment its effectiveness.[254] Studies using time-out in the treatment of SIB have used relatively long durations; the effects of shorter durations remain uninvestigated. Isolating a child for long durations obviously has the disadvantage of reducing the opportunities for adaptive learning in the given environment. This is not to say that time-out from a given environment necessarily punishes the child. As shown by Solnick et al.,[233] the punishing effects of time-out are a direct function of the reinforcing effects of time-in. As such, the usual institutional ward environment may not be reinforcing enough for certain children, and for them time-out from it may actually act as a reinforcer. One final consideration is that time-out may not prove effective with a child who is already withdrawn or has minimal interaction with others. In such cases, time-out only further isolates a socially withdrawn child.

EXTINCTION

Extinction refers to the withdrawal or withholding of positive reinforcement from a previously reinforced response. As a result, the given response eventually ceases to occur or occurs at a relatively low frequency.

In an experimental study Lovaas et al.[128] taught a nine-year-old schizophrenic girl a small repertoire of behaviors appropriate to music (e.g., clapping and rocking in rhythm with music). When music was played, experimenters reinforced the child's appropriate music behavior with social approval. In the second phase, social approval was not given following any behavior of the patient. That is, an extinction procedure was instituted. Both these phases were then repeated. The results showed that when the patient engaged in appropriate music behavior, her frequency of head- and arm-banging was at a low level. However, when extinction was introduced, her frequency of SIB increased dramatically. This suggests that the extinction of her appropriate behaviors was functionally related to the frequency of her SIB.

In another study, Lovaas and Simmons[129] used extinction to decrease the headhitting and headbanging of two severely retarded boys. The boys were placed in a room, one at a time, for 1.5 hours and the occurrence of their SIB was recorded. One patient exhibited 2,750 SIB acts in the first extinction session, but by the next session this declined to zero. This patient hit himself at least 9,000 times before his SIB was eliminated! The other patient required about 60 sessions before his SIB was brought under control. Similar results have been reported by Jones et al.,[101] who used extinction to treat a nine-year-old severely retarded autistic girl.[101] Twice a day the patient was isolated in a room for a period of two hours. Her SIB was eliminated within 18 weeks.

Myers[163] compared the effects of extinction, differential reinforcement of other behaviors (DRO), and a response-cost procedure in the treatment of self-biting in a 12-year-old boy. During extinction, the patient did not receive any attention for engaging in self-biting, attention being assumed to be the primary reinforcer for SIB in this case. During the DRO phase, the patient could earn 20–30 tokens per day for appropriate classroom behavior. However, tokens were withheld during the

SIB periods. And in the response-cost phase an additional requirement was that he lose one token each time he engaged in SIB. Myers[163] found the response-cost procedure more effective than either extinction or DRO. Of course, not all studies have found extinction to be the treatment of choice in the control of SIB or necessarily the most effective form of treatment. For example, Corte et al.[48] reported the failure of extinction to control SIB in two children. Extinction was used, however for only 12 sessions in this study, and had the treatment contingency been in effect for a larger number of sessions, it probably would have had positive results.

As with other punishment procedures, it has been suggested that positive reinforcement procedures should be used to augment the efficacy of extinction in the control of SIB in children. Duker[57] programmed the entire staff of a ward to ignore the self-biting of a patient with the Lesch-Nyhan syndrome but to reinforce him for engaging in adaptive social behavior. An almost complete suppression of self-biting was achieved.

In summary, these studies indicate that extinction may be one way to control SIB in some children. No definitive conclusions can be drawn about its efficacy, however, because current data is based on studies with basic methodological flaws (see Table 4). Several cautionary statements are in order at this point. Extinction usually results in an initial burst of response and potentially this could harm the patient more than his original problem. Depending on the topography, frequency, and intensity of the SIB, it may be dangerous to expose a patient, albeit temporarily, to an increase in SIB, which usually accompanies the onset of extinction. A related concern, particularly in institutional settings, is that the SIB could be accidentally reinforced during this temporary burst, thus leading to maintenance of SIB at a much higher rate than before. Spontaneous recovery, the temporary recurrence of the nonreinforced response during extinction, could also present similar problems. For example, SIB can be eliminated through extinction but after a few sessions or days it may reappear. If SIB is now accidentally reinforced, it effectively comes under a highly intermittent schedule of reinforcement that makes it much more resistant to extinction.[229]

As noted in the studies reviewed above, another concern is the length of treatment. Extinction usually requires a lengthy period to take effect and the speed with which SIB is reduced may depend on such factors as the schedule of reinforcement that maintained the SIB, the length of time the SIB has been reinforced, and the number of times extinction has been used in the past to reduce the given SIB.

A final consideration is the potential side effects of extinction. It has been noted that extinction may produce certain emotional responses, such as agitation, frustration, feelings of failure, rage,[228] or aggressive behavior.[96]

OVERCORRECTION

Overcorrection, a mild punishment procedure developed by Foxx and Azrin,[65] appears to be effective in the treatment of a variety of behavior problems in children. According to Foxx and Azrin,[66] the rationale of overcorrection is "to overcorrect the environmental effects of an inappropriate act and to require the disruptor intensively to practice overly correct forms of relevant behavior." Thus, the overcorrection procedure can be seen as consisting of two major components, restitution and positive practice. Positive practice has an advantage over other forms of punishment in that it specifically requires the patient to repeatedly practice the correct response within the same environment. Several studies have used variations of the basic overcorrection procedure to control SIB in children and adults.

Webster and Azrin[251] employed a procedure called required relaxation to control agitative-disruptive behavior in eight mentally retarded persons, two of whom exhibited a variety of SIB. Although required relaxation is basically an overcorrection technique, Webster and Azrin[251] see it as a procedure directed toward the agitated state rather than at the disruptive act that followed or resulted from the agitated state. In essence, required relaxation requires the patient to spend an extended period (a minimum of two hours) in relaxation, preferably in his own bed, following each episode of an agitative-disruptive act. Using a basic time-series design (AB), Webster and Azrin showed a reduction in SIB to near zero levels in two patients commensurate with the introduction of the required relaxation contingency. No generalization or follow-up data were reported.

In a second study, Azrin et al.[8] dealt specifically with the control of SIB through overcorrection procedures. However, in this study a multicomponent "educative" procedure, consisting of "autism reversal,"[10] required relaxation,[251] and "hand awareness training,"[11] was used. Again, using an AB-design, Azrin et al. showed a 90% reduction in the frequency of SIB within a single day when the educative procedure was made contingent on each occurrence of SIB in 11 mentally retarded patients. The mean number of SIB responses was reduced by about 99% by the end of three months of therapy; SIB was completely eliminated in 4 of the patients.

Freeman et al.[70] used overcorrection to treat nail-picking in a 6.5-year-old aphasic girl. The patient's hands were held by her side for one minute following each occurrence of nail-picking; positive reinforcement was given when she engaged in appropriate behavior. This treatment rapidly decreased the frequency of nail-picking from 10 to 24 bursts per 30-minute session to zero by the fourth day. Nail-picking was maintained at near zero levels for the next 21 days.

The data presented in the above three studies suggest that overcorrection procedures may be effective in controlling SIB in some patients. However, because of the methodological inadequacies inherent in these studies (e.g., lack of experimental controls and interobserver reliability), such a conclusion is tenuous.

In a somewhat better-designed study employing a multiple-baseline design across school and home settings, Harris and Romanczyk provided more conclusive evidence of the efficacy of overcorrection procedures.[91] Each instance of head- or chin-banging was followed by a ten-minute overcorrection procedure consisting of five minutes of up-down, left-right head movements and five of guided hand movements. SIB responses decreased from a mean of 32 responses per day at school to five and two per day in the first two weeks, respectively; only occasional bursts were observed thereafter. The frequency of SIB, however, remained unchanged at home until the overcorrection procedure was introduced there. The frequency of SIB decreased from a mean rate of 15.44 responses per day to two on the first day and zero on the second. Thereafter it was maintained at near zero levels at school and home for at least nine months. Overcorrection in the form of guided hand movements was also used by Zehr and Theobald[264] with two profoundly retarded girls in the treatment of headhitting and face-scratching.

Measel and Alfieri[148] used a combination of positive practice overcorrection and reinforcement of incompatible behavior with two profoundly retarded boys. These authors contend that reinforcement had no discernible effect on one of these boys, although when it was combined with positive practice, the behavior was immediately reduced and eventually eliminated. This reviewer does not agree with their contention because of methodological problems in their study. First, the reinforcement condition was introduced during session five in spite of a steeply decreasing baseline suggesting that the headslapping of this patient would have reached zero or near zero levels with a few more sessions. Second, the reinforcement condition was in operation for only four sessions, and again, in spite of a decreasing trend in the frequency of headslapping, this condition was terminated and overcorrection was added to the treatment procedure. Except for one data point, the frequency of SIB for individual sessions during the reinforcement phase appears to be less than the mean of the baseline condition. It is therefore suggested that the reinforcement condition was more effective than the authors maintained; in the absence of additional data it seems that the overcorrection procedure did little to augment the efficacy of the reinforcement procedure.

Measel and Alfieri[148] reported completely opposite effects of this treatment with a second patient who showed an increase in headbanging with reinforcement and, after an initial decrease, an increase with overcorrection and reinforcement. Again, the baseline and reinforcement conditions were in effect for three and two sessions, respectively, a period too short about which to make meaningful judgments. Furthermore, it is quite possible that since this subject used headbanging as an avoidance response, the termination of the reinforcement condition actually reinforced the patient. Although these investigators noted this possibility, they failed to test its validity by presenting only the overcorrection component of this procedure. If with both subjects the effects of the reinforcement condition was only to increase the rate of SIB, it seems countertherapeutic to include it with the overcorrection procedure in the next phase.

In a more recent study, Borreson[26] used positive practice overcorrection in the treatment of self-biting, which was used as an avoidance response by a profoundly retarded boy. This boy bit himself whenever he was required to engage in academic activities. When forced running was programmed following each self-biting response, SIB was virtually eliminated within a few months and the treatment gains were maintained for a two-year period.

Kelly and Drabman[107] used positive practice overcorrection to reduce high frequency eyepoking in a three-year-old visually handicapped boy. Every time he poked his eye his arm was raised and lowered 12 times. A DRO ten-second schedule of reinforcement was used in conjunction with this procedure, which meant that he was reinforced every ten seconds if no eyepoking had been observed. Each treatment session lasted ten minutes and generalization was assessed in a different setting during the 20 minutes immediately following termination of daily treatment sessions. Kelly and Drabman showed by means of a reversal design that this boy's eyepoking could be decreased and increased as a function of the implementation and withdrawal of the overcorrection procedure. It was further shown that response suppression generalized in the short term to another setting without explicit programming.

Matson et al.[142] used overcorrection techniques to control pica and hair-pulling in a profoundly retarded woman. Overcorrection for hair-pulling consisted of verbal reprimand and practice of an alternative behavior (appropriate hair brushing) for ten minutes. Hair pulling was reduced and maintained at near zero levels within a few days.

DeCatanzaro and Baldwin[50] used overcorrection in the form of repeated vertical arm movements, which is called forced arm exercise, to treat headhitting in two profoundly-retarded boys. Forced arm exercise in conjunction with a DRO schedule was found to be superior to forced arm exercise alone in the suppression of headhitting with these two patients. Singh et al.[224] successfully replicated this procedure in a study with a 16-year-old profoundly retarded girl.

In summary, current research suggests that overcorrection procedures may be effective in reducing SIB in certain patients. As noted above, the three initial studies using overcorrection[70, 251] used a case-study methodology and did not control for extraneous variables that could provide rival hypotheses regarding the demonstrated reduction of SIB in their subjects. However, some of the other studies used better experimental

TABLE 5—METHODOLOGICAL ANALYSIS OF STUDIES USING OVERCORRECTION PROCEDURES

AUTHOR	SUBJECT DESCRIPTION	TOPOGRAPHY	TREATMENT	DESIGN	INTEROBSERVER AGREEMENT	GENERALIZATION	FOLLOW-UP
Webster and Azrin[251]	21-yr-old profoundly retarded woman, 52-yr-old severely retarded woman	headbanging, self-kicking, self-hitting, running into walls and doors; self-biting	overcorrection (required relaxation)	AB	several observers: 100% agreement (informal measure)	—	—
Azrin et al.[8]	11 10–46-yr-old profoundly retarded persons; 5 males and 5 females, 1 schizophrenic male	headbanging, eyegouging, self-biting, self-hitting, face-slapping, and others	overcorrection, including required relaxation, hand control procedure, and hand awareness training, positive reinforcement for incompatible behaviors	AB	—	Yes. Treatment scheduled in several locations	—
Freeman et al.[70]	6.5-yr-old-girl	nail-picking	positive practice, overcorrection, positive reinforcement	AB	—	—	—
Harris and Romanczyk[91]	8-yr-old moderately retarded boy with autistic tendancies	headbanging, chinbanging	positive practice overcorrection	Multiple baseline across school and home settings	—	Yes. Treatment programmed across therapists and settings	9-mo anecdotal data
Measel and Alfieri[148]	14-yr-old profoundly retarded partially sighted boy	headslapping	positive practice overcorrection, positive reinforcement	ABCBC	2 observers: $r =$ .93	—	4-mo observational data
	16-yr-old profoundly retarded	headbanging	positive practice overcorrection, positive reinforcement	ABC	2 observers: 94.7% agreement	—	—

Study	Subject	Behavior	Treatment	Design	Reliability	Generalization	Follow-up
Kelly and Drabman[107]	3-yr-old visually handicapped boy	eyepoking	positive practice overcorrection, DRO	ABAB	2 observers: 98–100% agreement	Generalization to another setting was assessed	—
Matson et al.[142]	57-yr-old profoundly retarded woman	hair pulling	positive practice overcorrection	Multiresponse baseline	2 observers: 96–100% agreement	—	3-mo observational data
Zehr and Theobald[264]	24-yr-old profoundly retarded woman	headhitting	positive practice overcorrection	ABAB	2 observers: 94–100% agreement (assessed during baseline only)	—	—
	19-yr-old profoundly retarded woman	face-scratching					
DeCatanzaro and Baldwin[50]	8-yr-old profoundly retarded boy	headhitting	positive practice overcorrection, DRO	ABAD ABACD	—	Yes. Treatment programmed across ward staff and various settings	2-mo anecdotal information
	12-yr-old profoundly retarded boy						
Singh et al.[224] (experiment 2)	16-yr-old profoundly retarded girl	jawhitting	positive practice overcorrection, DRO	Multiple-baseline across settings and reversal ABAB	2 observers: 87–98% agreement	Yes. Treatment programmed across ward staff and various settings	6-mo observational data
Borreson[26]	22-yr-old profoundly retarded man	self-biting	positive practice overcorrection	ABAB	2 observers: 86–100% agreement	Yes. Treatment programmed in school and ward settings and across staff	2-yr observational data

421

controls that provided evidence attesting the efficacy of the procedure (Table 5). But it should be noted here that all but two studies[50, 224] used different components within their overcorrection package, thus rendering comparisons across experiments an extremely difficult exercise. Further research might well address itself to the question of replicability of these studies so that more general conclusions about the efficacy of the various overcorrection packages can be made.

A related problem concerns the differential effects of the various components used in overcorrection procedures. As noted elsewhere,[21] overcorrection consists of a number of distinct behavioral techniques, including extinction, time out from positive reinforcement, physical restraint, response prevention, prompting, and reinforcement of competing responses. If this procedure is to have general applicability in the treatment of behavioral disorders in children, then we need to know more about the facilitative effects of separate components.

DIFFERENTIAL REINFORCEMENT PROCEDURES

One way of suppressing or eliminating maladaptive behaviors in children is by increasing other, socially adaptive, behaviors. For example, Ayllon and Roberts[7] have shown that the reinforcement of correct performance on written assignments can be used to decrease discipline problems in fifth-grade boys. This technique for reducing maladaptive behaviors is commonly referred to as differential reinforcement. The basic requirement of this technique is that a reinforcer be delivered when the target response is *not* emitted for a specified time interval.[184] If the behavior being reinforced is other than the one that is being reduced (e.g., SIB), then the procedure is termed differential reinforcement of other behavior (DRO). A variation of this procedure specifies the reinforcement of a behavior incompatible with the target response. This procedure is termed differential reinforcement of incompatible behavior (DRI).

Peterson and Peterson[171] used DRO procedures to control headslapping and headbanging in an eight-year-old boy. Food and praise were used to reinforce periods without SIB (DRO) and their withdrawal for ten seconds was used to punish SIB. The frequency of SIB was reduced but it was found that pairing

DRO with a time out procedure (isolation) was much more effective, a finding noted in other studies.[27]

Lane and Domrath[121] in a study using case-study methodology reported the reduction of nail-pulling in a mentally retarded, psychotic patient. Sips of coffee were made contingent on the nonoccurrence of SIB for a brief interval. Since the pretreatment rate of SIB was very high, only 15-second intervals were scheduled. Later the time interval was progressively lengthened until the patient was able to be left by himself; sips of coffee were provided on an intermittent basis throughout the day.

Corte et al.[48] compared the effects of time out, DRO, and punishment via electric shock on the SIB of profoundly retarded adolescents. DRO was found to have no effect on the SIB of two patients. However, one patient responded well to DRO only when malt was used as the reinforcer and the patient had been deprived of the lunch that preceded the treatment sessions.

Candy was used to reinforce periods of time when a ten-year-old girl did not scratch her face in a study by Repp and Deitz.[181] Although the introduction of this procedure saw the immediate reduction of face-scratching, this study employed only a basic AB design from which no firm conclusions can be drawn. However, these investigators replicated the use of this procedure in another study that used adequate experimental controls and obtained similar results.[182] In this study praise was the only available reinforcement.

Several other studies using reversal designs have demonstrated the efficacy of DRO in the treatment of SIB (Table 6). Although there are minor variations in the programming of the DRO schedules in these studies, the general finding has been that self-injury in children can be reduced to near-zero levels with this procedure. Several topographically different forms of SIB have been treated with DRO schedules of reinforcement, including headbanging,[67, 179, 252] handbiting,[191] headslapping,[132] and scratching.[179]

One study used a multiple baseline across three classroom settings to treat wristbiting and fingerbiting in a ten-year-old boy. Primary reinforcers (e.g., pretzels, gumdrops, and mints) were used on a DRO schedule to reinforce periods when the patient did not indulge in self-biting.[131] SIB was rapidly brought under control in each setting with the introduction of the DRO contingency.

TABLE 6.—METHODOLOGICAL ANALYSIS OF STUDIES USING DIFFERENTIAL REINFORCEMENT PROCEDURES

AUTHOR	SUBJECT DESCRIPTION	TOPOGRAPHY	TREATMENT	DESIGN	INTEROBSERVER AGREEMENT	GENERALIZATION	FOLLOW UP
Peterson and Peterson[171]	8-yr-old mentally retarded boy	headslapping, headbanging	DRO, withdrawal of positive reinforcers	ABCAC	2 observers: 95% + agreement on 3 occasions	—	—
Bailey and Meyerson[15]	7-yr-old cribbound boy	headbanging, handchewing	DRI	ABCD	2 observers: 75–91% agreement	—	—
Lane and Domrath[121]	33-yr-old mentally retarded psychotic man	nailpulling	DRO	AB	—	Yes. Treatment programmed across ward staff and various settings	1-yr anecdotal information
Corte et al.[48]	2 profoundly retarded adolescents, 1 boy and 1 girl	headbanging, eyepoking	DRO	ABC	4 observers: 98–100% agreement	—	—
Repp and Deitz[181]	10-yr-old severely retarded girl	facescratching	DRO + verbal reprimand	AB	2 observers: 79–100% agreement	Yes. Treatment programmed across settings	—
Young and Wincze[261]	21-yr-old profoundly retarded woman	headbanging, headhitting	DRO, DRI	Multiple baseline	2 observers: 90–99% agreement	—	—
Weiher and Harman[252]	14-yr-old boy with Down's syndrome	headbanging	DRO	ABAB	2 observers: 100% agreement	—	2 weeks anecdotal information

Repp et al.[182]	14-yr-old severely retarded boy	handbiting	DRO	ABAB	2 observers: mean agreement of 83%	—	—
Ragain and Anson[179]	12-yr-old severely retarded girl	scratching, headbanging	DRO	ABAB	—	—	—
Frankel et al.[67]	6.7-yr-old profoundly retarded autistic girl	headbanging	extinction, DRO	ABABAC	2 observers: agreement over 90%	—	9-mo observational data
Luiselli it al.[131]	10-yr-old mentally retarded boy	wristbiting and fingerbiting	DRO	Multiple baseline	2 observers: 91.6–100% agreement	Yes. Treatment programmed across settings	—
Luiselli et al.[132]	10-yr-old moderately retarded boy	headslapping	DRO	ABAB	2 observers: 100% agreement	—	3.5-mo observational data
Rose[191]	9-yr-old schizophrenic girl	handbiting	DRO	ABABAB	2 observers: 92–100% agreement	—	—
Tarpley and Schroeder[242]	24-yr-old profoundly retarded man with Male Turner's syndrome 8-yr-old profoundly retarded boy with Down's syndrome 24-yr-old profoundly retarded woman	self-hitting	DRO, DRI	Multiple schedule	5 observers: 76–92% agreement	—	—

In a well-controlled experimental study, Tarpley and Schroeder[242] compared the effects of DRO and DRI schedules on SIB in three profoundly retarded patients. A multiple-schedule, within-subjects design was used. It was found that the two schedules produced differential effects; DRI proved more effective than DRO in reducing the rate of SIB in these patients. This does not support the findings of Young and Wincze,[261] who showed that the reinforcement of behavior compatible or incompatible with SIB was ineffective in decreasing the frequency of SIB in their own patient.

In summary, these studies attest to the efficacy of differential reinforcement procedures that suppress SIB by strengthening other, more adaptive, behaviors. Furthermore, differential reinforcement procedures follow the least restrictive treatment model and answer all current ethical concerns.[143]

PHYSICAL RESTRAINT

The SIB of institutionalized children is most frequently controlled by some form of physical restraint.[199] However, there is little empirical evidence to the efficacy of this procedure.[202] Schroeder et al. note[202] that when contingent restraint has been used it has been only as an adjunct to other procedures.[139, 161, 197, 201] Indeed, the therapeutic effects of response-contingent physical restraint when used by itself have yet to be demonstrated.

There has been some speculation in the literature that physical restraint may serve as a positive reinforcer in certain children.[21, 73, 243] Some empirical support for this view in the self-stimulation literature suggests a functional relationship between contingent restraint and self-stimulation.[64] Although there is also some support for this relationship in the self-injury literature,[61, 62, 189] the evidence is slim and needs further research.

COMBINED TREATMENT APPROACHES

Several investigators have used what is commonly termed a treatment package strategy in the behavioral literature.[105] This refers to treatment procedures that have multiple components and may or may not have a central conceptual focus. A good example of this approach is the voluminous literature on over-correction procedures that show that several distinct behavioral techniques can be combined to produce a procedure that rapidly brings an intractable behavioral problem under control. While this technique has limited value in analytical terms, its potential in practical terms has been realized in several studies that have reported excellent clinical control of SIB.*

OTHER APPROACHES

Several studies have reported other techniques that need to be replicated and verified before comments can be made about their efficacy. Such techniques include multifaceted behavior therapy (relaxation, thought-stopping, and desensitization),[41] desensitization,[33, 192] latent learning,[156] environmental manipulation,[158] and verbal control.[198]

Current Status and Future Directions

The research reviewed in this chapter, especially from the past decade, generally presents an optimistic prognosis for the treatment of self-injurious behavior in pediatric populations. Unfortunately, such optimism is not totally justified. While significant advances continue to be made in both our understanding of the nature and etiology of SIB and our ability to provide effective treatment, this chapter occasioned a number of concerns regarding the experimental research on which such optimism is based.

Although research on behavioral approaches to the treatment of SIB has been voluminous, much of it is scientifically uninterpretable because of poor experimental controls and, in some cases, lack of theoretical underpinnings. Furthermore, there has been an absence of sustained programmatic research, which has resulted in a small number of studies using a large number of techniques. Parametric studies of most behavioral techniques are virtually nonexistent. We simply do not know enough about the conditions under which our treatments work

---

*References 1, 164, 214–215, 226, 227, 237, 243, 246.

best, the impact of these techniques on the different topographies of SIB, or their effects with different populations. These areas need programmatic research in the future.

Another major concern has been the general lack of methodological rigor displayed in these studies, especially in most of the earlier literature. As noted elsewhere,[100] this situation has improved over the years, but even current research is notable for its violation of some of the methodological criteria outlined earlier. Studies often lack experimental controls considered standard for research on the outcome of treatment. For example, adequate baseline data are often not reported, weak experimental controls are used from which no conclusions about the efficacy of treatment can be evaluated, interobserver reliability data are not reported, and generalization and follow-up data are generally unavailable. Certainly, such methodological issues deserve greater attention, and future research must include the necessary controls.

Several investigators have mentioned the problems of producing generalized durable behavior change but few have provided data from programmed treatment. Despite the fact that generalization and maintenance of behavior change in extra-therapy settings has received considerable theoretical and experimental attention in the behavioral literature, this was found to be the area most neglected in the SIB literature. There have been almost no good data-based follow-up studies that have used observational procedures. Follow-up data is particularly crucial in this area of research because SIB is known to vary in terms of its frequency and intensity and to be quiescent over time. Future research could well address itself to the problems of generalization and maintenance of therapeutic effects across time and settings.

Summary

This chapter attempted to outline current trends and recent advances in the treatment of SIB. The major focus has been on the behavioral techniques, since it was obvious that at this stage other approaches have little to offer either diagnostically or therapeutically. It was pointed out, however, that these approaches and drug therapy in particular need further investigation before their role in the treatment of SIB can be adequately assessed.

This chapter critically evaluated the current behavioral approaches in some depth and advanced several recommendations for future work. The general impression gained from current research is that significant advances have been made in the last decade in our understanding of the problem and that a small number of well-controlled studies have shown that SIB in certain children can be controlled for up to three years. Yet a concerted research effort is required to overcome the methodological problems that appeared with disconcerting regularity in most of this research. It is sobering to note that no current prevalence studies of SIB report a major decline in the prevalence of SIB in pediatric populations despite our current ability to provide some form of meaningful treatment.

Acknowledgments

The author would like to thank Judy Singh, Heather King, and Karen Page for their assistance in the preparation of the manuscript for this chapter, and Dr. Ivan L. Beale for his editorial comments.

BIBLIOGRAPHY

1. Adam K.M., Klinge V., Keiser T.W.: The extinction of a self-injurious behavior in an epileptic child. *Behav. Res. Ther.* 11:351, 1973.
2. Allen K.E., Harris F.R.: Elimination of a child's excessive scratching by training the mother in reinforcement procedures. *Behav. Res. Ther.* 4:79, 1966.
3. Altman K., Haavik S., Cook J.W.: Punishment of self-injurious behavior in natural settings using contingent aromatic ammonia, *Behav. Res. Ther.* 16:85, 1978.
4. Aman M.G.: Psychoactive drugs in mental retardation, in Matson J.L. et al. (eds): *Treatment Issues and Innovations in Mental Retardation.* New York: Plenum Publishing Corp. In press.
5. Aman M.G., Singh N.N.: The usefulness of Thioridazine for treating childhood disorders: Fact or folklore? *Am. J. Ment. Defic.* 84:331, 1980.
6. Anderson L.T., Dancis J., Alpert M., et al.: Punishment learning and self-mutilation in Lesch-Nyhan disease. *Nature* 265:461, 1977.
7. Ayllon T., Roberts M.D.: Eliminating discipline problems by strengthening academic performance. *J. Appl. Behav. Anal.* 7:71, 1974.
8. Azrin N.H., Gottlieb L., Hughart L., et al.: Eliminating self-injurious behavior by educative procedures. *Behav. Res. Ther.* 13:101, 1975.
9. Azrin N.H., Holz W.C.: Punishment, in Honig W.K. (ed): *Operant Behavior: Areas of Research and Application.* New York: Appleton-Century-Crofts, 1966, p 380.
10. Azrin N.H., Kaplan S.J., Foxx R.M.: Autism reversal: Eliminating stereotyped self-stimulation of retarded individuals. *Am. J. Ment. Defic.* 78:241, 1973.

11. Azrin N.H., Nunn R.G.: Habit-reversal: A method of eliminating nervous habits and tics. *Behav. Res. Ther.* 11:619, 1973.
12. Bachman J.A.: Self-injurious behavior: A behavioral analysis. *J. Abnorm. Child Psychol.* 80:211, 1972.
13. Baer D.M.: Perhaps it would be better not to know everything. *J. Appl. Behav. Anal.* 10:167, 1977.
14. Baer D.M., Wolf M.M., Risley T.R.: Some current dimensions of applied behavior analysis. *J. Appl. Behav.* 1:91, 1968.
15. Bailey J., Meyerson L.: Effect of vibratory stimulation on a retardate's self-injurious behavior. *Psychol. Aspects Dis.* 17:133, 1970.
16. Balduzzi E.: Contributo alla psicopatologia degli stati ossessvi (A proposito di un caso clinica con impulsivita autolesiva). *Riv. Sper. Freniat.* 85:314, 1961.
17. Ball T.S., Sibbach L., Jones R., et al.: An accelerometer-activated device to control assaultive and self-destructive behaviors in retardates. *J. Behav. Ther. Exptl. Psychiat.* 6:223, 1975.
18. Ballinger B.R.: Minor self-injury. *Br. J. Psychiatry* 118:535, 1971.
19. Baroff G.S., Tate B.S.: The use of aversive stimulation in the treatment of chronic self-injurious behavior. *J. Am. Acad. Child. Psychiatry* 7:454, 1968.
20. Baumeister A.A.: Suppression of repetitive self-injurious behavior by contingent inhalation of aromatic ammonia. *J. Autism Child. Schizophr.* 8:71, 1978.
21. Baumeister A.A., Rollings J.P.: Self-injurious behavior, in Ellis N.R. (ed): *International Review of Research in Mental Retardation.* New York: Academic Press, 1976, vol 8, p 1.
22. Becker J.V., Turner S.M., Sajwaj T.E.: Multiple behavioral effects of the use of lemon juice with a ruminating toddler-age child. *Behav. Mod.* 2:267, 1978.
23. Bender L., Harnell H.: An observation nursery: A study of 250 children in the psychiatric division of Bellevue Hospital. *Am. J. Psychiatry* 97:1170, 1941.
24. Berkson G.: Stereotyped movements of mental defectives: VI. No effect of amphetamine or a barbiturate. *Percept. Mot. Skills* 21:698, 1965.
25. Berkson G., Mason W.A.: Stereotyped movements of mental defectives: IV. The effects of toys and the character of the acts. *Am. J. Ment. Defic.* 68:511, 1964.
26. Borreson P.M.: The elimination of a self-injurious avoidance response through a forced running sequence. *Ment. Retard.* 18:73, 1980.
27. Bostow D.E., Bailey J.B.: Modification of severe disruptive and aggressive behavior using brief timeout and reinforcement procedures. *J. Appl. Behav. Anal.* 2:31, 1969.
28. Brawley E.R., Harris F.R., Allen K.E., et al.: Behavior modification of an autistic child. *Behav. Sci.* 14:87, 1969.
29. Bright G.O., Whaley D.L.: Suppression of regurgitation and rumination with aversive events. *Mich. Ment. Health Res. Bull.* 2:17, 1968.
30. Browning R.M., Stover D.O.: *Behavior Modification in Child Treatment: An Experimental and Clinical Approach.* Chicago: Aldine-Atherton, 1977.
31. Bucher B., Lovaas O.I.: Use of aversive stimulation in behavior modification, in Jones M. (ed): *Miami Symposium on the Prediction of Behavior, 1967: Aversive Stimulation.* Coral Gables, Florida: University of Miami Press, 1968, p 77.
32. Buddenhagen R.G.: Until electric shocks are legal. *Ment. Retard.* 6:48, 1971.
33. Bull M., LaVecchio F.: Behavior therapy for a child with Lesch-Nyhan syndrome. *Develop. Med. Child Neurol.* 20:368, 1978.
34. Cain A.C.: The presuper-ego turning inward of aggression. *Psychoanal. Quart.* 30:171, 1961.
35. Callias M., Carr J., Corbett J.A., et al.: The use of behavior modification techniques in a community service for mentally handicapped children. *Proc. Royal. Soc. Med.* 66:1140, 1973.

36. Campbell D. T., Stanley J.C.: *Experimental and Quasi-Experimental Designs for Research.* Chicago: Rand McNally, 1966.
37. Carr E.G.: The motivation of self-injurious behavior: A review of some hypotheses. *Psychol. Bull.* 84:800, 1977.
38. Carr E.G., Newsom C.D., Binkoff J.A.: Stimulus control of self-destructive behavior in a psychotic child. *J. Abnorm. Child Psychol.* 4:139, 1976.
39. Carraz Y., Erhardt R.: L'Automutilation chez des enfants en institution. *Rev. Neuropsychiat. Infant.* 21:217, 1973.
40. Catel V.W., Schmidt J.: Uber familiare gichtische diathese in verdinung mit zerebalen und renalen symptomen bei einen kleinkind. *Dtsch. Med. Wochenschr.* 84:2145, 1959.
41. Cautela J.R., Baron M.G.: Multifaceted behavior therapy of self-injurious behavior. *J. Behav. Ther. Exptl. Psychiatry* 4:125, 1973.
42. Clark D.L., Krentzberg J.R., Chee F.K.W.: Vestibular stimulation influence on motor development in infants. *Science* 196:1228, 1977.
43. Clark F.H.: Rumination: A case report, *Arch. Gen. Psychiatry* 73:12, 1956.
44. Clark L.P., Uniker T.E.: An analytic study of stereotyped habit movements in children. *J. Nerv. Ment. Dis.* 66:46, 1927.
45. Cleland C.C., Clark C.: Sensory deprivation and aberrant behavior among idiots. *Am. J. Ment. Defic.* 71:213, 1966.
46. Cone J.D.: The relevance of reliability and validity for behavioral assessment. *Behav. Ther.* 8:411, 1977.
47. Corbett J.: Aversion for the treatment of self-injurious behavior. *J. Ment. Defic Res.* 19:79, 1975.
48. Corte H.E., Wolf M.M., Locket B.J.: A comparison of procedures for eliminating self-injurious behavior of retarded adolescents. *J. Appl. Behav. Anal.* 4:201, 1971.
49. Davenport R.K., Berkson G.: Stereotyped movements of mental defectives: II. Effects of novel objects. *Am. J. Ment. Defic.* 67:879, 1963.
50. DeCatanzaro D.A., Baldwin G.: Effective treatment of self-injurious behavior through a forced arm exercise. *Am. J. Ment. Defic.* 82:433, 1978.
51. De Lissovoy, V.: Headbanging in early childhood: A study of incidence. *J. Pediatr.* 58:803, 1961.
52. De Lissovoy V.: Headbanging in early childhood. *Child Develop.* 33:43, 1962.
53. De Lissovoy V.: Headbanging in early childhood: A suggested cause. *J. Genet. Psychol.* 102:109, 1963.
54. Dobrowski C.: Psychological basis of self-mutilation. *Genet. Psychol. Monogr.* 19:1, 1937.
55. Dorsey M.F.: *Reduction of Self-Injurious Behaviors in Retardates Using a Spray Mist.* Unpublished master's thesis, Western Michigan University, 1976.
56. Dorsey M.F., Iwata B.A., Ong P., et al.: Treatment of self-injurious behavior using a water mist: Initial response suppression and generalization. *J. Appl. Behav. Anal.* 13:343, 1980.
57. Duker P.C.: Behavior control of self-biting in a Lesch-Nyhan patient. *J. Ment. Defic. Res.* 19:11, 1975.
58. Duker P.C.: Behavior therapy for self-injurious behavior: Two case studies. *REAP* 1:223, 1975.
59. Duker P.C.: Remotely applied punishment versus avoidance conditioning in the treatment of self-injurious behaviors. *Europ. J. Behav. Anal. Mod.* 3:179, 1976.
60. Fabish W., Darbyshire R.: Report on an unusual case of self-induced epilepsy with comments on some psychological and therapeutic aspects. *Epilepsia* 6:335, 1965.
61. Favell J.E.: Current trends in the treatment of self-injury. Paper presented at the Annual Meeting and Conference of the National Society for Autistic Children, Dallas, Texas, 1978.
62. Favell J.E., McGimsey J.F., Jones M.L.: The use of physical restraint in the treat-

ment of self-injury and as positive reinforcement. *J. Appl. Behav. Anal.* 11:225, 1978.

63. Ferster C.B.: Positive reinforcement and behavioral deficits of autistic children. *Child Develop.* 32:437, 1961.

64. Forehand R., Baumeister A.A.: Bodyrocking and activity level as a function of prior movement restraint, in Gibson D., et al. (eds): *Managing the Severely Retarded: A Sampler,* Springfield Illinois: Charles C Thomas, Publisher, 1976, p 356.

65. Foxx R.M., Azrin N.H.: Restitution: A method of eliminating aggressive-disruptive behaviors of retarded and brain damaged patients. *Behav. Res. Ther.* 10:15, 1972.

66. Foxx R.M., Azrin N.H.: The elimination of autistic self-stimulatory behavior by overcorrection. *J. Appl. Behav. Anal.* 6:1, 1973.

67. Frankel F., Moss D., Schofield S., et al.: Case study: Use of differential reinforcement to suppress self-injurious and aggressive behavior, *Psychol. Rep.* 39:843, 1976.

68. Frankel F., Simmons J.Q.: Self-injurious behavior in schizophrenic and retarded children. *Am. J. Ment. Defic.* 80:512, 1976.

69. Freedman D.G., Boverman H., Freedman N.: Effects of kinesthetic stimulation on weight gain and on smiling in premature infants. Paper presented at the Meeting of the American Orthopsychiatric Association, San Francisco, 1966.

70. Freeman B.J., Graham V., Ritvo E.R.: Reduction of self-destructive behavior by overcorrection. *Psychol. Rep.* 37:446, 1975.

71. Freud A.: *Three Contributions to the Theory of Sex.* New York: Modern Library, 1938.

72. Freud A., Burlingham D.G.: *Infants Without Families.* New York: International Universities Press, 1944.

73. Friedin B.: Clinical issues on the physical restraint experience with self-injurious children. *Res. Retard.* 4:1, 1977.

74. Frith C.D., Johnstone E.C. Joseph M.H., et al.: Double-blind clinical trial of 5-hydroxytryptophan in a case of Lesch-Nyhan syndrome. *J. Neurol. Neurosurg. Psychiatry* 39:656, 1976.

75. Fritz-Herbert J.: The origin of headbanging: A suggested explanation with an illustrated case history. *J. Ment. Sci.* 96:793, 1950.

76. Fritz-Herbert J.: Headbanging and allied behavior: Further observations. *J. Ment. Sci.* 98:330, 1952.

77. Gaylord-Ross R.J., Weeks M., Lipner C.: An analysis of antecedents, response, and consequent events in the treatment of self-injurious behavior. *Educ. Train. Ment. Retard.* 15:35, 1980.

78. Gee S.: Miscellanies. *St. Bartholomew's Hosp. Rep.* 22:96, 1886.

79. Genovese E., Napoli P.A., Bolego-Zonta N.: Self-aggressiveness: A new type of behavior change induced by pemoline. *Life Sci.* 8:513, 1969.

80. Gesell A., Ilg F.L.: *Infant and Child in the Culture of Today.* New York: Harper, 1943.

81. Glass G.V., Willson V.L., Gottman J.M.: *Design and Analysis of Time-Series Experiments.* Boulder, Colorado: University of Colorado Press, 1975.

82. Goodenough F.: *Anger in Young Children.* Minneapolis: University of Minnesota Press, 1931.

83. Green A.H.: Self-mutilation in schizophrenic children. *Arch. Gen. Psychiatry* 17:234, 1967.

84. Green A.H.: Self-destructive behavior in physically abused schizophrenic children: Report of case. *Arch. Gen. Psychiatry* 19:171, 1968.

85. Green A.H.: Self-destructive behavior in battered children. *Am. J. Psychiatry* 135:579, 1978.

86. Greenacre P.: Problems of infantile neurosis: A discussion. *Psychoanal. Study Child.* 9:37, 1954.
87. Griffin J.C., Locke B.J., Landers W.F.: Manipulation of potential punishment parameters in the treatment of self-injury. *J. Appl. Behav. Anal.* 8:458, 1975.
88. Hall G.S.: A study of anger. *Am. J. Psychol.* 10:516, 1899.
89. Hall H., Thorne D.E., Shinedling M., et al.: Overcoming situation-specific problems associated with typical institutional attempts to suppress self-mutilative behavior. *Train. Sch. Bull.* 70:111, 1973.
90. Hamilton J., Stephens L., Allen P.: Controlling aggressive and destructive behavior in severely retarded institutionalized residents. *Am. J. Ment. Defic.* 71:852, 1967.
91. Harris S.L., Romanczyk R.G.: Treating self-injurious behavior of a retarded child by overcorrection. *Behav. Ther.* 7:235, 1976.
92. Hersen M., Barlow D.H.: *Single Case Experimental Designs: Strategies for Studying Behavior Change in the Individual.* New York: Pergamon Press, 1976.
93. Hollis J.H.: The effects of social and nonsocial stimuli on the behavior of profoundly retarded children: Part I. *Am. J. Ment. Defic.* 69:755, 1965.
94. Hollis J.H.: The effects of social and nonsocial stimuli on the behavior of profoundly retarded children: Part II. *Am. J. Ment. Defic.* 69:722, 1965.
95. Horner R.D., Barton E.S.: Operant techniques in the analysis and modification of self-injurious behavior. *Behav. Res. Sev. Develop. Dis.* 1:61, 1980.
96. Hutchinson R.R., Azrin N.H., Hunt G.M.: Attack produced by intermittent reinforcement of a concurrent operant response. *J. Expt. Anal. Behav.* 11:489, 1968.
97. Ilg F.L., Ames L.B.: *Child Behavior.* New York: Harper, 1955.
98. Jenkins J., Becker J.: Positive reinforcement, overcorrection, and punishment in the management of out-of-seat behavior. Paper presented at the Meeting of the Southeastern Psychological Association, Atlanta, Georgia, 1975.
99. Jervis G.A., Stimson C.W.: De Lange Syndrome. *J. Pediatr.* 63:634, 1963.
100. Johnson W.L., Baumeister A.A.: Self-injurious behavior: A review and analysis of methodological details of published studies. *Behav. Mod.* 2:465, 1978.
101. Jones F.H., Simmons J.Q., Frankel F.: An extinction procedure for eliminating self-destructive behavior in a 9-year-old autistic girl. *J. Autism Child. Schizophr.* 4:241, 1974.
102. Kazdin A.E.: Characteristics and trends in applied behavior analysis. *J. Appl. Behav. Anal.* 8:332, 1975.
103. Kazdin A.E.: *Behavior Modification in Applied Settings.* Homewood, Illinois: Dorsey Press, 1975.
104. Kazdin A.E.: Artifact, bias, and complexity of assessment: The ABC's of reliability. *J. Appl. Behav. Anal.* 10:141, 1977.
105. Kazdin A.E.: Therapy outcome questions requiring control of credibility and treatment-generated expectancies. *Behav. Res. Ther.* 10:81, 1979.
106. Kazdin A.E., Kopel S.A.: On resolving ambiguities of the multiple-baseline design: Problems and recommendations. *Behav. Ther.* 6:601, 1975.
107. Kelly J.A., Drabman R.S.: Generalizing response suppression of self-injurious behavior through an overcorrection punishment procedure: A case study. *Behav. Ther.* 8:468, 1977.
108. Kent R.N., Foster S.L.: Direct observational procedures: Methodological issues in naturalistic settings, in Ciminero A.R., et al. (eds): *Handbook of Behavioral Assessment.* New York: John Wiley & Sons, 1977, p 279.
109. Kiloh L.G., Aye R.S., Rushwortz R.G., et al.: Stereotactic amygdaloidotomy for aggressive behavior. *J. Neurol. Neurosurg. Psychiatry* 37:437, 1974.
110. Knepler K.N., Sewall S.: Negative practice paired with smelling salts in the treatment of a tic. *J. Behav. Ther. Exptl. Psychiatry* 5:189, 1974.
111. Kohlenberg R.J., Levin M., Belcher S.: Skin conductance changes and the pun-

ishment of self-destructive behavior: A case study. *Ment. Retard.* 10:11, 1973.
112. Korner A.F., Thoman E.B.: Visual alertness in neonates as evoked by maternal care. *J. Exptl. Child. Psychol.* 10:67, 1970.
113. Korner A.F., Thoman E.B.: The relative efficacy of contact and vestibular-proprioceptive stimulation in soothing neonates. *Child Develop.* 43:443, 1972.
114. Korten J.J., Van Dorp A., Hustinx Th.W.J., et al.: Self-mutilation in a case of 49 XXXXY chromosomal constitution. *J. Ment. Defic. Res.* 19:63, 1975.
115. Kratochwill T.R. (ed): *Single Subject Research: Strategies for Evaluating Change.* New York: Academic Press, 1978.
116. Kratochwill T.R., Wetzel R.J.: Observer agreement, credibility, and judgment: Some considerations in presenting observer agreement data. *J. Appl. Behav. Anal.* 10:133, 1977.
117. Kravitz H., Boehm S.: Rhythmic habit patterns in infancy: Their sequence, age of onset, and frequency, *Child Develop.* 42:399, 1971.
118. Kravitz H., Rosenthal V., Teplitz Z., et al.: A study of headbanging in infants and children. *Dis. Nerv. Syst.* 21:203, 1960.
119. Kulka A., Fry C., Goldstein F.J.: Kinesthetic needs in infancy. *Am. J. Orthopsychiatry* 30:562, 1960.
120. Lammers A.J.J.C., van Rossum J.M.: Bizarre social behavior in rats induced by a combination of peripheral decarboxylase inhibitor and dopa. *Europ. J. Pharmacol.* 5:103,1968.
121. Lane R.G., Domrath R.P.: Behavior therapy: A case study. *Hosp. Community Psychiatry* 21:150, 1970.
122. Lesch M., Nyhan W.L.: A familial disorder of uric acid and central nervous system function. *Am. J. Med.* 36:561, 1964.
123. Lester D.: Self-mutilating behavior. *Psychol. Bull.* 78:119, 1972.
124. Letts R.M., Hobson D.A.: Special devices as aids in the management of child self-mutilation in the Lesch-Nylan syndrome. *Pediatrics* 55:852, 1975.
125. Levy D.M.: On the problem of movement restraint. *Am. J. Orthopsychiatry* 14:644, 1944.
126. Levy D.M., Patrick H.T.: Relation of infantile convulsions, headbanging, and breath-holding to fainting and headaches in the parents. *Arch. Neurol. Psychiatry* 19:865, 1928.
127. Lourie R.S.: The role of rhythmic patterns in childhood. *Am. J. Psychiatry* 105:653, 1949.
128. Lovaas O.I., Freitag G., Gold V.J., et al.: Experimental studies in childhood schizophrenia: I. Analysis of self-destructive behavior. *J. Exptl. Child. Psychol.* 2:67, 1965.
129. Lovaas O.I., Simmons J.Q.: Manipulation of self-destruction in three retarded children. *J. Appl. Behav. Anal.* 2:143, 1969.
130. Lucero W.J., Frieman J., Spoering K., et al.: Comparison of three procedures in reducing self-injurious behavior. *Am. J. Ment. Defic.* 5:548, 1976.
131. Luiselli J.K., Helfen C., Collozzi G., et al.: Controlling self-inflicted biting of a retarded child by the differential reinforcement of other behavior. *Psychol. Rep.* 42:435, 1978.
132. Luiselli J.K., Pemberton B.W., Helfen C.S.: Effects and side-effects of a brief overcorrection procedure in reducing multiple self-stimulatory behavior: A single case analysis. *J. Ment. Defic. Res.* 22:287, 1978.
133. Lutzker J.R.: Reducing self-injurious behavior by facial screening. *Am. J. Ment. Defic.* 82:510, 1978.
134. Lutzker J.R., Spencer T.: Punishment of self-injurious behavior in retardates by brief application of a harmless face cover. Paper presented at the Meeting of the American Psychological Association, New Orleans, 1974.

135. MacKay D., McDonald G., Morrisey M.: Self-mutilation in the mentally subnormal. *J. Psychol. Res. Ment. Subnorm.* 1:25, 1974.
136. Maisto C.R., Baumeister A.A., Maisto A.A.: An analysis of variables related to self-injurious behavior among institutionalized retarded persons, *J. Ment. Defic. Res.* 22:27, 1978.
137. Marholin II D., Siegel L.J.: Beyond the law of effect: Programming for the maintenance of behavioral change, in Marholin II D. (ed): *Child Behavior Therapy.* New York: Gardner Press, 1978, p 397.
138. Marholin II D., Siegel L.J., Phillips D.: Transfer and treatment: A search for empirical procedures, in Hersen M., et al.(eds): *Progress in Behavior Modification.* New York: Academic Press, 1976, vol 3, p 293.
139. Marholin II D., Townsend N.M.: An experimental analysis of side effects and response maintenance of a modified overcorrection procedure: The case of the persistent twiddler. *Behav. Ther.* 9:383, 1978.
140. Marks J.F., Baum J., Keele D.K., et al.: Lesch-Nyhan syndrome treated from the early neonatal period. *Pediatrics* 42:357, 1968.
141. Martin R.: *Legal Challenges to Behavior Modification.* Champaign, Illinois: Research Press, 1975.
142. Matson J.L., Stephens R.M., Smith C.: Treatment of self-injurious behavior with overcorrection. *J. Ment. Defic. Res.* 22:175, 1978.
143. May J.G., Risley T.R., Twardosz S., et al.: Guidelines for the use of behavioral procedures in state programs for retarded persons. *Mental Retardation Res.* 1:1, 1975.
144. Mayhew G., Harris F.: Decreasing self-injurious behavior: Punishment with citric acid and reinforcement of alternative behavior. *Behav. Mod.* 3:322, 1979.
145. McCoull G.: Report on the Newcastle-upon-Tyne Regional Aetiological Survey of Mental Retardation 1966–71. Unpublished research report. Quoted in Corbett J.: Aversion for the treatment of self-injurious behavior, *J. Ment. Defic. Res.* 19:79, 1975.
146. McFarlain R.A., Andy O.J., Scott R.W., et al.: Suppression of headbanging on the ward. *Psychol. Rep.* 36:515, 1975.
147. McPherson L., Joachim R.: The use of electric shock to reduce headbanging in a mentally retarded boy: A case study. *Aust. J. Ment. Retard.* 3:20, 1974.
148. Measel C.J., Alfieri P.A.: Treatment of self-injurious behavior by a combination of reinforcement for incompatible behavior and overcorrection. *Am. J. Ment. Defic.* 81:147, 1976.
149. Merbaum M.: The modification of self-destructive behavior by a mother-therapist using aversive stimulation. *Behav. Ther.* 4:442, 1973.
150. Merwin G.A., Kornegay C.L.: Reduction of three self-injurious behaviors of a mentally retarded female through contingent water spray mist to the face. Paper presented to the 23rd Annual Convention of the Southeastern Regional American Association on Mental Deficiency, St. Petersburg, Florida, 1977.
151. Miron N.B.: The primary ethical consideration. *Hosp. Comm. Psychiatry* 19:226, 1968.
152. Miron N.B.: Behavior modification techniques in the treatment of self-injurious behavior in institutionalized retardates. *Suicidology* 8:64, 1971.
153. Milttleman B.; Psychodynamics of motility. *Int. J. Psychoanal.* 38:197, 1958.
154. Mizuno T., Yugari Y.: Self-mutilation in Lesch-Nyhan Syndrome. *Lancet* 1:761, 1974.
155. Mizuno T., Yugari Y.: Prophylactic effect of L-5-hydroxytryptophan on self-mutilation in the Lesch-Nyhan syndrome. *Neuropaediatrie* 6:13, 1975.
156. Mogel S., Schiff W.: Extinction of a headbanging symptom of eight years' duration in two minutes: A case report. *Behav. Res. Ther.* 5:131, 1967.

157. Mowrer O.H.: *Learning Theory and Behavior*. New York: John Wiley & Sons, 1960.
158. Mulick J.A., Hoyt P., Rojahn J., et al.: Reduction of a "nervous habit" in a profoundly retarded youth by increasing toy play. *J. Behav. Ther. Exptl. Psychiatry* 9:381, 1978.
159. Munkvad I., Randrupp A.: The persistence of amphetamine stereotypes of rats in spite of strong sensation. *Acta Psychiatr. Scand.* 42(suppl) 191:178, 1966.
160. Murphy R.J., Ruprecht M.J., Baggio P., et al.: The use of mild punishment in combination with reinforcement of alternative behaviors to reduce the self-injurious behavior of a profoundly retarded individual. *Am. Assoc. Educ. Severely Profoundly Handicapped Rev.* 4:187, 1979.
161. Murphy R.J., Ruprecht M., Nunes D.L.: Elimination of self-injurious behavior in a profoundly retarded adolescent using intermittent timeout, restraint, and blindfold procedures. *Am. Assoc. Educ. Severely Profoundly Handicapped Rev.* 4:334, 1979.
162. Muttar A.K., Peck D., Whitlow D., et al.: Reversal of a severe case of self-mutilation. *J. Ment. Defic. Res.* 19:3, 1975.
163. Myers D.V.: Extinction, DRO, and response-cost procedures for eliminating self-injurious behavior: A case study. *Behav. Ther.* 13:189, 1975.
164. Myers J.J., Deibert A.N.: Reduction of self-abusive behavior in a blind child by using a feeding response. *J. Behav. Ther. Exp. Psychiatry* 2:141, 1971.
165. Nelson R.O., Hayes S.C.: The nature of behavioral assessment: A commentary. *J. Appl. Behav. Anal.* 12:491, 1979.
166. Nunes D.L., Murphy R.J., Ruprecht M.L.: Reducing self-injurious behavior of severely retarded individuals through withdrawal of reinforcement procedures. *Behav. Mod.* 1:499, 1977.
167. Nyhan W.L.: Lesch-Nyhan syndrome: Summary of clinical features. *Fed. Proc.* 27:1034, 1968.
168. Nyhan W.L.: The Lesch-Nyhan syndrome. *Dev. Med. Child Neurol.* 20:376, 1978.
169. Parker C.E., Mavalwala J., Weise P., et al.: The 47XYY syndrome in a boy with behavior problems and mental deficiency. *Am. J. Ment. Defic.* 74:660, 1970.
170. Paul H.A., Romanczyk R.G.: The use of air splints in the treatment of self injurious behavior. *Behav. Ther.* 4:320, 1973.
171. Peterson R.F., Peterson L.R.: The use of positive reinforcement in the control of self-destructive behavior in a retarded boy. *J. Exp. Child Psychol.* 6:351, 1968.
172. Peterson R.F., Peterson L.W.: Hydropsychotherapy: Water as a punishing stimulus in the treatment of a problem parent-child relationship, in Etzel B.C., et al. (eds): *New Developments in Behavioral Research: Theory, Method, and Application*. New Jersey: Lawrence Earlbaum Associates, 1977, p 247.
173. Phillips R.H., Muzaffer A.: Some aspects of self-mutilation in the general population of a large psychiatric hospital. *Psychiatr. Q.* 35:421, 1961.
174. Picker M., Poling A., Parker A.: A review of children's self-injurious behavior. *Psychol. Rec.* 29:435, 1979.
175. Pinsky L., Digeorge A.M.: Congenital familial sensory neuropathy with anhidrosis. *J. Pediatr.* 68:1, 1966.
176. Podolsky E.: *Encyclopedia of Aberrations*. New York: Philosophical Library, 1953.
177. Primrose D.A.: Treatment of self-injurious behavior with GABA (γ-amino butyric acid) analogue. *J. Ment. Defic. Res.* 23:163, 1979.
178. Prochaska J., Smith N., Marzilla R., et al.: Remote-control aversive stimulation in the treatment of headbanging in a retarded child. *J. Behav. Ther. Exp. Psychiatry* 5:285, 1974.
179. Ragain R.D., Anson J.E.: The control of self-mutilating behavior with positive reinforcement. *Ment. Retard.* 14:22, 1976.

180. Rechter E., Vrablic M.: The right to treatment including aversive stimuli. *Psychiatry Q.* 48:445, 1964.
181. Repp A.C., Deitz S.M.: Reducing aggressive and self-injurious behavior of institutionalized retarded children through reinforcement of other behaviors. *J. Appl. Behav. Anal.* 7:313, 1974.
182. Repp A.C., Deitz S.M., Deitz D.E.D.: Reducing inappropriate behaviors in classrooms and in individual sessions through DRO schedules of reinforcement. *Ment. Retard.* 14:11, 1976.
183. Ressman A.C., Butterworth T.: Localized acquired hypertrichosis. *Arch. Dermatol. Syphilis* 65:418, 1952.
184. Reynolds G.S.: Behavioral contrast. J. Exp. Anal. Behav. 4:57, 1961.
185. Ribble M.A.: *The Rights of Infants: Early Psychological Needs and Their Satisfaction.* New York: Columbia University Press, 1943.
186. Rincover A., Koegel R.L.: Research on the education of autistic children: Recent advances and future directions, in Lahey B.B., et al. (eds): *Advances in Clinical Child Psychology.* New York: Plenum Press, 1977, vol 1, p 329.
187. Risley T.R.: The effects and side effects of punishing the autistic behaviors of a deviant child. *J. Appl. Behav. Anal.* 1:21, 1968.
188. Risley T.R., Wolf M.M.: Strategies for analyzing behavioral change over time, in Nesserole J., et al. (eds): *Life-Span Developmental Psychology: Methodological Issues.* New York: Academic Press, 1972, p 175.
189. Rojahn J., Mulick J.A., McCoy D., et al.: Setting effects, adaptive clothing, and the modification of headbanging and self-restraint in two profoundly retarded adults. *Behav. Anal. Mod.* 2:185, 1978.
190. Romanczyk R.G., Goren E.R.: Severe self-injurious behavior: The problem of clinical control. *J. Consult. Clin. Psychol.* 43:730, 1975.
191. Rose T.L.: Reducing self-injurious behavior by differentially reinforcing other behaviors. *Am. Assoc. Educ. Severely Profoundly Handicapped Rev.* 4:179, 1979.
192. Ross R.R., Meichenbaum D.H., Humphrey C.: Treatment of nocturnal headbanging by behavior modification techniques: A case report. *Behav. Res. Ther.* 9:151, 1971.
193. Ross R.T.: Behavioral correlates of levels of intelligence. *Am. J. Ment. Defic.* 76:515, 1972.
194. Russo D.C., Carr E.G., Lovaas O.I.: Self-injury in pediatric populations, in Ferguson J., et al. (eds): *Advances in Behavioral Medicine.* New York: Spectrum Publications. In press.
195. Sajwaj T., Libet J., Agras S.: Lemon-juice therapy: The control of life-threatening rumination in a six-month-old infant. *J. Appl. Behav. Anal.* 7:557, 1974.
196. Sallustro F., Atwell C.W.: Body rocking, headbanging, and headrolling in normal children. *J. Pediatr.* 93:704, 1978.
197. Saposnek D.T., Watson L.S.: The elimination of the self-destructive behavior of a psychotic child: A case study. *Behav. Ther.* 5:79, 1974.
198. Schneider H.C., Ross J.S.G., Dubin W.J.: A practical alternative for the treatment of tantrum and self-injurious behavior. *J. Behav. Ther. Exp. Psychiatry* 10:73, 1979.
199. Schroeder S.R.: The analysis of self-injurious behavior: Pathogenesis and treatment. Unpublished study, University of North Carolina and Murdock Center, 1974.
200. Schroeder S.R., Humphrey R.H.: Environmental context effects and contingent restraint time-out of self-injurious behavior in a deaf-blind profoundly retarded woman. Paper presented at the 101st Annual Meeting of the American Association on Mental Deficiency, New Orleans, La., 1977.
201. Schroeder S.R., Peterson C.R., Soloman L.J., et al.: EMG feedback and the contin-

gent restraint of self-injurious behavior among the severely retarded: Two case illustrations. *Behav. Ther.* 8:738, 1977.

202. Schroeder S.R., Rojahn J., Mulick J.A.: On the ethical and unethical use of timeout: Appearances can be deceiving. *Behav. Anal. Mod.* 2:200, 1978.

203. Schroeder S.R., Rojahn J., Mulick J.A.: Ecobehavioral organization of developmental day care for the chronically self-injurious. *J. Pediatr. Psychol.* 3:81, 1978.

204. Schroeder S.R., Schroeder C.S., Smith B., et al.: Prevalence of self-injurious behaviors in a large state facility for the retarded: A three-year followup study. *J. Aut. Child. Schizophr.* 8:261, 1978.

205. Sears R.: Relation of early socialization experience to aggression. *J. Abnorm. Psychol.* 63:466, 1961.

206. Seegmiller J.E.: Diseases of purine and pyrimidine metabolism, in Bondy P.K. (ed): *Duncan's Diseases of Metabolism,* ed 6. Philadelphia: W.B. Saunders Co., 1969.

207. Seegmiller J.E.: Lesch-Nyhan syndrome and the X-linked uric acidurias. *Hosp. Pract.* 7:79, 1972.

208. Shear C.S., Nyhan W.L., Kirman B.H., et al.: Self-mutilative behavior as a feature of the de Lange syndrome. *J. Pediatr.* 78:506, 1971.

209. Shintoub S.A., Soulairac A.: L'Enfant automutilateur. *Psychiatr. Enfant* 3:119, 1961.

210. Shodell M., Reiter H.: Self-mutilative behavior in verbal and nonverbal schizophrenic children. *Arch. Gen. Psychiatry* 19:453, 1968.

211. Sifneos P.E.: Is dynamic psychotherapy contraindicated for a large number of patients with psychosomatic diseases? *Psychother. Psychosomatol.* 21:133, 1972.

212. Silverstein R., Blackman S., Mandell W.: Autoerotic headbanging: A reflection of the opportunism of infants. *J. Child Psychiatry* 5:235, 1966.

213. Simmons J.Q., Reed B.J.: Therapeutic punishment in severely disturbed children. *Curr. Psychiatr. Ther.* 9:11, 1969.

214. Singh N.N.: Psychological treatment of self-injury. *N.Z. Med. J.* 84:484, 1976.

215. Singh N.N.: Prevalence of self-injury in institutionalized retarded children. *N.Z. Med. J.* 86:325, 1977.

216. Singh N.N.: Behavioral control of self-injury in the mentally retarded. *N.Z. Psychol.* 6:52, 1977.

217. Singh N.N.: Aversive control of running away, in Glynn T., et al. (eds): *Behavior Analysis in New Zealand.* Auckland: University of Auckland, 1978, p 69.

218. Singh N.N.: Aversive control of breath-holding. *J. Behav. Ther. Exp. Psychiatry* 10:147, 1979.

219. Singh N.N.: Aversive control of rumination in the mentally retarded. *J. Pract. Approach Develop. Handicap.* 3:2, 1979.

220. Singh N.N.: The effects of facial screening on infant self-injury. *J. Behav. Ther. Exp. Psychiatry* 11:131, 1980.

221. Singh N.N.: Rumination, in Ellis N.R. (ed): *International Review of Research in Mental Retardation.* New York: Academic Press, 1981, vol 10, p 139.

222. Singh N.N., Beale I.L., Dawson M.J.: Duration of facial screening and suppression of self-injurious behavior: Analysis using an alternating treatments design. *Behav. Assess.* 3:411, 1981.

223. Singh N.N., Dawson M.J., Gregory P.R.: Suppression of chronic hyperventilation through response-contingent aromatic ammonia. *Behav. Ther.* 11:561, 1980.

224. Singh N.N., Dawson M.J., Gregory P.R.: Self-injury in the profoundly retarded: Clinically significant versus therapeutic control. *J. Ment. Defic. Res.* 24:87, 1980.

225. Singh N.N., Dawson M.J., Manning P.: Treatment of self-injurious behavior by facial screening: Is visual blocking a necessary component? Submitted for publication.

226. Singh N.N., Gregory P.R., Pulman R.M.: Treatment of self-injurious behavior: A three-year followup. *N.Z. Psychol.* 9:65, 1980.
227. Singh N.N., Pulman R.M.: Self-injury in the de Lange syndrome. *J. Ment. Defic. Res.* 23:79, 1979.
228. Skinner B.F.: *Science and Human Behavior.* New York: Free Press, 1953.
229. Slamecka N.J.: Tests of the discrimination hypothesis. *J. Gen. Psychol.* 63:63, 1960.
230. Slawson P.F., Davidson P.W.: Hysterical self-mutilation of the tongue. *Arch. Gen. Psychiatry* 11:581, 1964.
231. Smeets P.M.: Some characteristics of mental defectives displaying self-mutilative behaviors. *Train. Sch. Bull.* 68:131, 1971.
232. Smolev S.R.: The use of operant techniques for the modification of self-injurious behavior. *Am. J. Ment. Defic.* 76:295, 1971.
233. Solnick J.V., Rincover A., Peterson C.R.: Some determinants of the reinforcing and punishing effects of timeout. *J. Appl. Behav. Anal.* 10:415, 1977.
234. Soule D., O'Brien D.: Self-injurious behavior in a state centre for the retarded: Incidence. *Res. Retard.* 1:1, 1974.
235. Spitz R., Wolf K.M.: Autoerotism: Some empirical findings and hypotheses on three of its manifestations in the first year of life. *Psychoanal. Study Child* 3–4:85, 1949.
236. Sprague R.L., Werry J.S.: Methodology of psychopharmacological studies with the retarded, in Ellis N.R. (ed): *International Review of Research in Mental Retardation.* New York: Academic Press, 1971, vol 5, p 147.
237. Steen P.L., Zuriff G.E.: The use of relaxation in the treatment of self-injurious behavior. *J. Behav. Ther. Exp. Psychiatry* 8:447, 1977.
238. Stinnett J.L., Hollender M.H.: Compulsive self-mutilation. *J. Nerv. Ment. Dis.* 150:371, 1970.
239. Stokes T.F., Baer D.M.: An implicit technology of generalization. *J. Appl. Behav. Anal.* 10:349, 1977.
240. Storkvis B.: Possibilités et limitations de la relaxation dans la médecine psychosomatique. *Rev. Med. Psychosomatol.* 2:142, 1960.
241. Tanner B.A., Zeiler M.: Punishment of self-injurious behavior using aromatic ammonia as the aversive stimulus. *J. Appl. Behav. Anal.* 8:53, 1975.
242. Tarpley H.D., Schroeder S.R.: Comparison of DRO and DRI on rate of suppression of self-injurious behavior. *Am. J. Ment. Defic.* 84:188, 1979.
243. Tate B.G.: Case study: Control of chronic self-injurious behavior by conditioning procedures. *Behav. Ther.* 3:72, 1972.
244. Tate B.G., Baroff G.S.: Aversive control of self-injurious behavior in a psychotic boy. *Behav. Res. Ther.* 4:281, 1966.
245. Ter Vrugt D., Pederson D.R.: The effects of vertical rocking frequencies on the arousal level in two-month-old infants. *Child Dev.* 44:205, 1973.
246. Thomas R.L., Howard G.A.: A treatment program for a self-destructive child. *Ment. Retard.* 9:16, 1971.
247. Thompson J.: *The Clinical Study and Treatment of Sick Children.* Edinburgh: Oliver and Boyd, 1933.
248. Van Velzen W.J.: Autoplexy or self-destructive behavior in mental retardation, in Primrose D.A. (ed): *Proceedings of the Third Congress of the IASSMD.* Warsaw: Polish Medical Publishers, 1975, p 734.
249. Varga E., Simpson G.M.: Loxapine succinate in the treatment of uncontrollable destructive behavior. *Cur. Ther. Res.* 13:737, 1971.
250. Wahler R.G., Berland R.M., Coe T.D.: Generalization processes in child behavior change, in Lahey B.B., et al. (eds): *Advances in Clinical Child Psychology.* New York: Plenum Press, 1979 vol 2, p 35.

251. Webster D.R., Azrin N.H.: Required relaxation: A method of inhibiting agitative-disruptive behavior of retardates. *Behav. Res. Ther.* 11:67, 1973.
252. Weiher R.G., Harman R.E.: The use of omission training to reduce self-injurious behavior in a retarded child. *Behav. Ther.* 6:261, 1975.
253. Whaley D.L., Tough J.: Treatment of a self-injuring mongoloid with shock-induced suppression and avoidance. *Mich. Ment. Health Res. Bull.* 2:33, 1968.
254. White G.D., Neilson G., Johnson S.M.: Timeout duration and the suppression of deviant behavior in children. *J. Appl. Behav. Anal.* 5:111, 1972.
255. Whitney L.R.: The effects of operant conditioning on the self-destructive behavior of retarded children, cited in Smeets P.M.: Some characteristics of mental defectives displaying self-mutilative behaviors, *Train. Sch. Bull.* 68:131, 1971.
256. Wilbur R.L., Chandler P.J., Carpenter B.L.: Modification of self-mutilative behavior by aversive conditioning. *Biomed. Sci. Instru.* 11:185, 1975.
257. Wolf M., Risley T., Johnston M., et al.: Application of operant conditioning procedures to the behavior problems of an autistic child: A follow-up and extension. *Behav. Res. Ther.* 5:103, 1967.
258. Wolf M., Risley T., Mees H.: Application of operant conditioning procedures to the behavior problems of an autistic child. *Behav. Res. Ther.* 1:305, 1964.
259. Wright L.: Aversive conditioning of self-induced seizures. *Behav. Ther.* 4:712, 1973.
260. Yeakel M.H., Salisbury L.L., Greer S.L., et al.: An appliance for autoinduced aversive control of self-injurious behavior. *J. Exp. Child Psychol.* 10:159, 1970.
261. Young J.A., Wincze J.P.: The effects of the reinforcement of compatible and incompatible alternative behaviors on the self-injurious and related behaviors of a profoundly retarded female adult. *Behav. Ther.* 5:614, 1974.
262. Zegiob L., Alford G.S., House A.: Response suppressive and generalization effects of facial screening on multiple self-injurious behavior in a retarded boy. *Behav. Ther.* 9:688, 1978.
263. Zegiob L.E., Jenkins J., Becker J., et al: Facial screening: Effects on appropriate and inappropriate behaviors. *J. Behav. Ther. Exp. Psychiatry* 7:355, 1976.
264. Zehr M.D., Theobald D.E.: Manual guidance used in a punishment procedure: The active ingredient in overcorrection. *J. Ment. Defic. Res.* 22:263, 1978.
265. Zuk G.H.: Psychodynamic implications of self-injury in defective children and adults. *J. Clin. Psychol.* 16:58, 1960.

Seizures and Other Paroxysmal Disorders

CHARLES B. BRILL, M.D.

Associate Professor
Departments of Pediatrics and Neurology
Director, Division of Pediatric Neurology
Hahnemann Medical College and Hospital
Philadelphia, Pennsylvania

AND

MICHAEL H. MITCHELL, M.D.

Lt. Col. U. S. Army Medical Corps
Chief of Pediatric Neurology
Letterman Army Medical Center
Presidio of San Francisco, California

PAROXYSMAL DISORDERS are recurrent, reversible alterations of brain function. Several occur frequently in children, particularly seizures, status epilepticus, migraine, syncope, and breath-holding spells. Others include paroxysmal vertigo, hypoglycemia, psychiatric disorders, drug abuse, and certain congenital errors of metabolism.

Seizure Disorders

Seizures are clinical manifestations of hypersynchronous firing of cerebral cortical neurons. Although there are many types of seizures, they share in common their abrupt onset and cessation, usually brief duration, alteration in consciousness, and an abnormality of the EEG during the attack. Seizures are a sign of brain dysfunction just as tachypnea is a sign of pulmonary dysfunction. Seizure or epilepsy is not a disease in itself:

441

0065-3101/81/0028-0441-0489-$03.75

a seizure is a symptom, the cause of which must be sought and corrected if possible. Seizures are more frequent in children than adults and are among the commonest neurologic disorders in pediatrics. Somewhat above 4% of all children experience one or more seizures between infancy and adolescence. This higher frequency of seizures in childhood reflects a greater seizure susceptibility in the immature brain that many children eventually outgrow, particularly when they are otherwise neurologically normal.

The stage of cerebral development strongly influences seizures. Examples are neonatal seizures, infantile spasms, and febrile convulsions where the onset, types, and duration of seizures are remarkably age-dependent. Cerebral maturation and the presence or absence of demonstrable brain pathology are major factors that determine whether seizures will be outgrown, change in type, or persist to become epilepsy in adulthood.

DESCRIPTION AND CLASSIFICATION OF SEIZURES

Hughlings Jackson's 1880 definition of seizures remains one of the best: "A seizure is an occasional, excessive and disorderly discharge of neurons resulting in an excess, distortion or deficit or central nervous system function. These disruptions of CNS function will vary according to the area of seizure onset and pathways of spread within the brain."[1]

Our description of seizures (Table 1) is derived from the International Classification, which is based on both clinical and EEG abnormalities.[2] This description successfully characterizes most childhood seizures.

Epilepsy, a Greek word meaning "seizure," is a heterogeneous group of disorders having in common a susceptibility to recurring seizures caused by intrinsic congenital or acquired brain abnormalities that may or may not be demonstrable by present-day diagnostic techniques[3, 4] (Figs 1–6). The types of seizures and the presence or absence of nonseizure neurologic abnormalities such as mental retardation or cerebral palsy depends on what brain disease is present in each patient and the amount and distribution of the pathology. Frequently, seizures occur in children who are otherwise neurologically and developmentally normal. When seizures are completely or nearly

TABLE 1.—Seizure Classification with Examples of Clinical and EEG Findings

SEIZURE TYPE	EXAMPLES OF SEIZURE ACTIVITY	TYPICAL EEG FINDINGS
Partial seizures	Some memory or consciousness maintained. Attacks may secondarily generalize to a major motor (rarely, absence) seizure	Focal abnormality-frontal* Normal†
Motor (Focal motor)	Jacksonian march, adversive, speech arrest	Focal abnormality-parietal,* occipital or temporal* Normal†
Sensory (Focal sensory)	Localized cutaneous, visual, auditory, smell, taste, or vertiginous sensations	Focal abnormality* Normal† (especially if drowsiness/light sleep not recorded)
Complex (Psychomotor)	Impaired consciousness, visual or auditory misperceptions or hallucinations, anxiety, automatisms, déja vu, visceral sensations, aura (warning). (Note: typical postictal lethargy and headache)	Focal abnormality-temporal* Normal
Multifocal	Multiple partial seizures	Multifocal abnormalities
Generalized seizures	Memory and consciousness lost	
Major motor ("Convulsion" or grand mal)	Tonic-clonic. Sometimes purely clonic or tonic. "Secondary generalized major motor seizures" are very common, manifested by aura, initial partial seizure or focal interictal EEG abnormality	Focal or generalized Normal† Bilaterally synchronous discharges‡
Absence (Petit mal)	Brief loss of consciousness with or without eye blinking, automatism, clonic jerks or changes in tone. (Note: no postictal symptoms)	Bilaterally synchronous discharges especially 3/second spike-wave. Activated with hyperventilation or photic stimulation
Myoclonic	Massive or localized single jerks, often occurring in clusters. One characteristic type is infantile spasm	Various bilateral discharges‡ (Hypsarrhythmia in infantile spasms)
Atonic (astatic or "drop seizures")	Abrupt loss of tone, resultant fall frequently causing facial injury. Often associated with myoclonic seizures	Various bilateral discharges‡

*Focal paroxysmal discharges or disturbances of background rhythms (see Fig 7).
†EEG may become positive with special techniques (e.g., sleep recording or nasopharyngeal leads).
‡Such as spike-wave, polyspike, or paroxysmal slow waves (see Figure 9).

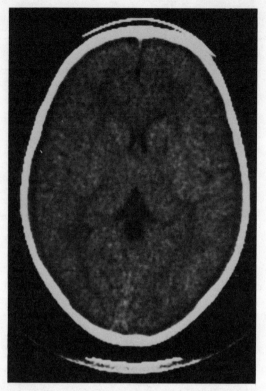

Fig 1.—Two-and-a-half-year-old boy with developmental delay and hypotonia. He had a 12-minute generalized seizure associated with a fever of 102 F. Normal CAT scan. Note that this is a symptomatic seizure, because of the prolonged duration, low fever and abnormal neurodevelopmental status, and not a simple febrile seizure.

completely controlled through good medical management, a large portion of epileptic children live unhampered lives, do well in school, get a driver's license, and pursue a satisfying adult career. Although we do not ignore the terms "epilepsy" and "epileptic," we do prefer the official label "seizure disorder," which is more objective, more comprehensible to laymen, and far less prejudicial when it appears in a child's school or medical records. In nonepileptics, sudden onset of seizures frequently indicates such serious acute brain diseases as intracranial infection, head injury, and various toxic/metabolic disorders. Also, about 4% of small children have seizures triggered by high fever[5] (see "Febrile Convulsions" below), as opposed to epilepsy, which affects only 0.5% of children in the same age group.[6]

PARTIAL SEIZURES

"Partial seizures" is a relatively new term encompassing manifestations of localized seizure involvement of the brain (Figure 7). The cerebral localization can be inferred by history or observations of the initial symptoms or motor phenomena. Often a description by the parent or other observer must be sought, since the patient may have partial or complete amnesia after the attack. Sometimes the history will give a better localization for the origin of partial seizures than the EEG.

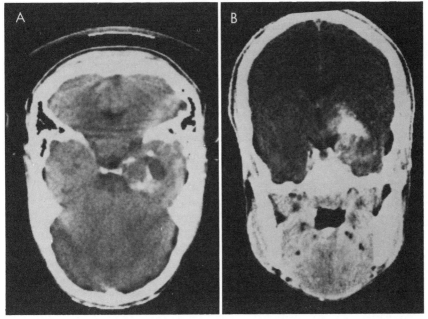

Fig 2.—Twelve-year-old boy with a severe behavior disorder and generalized seizures, preceded by an aura of vague upper abdominal discomfort. CT scan, done in axial plane, without contrast enhancement (**A**), shows a densely calcified, partly cystic temporal lobe tumor. Views in coronal plane, done with contrast enhancement (**B**), shows extension into thalamus and hypothalamus, with slight midline shift, and compression of ipsilateral lateral ventricle.

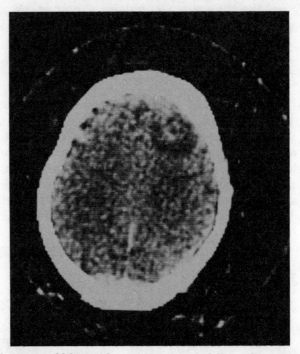

Fig 3.—A 14-year-old boy with cyanotic congenital heart disease who presented with fever, obtundation, and a left focal seizure. Examination showed a left hemiparesis and papilledema. CAT scan showed a right frontal contrast enhancing lesion, with central lucency and surrounding edema. Surgical diagnosis was brain abscess.

PARTIAL MOTOR SEIZURES.—The most typical "focal" or partial motor seizure is tonic stiffening and/or clonic jerking of the face or extremity contralateral to the cerebral focus. Most often the initial involvement is rather diffuse, for example an entire extremity or the face and an arm. Relatively rare are Jacksonian seizures, which begin in a highly localized part and then "march" in a way predictable from the functional anatomy of the motor strip: for example, an initial twitching of the thumb spreading to the fingers, hand, and arm, and then simultaneously to the face and lower extremity. These seizures indicate a focus in or near the contralateral precentral gyrus (motor strip).

Adversive seizures are also common.[7] The head and eyes are turned contralaterally from the focus, and the extremities on both sides may assume characteristic postures, particularly extension of the contralateral and flexion of the ipsilateral extremities in a manner similar to the infantile tonic neck reflex. Sometimes the contralateral rotation of the head and trunk is so strong that the patient actually turns in circles. Adversive seizures usually arise from contralateral cerebral foci but they may arise anywhere in the hemisphere, particularly in frontal areas.[8]

Purely inhibitory seizures causing only temporary paralysis of the affected part are rare. When the hemisphere dominant for speech (usually the left) is involved, speech arrest or aphasia may accompany or represent a partial seizure. Postictal (Todd's) paralysis of the involved parts may follow a partial

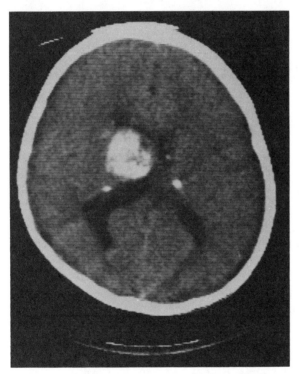

Fig 4.—An eight-year-old boy with severe, mixed seizure disorder, mental retardation, and hypotonic quadraparesis. Skin showed multiple vitiliginous spots and adenomata sebaceum. CAT scan, without contrast, shows multiple subependymal calcific masses, with a large mass in the region of the right foramen of Monro. Diagnosis—tuberous sclerosis.

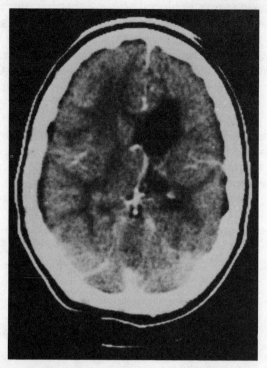

Fig 5.—A 12-year-old girl with spastic right hemiparesis and brief right focal sei-zures, both with and without loss of consciousness. CAT scan shows a porencephalic cyst of frontal horn of lateral ventricle. The entire left hemisphere is smaller than the right.

or generalized motor seizure and usually clears within several hours to days. The paralysis comes from excessive inhibitory influences from the brain.

In children, partial motor seizures, focal or multifocal, often accompany acute generalized diffuse disturbances in brain function, as in meningitis or hyponatremia, or reflect underlying diffuse brain damage. Although each patient must be evaluated carefully, partial seizures in these situations may not indicate permanent localized brain damage, particularly in children younger than 8 years of age. Epileptic children with stereotyped partial seizures and well-defined EEG foci (see Fig 7) can be assumed to have a cortical lesion, which may be demonstrated by a computerized axial tomography (CAT) scan.

When demonstrable, examples of lesions causing chronic partial seizures are cysts, vascular anomalies, brain abscesses, and tumors. Figures 2, A and B, and 3, 4, and 5 show several examples demonstrated by CAT scans.

PARTIAL SENSORY SEIZURES.—Partial sensory seizures occur when irritative foci affect cerebral cortical sensory areas; thus they can be categorized as somatic and special sensory seizures. Somatic sensory seizures arise from the contralateral postcentral gyrus (sensory strip) and are most frequently described as elemental sensations such as numbness or tingling, pins and needles, movement, warmth, or other sensations. The initial localized sensations may spread on the involved side, as does a Jacksonian motor seizure. Due to the proximity and overlap of the Rolandic motor and sensory strips, motor seizure phenomena often occur concurrently.

A common type of partial sensory, or partial motor, seizure

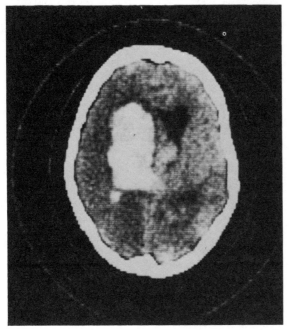

Fig 6.—An 18-year-old girl with a history of right focal seizures. She had sudden onset of a similar seizure with headache, right hemiparesis, and coma. CAT scan without contrast showed a large thalamic hemorrhage. Post-mortem examination showed an arteriovenous malformation as cause of hemorrhage.

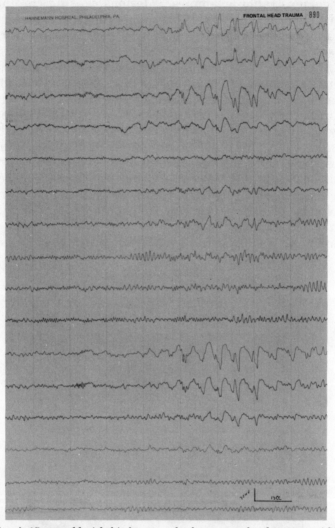

Fig 7.—A 15-year-old girl, hit by car, who has severe head trauma with loss of consciousness, seizures, and frontal lobe contusion. EEG shows left frontal spike and spike wave abnormality (T_3–F_7, F_7–FP_1, FP_1–FP_2, and F_3–C_3, C_3–P_3). Note that location of abnormality is more important than configuration of abnormality, spike-wave configuration in this case. Patient also shows that spike-wave abnormality is seen in focal epilepsy, and not only in absence seizures.

is benign focal epilepsy with Rolandic spikes. The sensory aura or motor activity frequently involves the facial structures. Those seizures often occur during sleep. The EEG shows Rolandic or midtemporal spikes[9] (Fig 8). The benign nature of this type of seizure is shown by the excellent control with anticonvulsants and disappearance of seizures with normalization of the EEG in the early teens.

Special sensory seizures arise from the occipital visual, temporal auditory-vestibular and olfactory, and Sylvian taste areas. Occipital visual seizures are usually elementary phe-

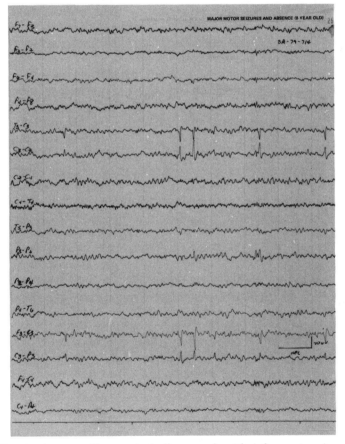

Fig 8.—A nine-year-old, neurologically normal, with infrequent major and absence seizures. EEG shows rolandic vertex spikes (T_3–C_3, C_3–C_2 and F_3–C_3, C_3–P_3). Note that there is a small wave following each spike. Slow waves are inhibitory.

nomena such as flashing lights and need to be differentiated from migraine attacks. More complex visual seizures, such as a change in size or color of objects seen, usually arise from temporal lobe association areas. Seizures from the other sensory areas produce hallucinations of sound, motion, smell, or taste, which, because of their close proximity to other temporal lobe structures, are very frequently the aura to a complex seizure. Seizures with an aura of an odor, usually unpleasant (unciate fits), have a 40% association with temporal lobe tumors.[10]

COMPLEX PARTIAL SEIZURES.—Complex partial seizures (also commonly called "psychomotor" or "temporal lobe" seizures) are fascinating, particularly because they affect areas of the cerebral cortex serving such complex functions as emotion, memory, other intellectual activities, and the highest levels of autonomic system integration.

Although the pattern of seizure phenomena varies greatly from patient to patient, the attacks are usually characteristic and indicative of origin in one or the other temporal lobes, especially the anterior and medial "limbic" portions. These seizures may be the result of hypoxia due to birth trauma or prolonged infantile febrile seizures or hamartomatous malformations in the temporal lobes.[11] Adolescence is a particularly important time for the development of complex partial seizures, most likely due to the combination of preexisting lesions and maturational characteristics of the temporal lobe.

Complex partial seizures often start with a warning (aura), and can be described as five general types: (1) arrest of activity with staring only, (2) arrest of activity with staring followed by automatisms, (3) psychic seizures, (4) seizures with visceral phenomena, and (5) progression to secondary generalized seizures. These seizures are frequently considered in the differential diagnosis of childhood behavioral and psychiatric disorders.[12]

Attacks causing arrest of activity with staring typically last one to two minutes, rarely longer than five. Consciousness is impaired and the patient usually cannot remember the attack.[13] These "psychomotor lapses" are frequently misdiagnosed as simple absences (petit mal) but they are different due to their longer duration, postictal confusion, and EEG findings. Psychomotor spells typically start with an arrest of activity with staring, followed by simple or complex automatisms. Automatisms are repetitive, automatic-appearing movements. Simple automatisms include various orofacial movements, such as lip-smacking, chewing, or mumbling, and movements of the hands, such as pulling at clothing, rubbing the face, or fumbling with objects. Because simple automatisms also occur in absences, there is further potential confusion between these two different seizure disorders (see also "Generalized Seizures" below).

Complex automatisms encompass more integrated motor activity, such as running in circles, removal of clothing, or continuing, in a rather aimless way, some voluntary activity that was in progress before the seizure. Often the automatic behavior reflects a partial awareness of the environment.

In psychic seizures auras (psychic phenomena) are consciously experienced by the patient. Affective components are common, usually fear or anxiety, and are generally recognized by the patients as not being real. Only a few patients describe the affective experiences as being pleasant. Memory phenomena include the famous déja vu, a peculiar and inappropriate sense of familiarity, jamais vu, a sudden feeling of strangeness of the current environment, or a recollection from the past. Perceptual distortions of sight or sound can be striking, such as the "zoom lens" phenomenon, where objects in the environment seem to shrink or enlarge (this occurs in the Alice in Wonderland syndrome; see "Migraine" below). Hallucinations, such as formed visual or auditory images or reliving a past experience, can be stereotyped or vary from attack to attack.

MULTIFOCAL SEIZURES

Children with multifocal seizures fall into two large groups: those with acute brain disturbances, such as anoxia, bacterial meningitis, encephalitis, hypoglycemia, hyponatremia, hypocalcemia, or lead intoxication, whose prognosis depends on whether the acute cerebral insults are fully reversible or not, and those epileptic children who usually have other signs of diffuse brain injury, particularly mental retardation, and/or cerebral palsy. Seizures in the latter children consist of various partial motor disturbances, such as jerky eye movements, tonic adversive posturing, and localized clonus, and are often difficult or impossible to fully control. Frequently these children also suffer generalized attacks, such as major motor, myoclonic, atypical absence, and atonic seizures.

GENERALIZED SEIZURES

The several types of generalized seizures imply diffuse discharges that occur synchronously in both cerebral hemispheres. Apparently all of us have cerebral mechanisms for the most common type of generalized seizure, the major motor seizure, so it is not surprising that major motor seizures are common and occur in many different clinical settings. Probably most major seizures are secondary generalized seizures resulting when initially localized discharges in a diseased brain rapidly become diffuse. On the other hand, certain epilepsies, particularly typical absences and a few major motor seizures, are called primary generalized seizures because at present no localized "generator" has been found to explain the bilaterally synchronous EEG discharges in these patients.

MAJOR MOTOR SEIZURES

After early infancy major motor seizures are by far the most common type of seizure, occurring in about 80% of epileptic children and children with simple febrile convulsions. Of epileptic children with major motor seizures, about half also have other seizure types. When parents say "convulsion" they usually mean a major motor seizure and, when asked, will usually recall their fear that their child was dying when the convulsion began.

The attack may occur abruptly or be preceded by an aura or by nonspecific prodromal behavioral changes such as irritability. When an aura is experienced beforehand, there definitely is a focal origin of the convulsion. In this setting, auras are initial partial sensory or partial complex seizures progressing immediately to a secondary generalized major motor seizure.

Next there is a sudden loss of consciousness, a fall if the child is not supported, and a generalized muscle contraction resulting in the tonic phase of diffuse rigidity, arrest of breathing, cyanosis, and upward deviation of the eyes. Sometimes there is a piercing cry, biting of the tongue or cheek, and loss of urine or stool. The tonic phase is followed by a clonic phase of repeated flexor spasms of the entire body as the brain's inhibitory influences start to damp out the excessive excitation. Jerking respirations now resume and the intervals between clonic jerks lengthen until clonus ceases. Pooling of pharyngeal secretions is prominent. Autonomic phenomena also occur, including pupillary dilatation, skin vasomotor changes, piloerection, sweating, tachycardia, and hypertension.

Clonic jerks are followed by the postictal phase, with unconsciousness, flaccid muscles, and loss of tendon and extensor plantar reflexes. As patients awaken, they are confused and frequently so irritable that they become combative. Often there is postictal headache and a desire to sleep. Unfortunate consequences can occur if the postictal state is mistaken for intoxication or some sort of antisocial behavior. The patient cannot remember the attack, but knows that it occurred because of the postictal discomfort.

In children there is considerable variation in the severity and duration of the convulsive phase as well as the length of postictal CNS depression. Typically the tonic and clonic phases together last about two minutes, but often may range from 30 seconds to 5 minutes in length. Although most children suffer no discernible brain injury from occasional brief major motor seizures, there is always the risk of anoxia, especially if status epilepticus develops. Major motor status epilepticus refers to convulsions prolonged over 15 minutes or those that recur so frequently that the patient does not recover consciousness in between; it is a true medical emergency.

Besides typical tonic-clonic major motor seizures, there are purely tonic or clonic variants. As a rule, tonic seizures are brief and often occur during sleep. Purely clonic generalized seizures occur mostly in small children, especially in febrile convulsions.

The EEG during a major seizure reveals generalized high-frequency discharges during the tonic phase and spike-wave discharges in the clonic phase. The waves represent inhibitory neural activity. During the postictal phase, brain waves are initially depressed in amplitude and then are abnormally slow. The postictal slowing subsides gradually and will sometimes require seven to ten days to completely disappear.

Pseudoseizures or hysterical seizures may be confused with grand mal spells. These seizures frequently occur in adolescent females who have a history of being sexually threatened. An aura is absent or has the quality of anxiety. Consciousness is not completely lost. The movements are more coordinated and less jerky than those of a typical grand mal spell. Opisthotonos or pelvic thrusting are prominent. Incontinence and tongue biting are rarely if ever seen and there is no postictal confusion or drowsiness.[14] Pseudoseizures are a prime indication for the use of simultaneous EEG and videotape monitoring of the patient's "seizures." During an episode the visualized movements may appear to be clearly nonepileptic and the EEG will not show bursts of paroxysmal or spike activity.

ABSENCE SEIZURES

Absence or petit mal seizures are in essence "blank stares" with sudden, brief interruptions of consciousness.

Typical absences form a relatively distinctive, and well-known entity in epilepsy, that is largely confined to children over five years of age and adolescence. However, it is found in only about 5% of all childhood epilepsy patients. The term petit mal should probably be avoided because many laymen, and some physicians, use it to describe any seizure other than a generalized convulsion.

Absences commonly last less than ten seconds and infrequently more than 30 seconds. They are subdivided into simple and complex forms; both can occur in the same person. In a simple absence the patient suddenly stares blankly, stops verbal or motor activity, and is unconscious but does not fall. There is no warning (aura). The attack begins and ends abruptly; the patient is fully alert afterwards. Although typically unaware of the seizure itself, the patient may detect it from the interruption of ongoing events. Attacks that last over ten seconds tend to be complex, with additional features such as eyelid fluttering, drooping of the head, myoclonic jerks, and automatisms such as fumbling of the hands, lip-smacking, or verbal stuttering. Repetitive movements tend to occur at a rate of three per second. These longer spells may be confused with complex partial seizures.

In the untreated patient with typical absences, the attacks

are extremely frequent; 20 to 40 attacks per day are common, and there may be hundreds of them. The EEG is virtually always abnormal, displaying sudden generalized bursts of three-per-second spike-wave complexes (Fig 9) during and between attacks. Clinical attacks and EEG discharges can often be induced by asking the patient to hyperventilate, or by stroboscopic light stimulation or emotional tension (e.g., the normal anxiety of being called upon in class). When the EEG dis-

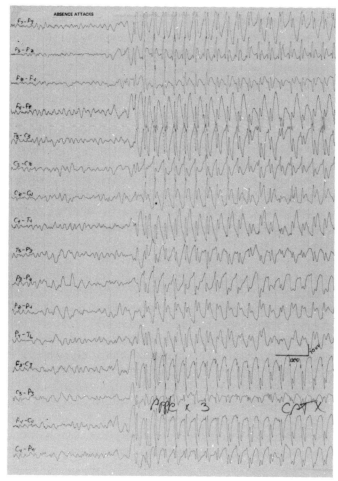

Fig 9.—A five-year-old neurologically normal girl with staring spells. Note generalized 3-Hz spike-wave bursts, with normal preceeding background activity.

458   CHARLES B. BRILL AND MICHAEL H. MITCHELL

charges last four seconds or longer, consciousness is transiently impaired and the clinical attack is usually obvious. Since absences typically begin in children aged five to ten, teachers or parents frequently misinterpret them initially as daydreaming or peculiar mannerisms.

Children with typical absences are, except for their "spells," usually neurologically normal. A few show learning disabilities, at the onset of the seizure disorder or when seizure control is difficult.[15] Less than 5% are retarded. In many patients a positive family history suggests an autosomal dominant genetic inheritance pattern.[16]

It is important to differentiate absences from brief, complex partial (psychomotor) seizures because of the occurrence of staring and partial automatisms in both. As opposed to absences, brief psychomotor seizures generally last longer than 30 seconds, are often preceded by an aura, may cause only partial alteration of consciousness, produce postictal confusion and often headache, and usually show localized EEG abnormalities. This differentiation is important because of significant differences in etiology and drug therapy.

Usually the prognosis for seizure control and outgrowing absence seizures in adolescence or young adulthood is good. However, about 50% of patients have one or several major motor seizures during their course and a minority remain epileptics in adult life.[17]

Petit mal status or "spike-wave stupor" is a prolonged confusional state lasting hours or even days, with associated continuous spike-wave discharges. This may occur in atypical or typical absence seizure states. The diagnosis is confirmed by obtaining an immediate EEG (Fig 10).

"Atypical" absence seizures are clinically similar to "typical" absences but are very different in the total clinical picture and EEG findings. Children in this category are heterogeneous but the majority are retarded or borderline retarded. One large group, called "petit mal variant" or Lennox-Gasteaut syndrome, exhibits mental retardation, "slow" (two per second) spike-wave discharges, and multiple types of seizures, including absences, tonic seizures in sleep, multifocal, and myoclonic/atonic seizures (see below). Most of these patients have secondary generalized seizures; their underlying neurologic substrate is abnormal.

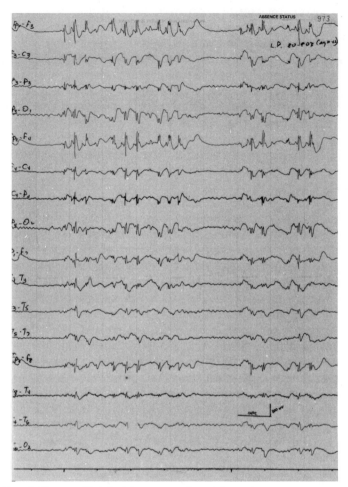

Fig 10.—A 12-year-old girl with stupor and eyelid twitches who was noted on EEG to have trains of generalized, irregular spike-wave bursts consistent with absence status. She responded promptly to diazepam given intravenously.

MYOCLONIC AND ATONIC SEIZURES

Myoclonic and atonic seizures are difficult problems in childhood epilepsy because affected children (1) are often difficult to classify due to multiple seizure manifestations and types, (2) have a high incidence of other neurologic problems, and (3) are very difficult to control. Their ultimate neurologic outcome tends to be poor in terms of mental retardation and subsequent epilepsy. Many patients with myoclonic/atonic seizures experience other seizure types as well, particularly atypical absences, multifocal and major motor seizures.

Myoclonus is a sudden involuntary jerk that may be generalized or localized to one body part. Patterns of seizure myoclonus vary; some forms of myoclonus are not seizures, such as the normal myoclonic jerks that occur when one is falling asleep, called hypnogogic jerks.

Atonic seizures cause a sudden tonal loss of a few seconds' duration. As "epileptic drop attacks," atonic seizures often result in serious facial injury because of their sudden, unpredictable loss of tone and lack of protective responses. The EEG in this group of patients shows a slow spike and wave pattern, at a rate slower than 2.5 Hz.

Infantile spasms are the most characteristic syndrome of myoclonic epilepsy in infancy. They are often the first recognized neurologic symptoms in a baby who will later be retarded. They are frequently responsive to a unique treatment, e.g., ACTH or corticosteroids. They characteristically begin around the sixth month and usually cease by the second birthday. The attacks are a two- to three-second generalized muscle contraction causing flexion of the trunk and extension of the arms and legs; hence the descriptive names, infantile spasm, salaam attack, or lightning spasm. Like other myoclonic seizures, infantile spasms tend to occur in clusters, particularly during drowsiness or arousal. Usually the EEG shows a continuously abnormal pattern called "hypsarrhythmia," a totally disorganized record with high-voltage slow waves, and random, interictal spikes.

SPECIFIC CAUSES OF SEIZURES

Table 2 lists causes of seizures in three critical age groups. This diversity of causes emphasizes the importance of considering seizures as symptoms of CNS involvement and the need to treat the underlying cause, if possible, as well as the symptom.

PATHOGENESIS OF SEIZURES

METABOLIC FACTORS.—Neurons function by conducting electrochemical impulses along their membranes and affecting

TABLE 2.—CAUSES OF SEIZURES BY AGE GROUP*

NEWBORN PERIOD	INFANCY-CHILDHOOD	ADOLESCENCE

Anoxia or ischemia
  Antepartum
  Intrapartum
  Postpartum
	Febrile convulsions
	
	Perinatal insult
	
	Cerebral malformation
		Unknown
		
		Trauma
		
		Anoxia or ischemia

Prematurity
  Intraventricular or
    germinal matrix
    hemorrhage
Metabolic derangement (see
  Table 3)
	Trauma
	  Accidents
	  Child abuse
	Anoxia or ischemia
		Infection
		
		Drug abuse
		
		Perinatal insult

Intrauterine growth retardation
  Poor brain growth
	Infection
	  Meningitis
	  Brain abscess
	  Encephalitis
		Genetic
		
		Brain tumor

Infection
  Meningitis
  Sepsis
  Encephalitis
    (Herpes simplex)
    Enteroviruses
Prenatal abnormality
  Cerebral malformations
  Intrauterine infections
    Rubella
    Cytomegalovirus
    Toxoplasmosis
    Syphilis and others
    Tuberous sclerosis
	Genetic
	  Nondegenerative, e.g., classic
	    absences
	  Neurocutaneous syndromes
	  Inborn errors
	  Aminoacidurias
	  Hypoglycemia
	  Lipid storage diseases
	  Hemoglobinopathies, etc.
	
	Metabolic derangement
	  Hypocalcemia
	  Hypoglycemia
	  Hyper- and hyponatremia
	  Uremia
	  Reye's syndrome
		Vascular malformation
		  or disease

Birth injury	Intoxication Drug ingestion	

Drug withdrawal
  Barbiturates
  Narcotics
Unknown
Inborn errors of metabolism
  (see Table 3)
Benign neonatal seizures
	Lead poisoning
	
	Brain tumor
	Vascular malformation or disease	

*Listed by approximate order of frequency.

other neurons through synaptic neurotransmitters. If there is a reduction in the difference between the resting potential and the action potential of the membrane, the seizure threshold is lowered. Derangement of these neuronal membrane functions is the physiologic hallmark of seizure activity. Normally, the CNS depends on a continuous blood oxygen and glucose supply because CNS stores of glycogen and high-energy compounds are very limited and the brain has a very high metabolic rate. During a prolonged major motor seizure, cerebral energy metabolism increases while cerebral blood flow and oxygen and glucose supplies tend to remain the same or decrease due to impaired cardiorespiratory function from the convulsive activity. Cerebral anoxia, acidosis, and circulatory disturbance pose serious threats for further brain damage during convulsive status epilepticus.[18]

Normal neuronal energy metabolism produces high-energy compounds, particularly adenosine triphosphate (ATP), which maintain the neuronal resting potential and repolarization through the $Na+ - K+$ ATPase membrane "pump." During both normal and seizure-induced neuronal depolarization, $Na+$ rushes into the neuron. Repolarization is rapidly accomplished by curtailment of the $Na+$ influx and a transient $K+$ outflow. Then the $Na+ - K+$ ATPase pump reestablishes the resting ion gradients (low intracellular $Na+$, high intracellular $K+$ by pumping $Na+$ out in exchange for $K+$). A deficiency in the activity of cortical $Na+ - K+$ ATPase has been found in seizure foci.[19] Other factors influencing depolarization/repolarization include: (1) $Ca++$ and $Mg++$, which seem to modulate $Na+ - K+$ permeabilities, (2) neurotransmitters, such as the excitatory transmitter acetycholine that increases $Na+$ permeability and the inhibitory transmitter γ-aminobutyric acid (GABA), which appears to increase $Cl-$ permeability,[20] (3) $Cl-$, which affects membrane potentials, (4) glial cells, which may stabilize neurons by taking up excess extracellular $K+$, and (5) many other possible factors, including structural characteristics of the membrane macromolecules, actions of other neurotransmitters, and influences of trace metals.

A number of systemic metabolic disturbances are routinely complicated by seizures. Anoxia and hypoglycemia destabilize neuronal membranes through impaired energy metabolism. Seizures typically accompany states of hyponatremia, hypocalcemia, and hypomagnesemia. Striking seizures and EEG changes occur in infants who are vitamin B_6 deficient, probably through insufficiency of GABA, whose synthesis is B_6-dependent.[21]

CELLULAR AND PHYSIOLOGIC FACTORS.—The intrinsic cerebral abnormalities underlying chronic seizure states appear multiple, especially when the great diversity of epilepsy in childhood is considered. Some theories suggest that neuronal groups become hypersensitive as the result of loss of afferent connections, abnormal postsynaptic receptors, or mechanical distortion of neuronal processes. Another theory suggests a glial cell abnormality, such as defective glial K+ uptake,[22] resulting in neuronal depolarization from excessive extracellular K+, which is liberated in large amounts by the depolarization of epileptic cells.[23] Such pathogenic processes might be seen in abnormally functioning neurons surrounding an area of brain damage, as are found in temporal lobe resections for complex partial seizures[24] that show glial cell proliferations, partial loss of neurons, and partial loss of synapses from the remaining neurons.

In some patients the focus is a definite pathologic lesion (see Figs 2–6), examples of which are (1) localized malformation of cortical blood vessels, (2) scars from old injuries such as head trauma, hemorrhage, anoxia, or infection, (3) cysts, (4) foci of active infection, (5) the malformations of neurocutaneous diseases such as neurofibromatosis or tuberous sclerosis, and (6) space-occupying lesions such as brain tumors, abscesses, and subdural hematomas from child abuse. Virtually all epileptogenic foci lie in the cerebral cortex, although foci in deep neuronal groups can occur. Electric recordings from cortical foci reveal characteristic autonomous, rhythmic, highly synchronized discharges that represent bursts of action potentials and activity of both excitatory and inhibitory synapses. If the firing of these cells becomes sufficiently synchronized, the scalp EEG shows typical discharges such as spikes, as in Figures 7–10. However, the scalp EEG fails to record some foci because of remote location or insufficient synchronization.[25] Through their axonal processes, the neurons of the focus propagate their abnormal discharges to other areas of the brain, and it is the balance of inhibitory versus excitatory impulses that determines whether or not a clinical seizure results. Present evidence indicates that secondary generalized seizures occur when an excitatory feedback circuit is set up from a cortical focus to deep neuronal masses such as the thalamus and basal ganglia, from which they are relayed back to the entire cortex.[26]

The "primary generalized epilepsies" are less common and more poorly understood than focal epilepsy. The most characteristic generalized epilepsy in childhood is typical absences (petit mal), where genetic and maturational factors suggest a neuronal biochemical disorder.[16] In absence, excitatory stimuli may be relayed from the intralaminar nuclei of the thalamus to the cortex, causing the 3-Hz EEG pattern.

GENETIC AND MATURATIONAL FACTORS.—Genetic influences can be principal or contributing causes of seizures and are of greater importance in childhood than adults. Autosomal dominant inheritance, with incomplete penetrance, is implicated in classic absences. In EEG studies of nonepileptic relatives of children with typical absence seizures, the three-per-second spike-wave discharge is asymptomatically expressed in an autosomal dominant fashion. Genetic predisposition is also seen in posttraumatic epilepsy, where the likelihood of a seizure disorder resulting from serious head injury is up to five times greater in those patients having a positive family history of epilepsy. Family history is often positive in simple febrile seizures. Seizures are common in neurofibromatosis and tuberous sclerosis, both of which are inherited in an autosomal dominant fashion.

Maturational factors strongly influence seizure type in the neonatal period and infancy (see "Neonatal Seizures" and "Febrile Convulsions" below, and Table 2). Adolescence is also a critical time for the expression of maturational factors: a long-standing cerebral lesion may first manifest itself with seizures, or a preexisting seizure disorder may be "outgrown" or become worse.

CEREBRAL DAMAGE FROM SEIZURES.—It has already been emphasized that anoxic brain damage may occur when ventilation is impaired, as in prolonged major motor seizures or newborn apneic seizures. Another concern is that the abnormal neuronal activity of seizures might injure brain cells, particularly in infancy, when cell maturation and growth are very active. In neonatal rats, brief electroshock seizures (less than half a second of convulsive activity once daily for ten days) reduces brain size, cell number, and rate of early motor-reflex development. In animals, normal neuronal groups can become "epileptic cells" after frequent low-intensity stimulation (kindling)[28] or after bombardment of a distant epileptic focus (mirror focus).[29] Both of these phenomena can be prevented by phenobarbital treatment.

Parents frequently raise the question of whether seizures cause additional brain damage or retardation. The answer is not clear-cut, and multiple factors are involved. A patient with frequent seizures and resultant postictal depression would function poorly if the sum of the ictal and postictal times represents a significant portion of the patient's waking day. In addition, some of the drugs used to treat seizures, particularly phenobarbital and phenytoin, are mental depressants and interfere with cognitive function and learning. These factors are examples of pseudoretardation; if the seizures were controlled with a nontoxic drug the patient might have improved or have normal intellectual function. A patient with uncontrolled seizures may have a progressive cerebral disease of grey matter, e.g., infantile Gaucher's disease or Niemann-Pick disease, type A, that causes both seizures and dementia. A chronically brain-damaged patient (for example status postanoxia with cerebral palsy and mental retardation) may have seizures and retardation as results independent of the insult that leads to the severe static encephalopathy. Major motor status epilepticus can lead to brain damage due to increased cerebral metabolic rate and hypoxia, hyperthermia, and acidosis during the prolonged seizures (see the section on status epilepticus). Infantile spasms and other seizures in the atonic/myoclonic group have a very high association of preceeding or subsequent mental retardation. Both effects are probably due to the encephalopathy that caused the seizures.

Pathologically, the brains of many chronic epileptics show no gross abnormality, so that a history of recurrent spells need not imply increased brain damage. However, patients with a history of status epilepticus may have evidence of hypoxic brain damage.

Patients with uncontrolled seizure disorders occasionally have intellectual deterioration.[30] This is particularly true if there is a known insult or etiology for the seizures (26%) as opposed to patients with "idiopathic" epilepsy (10%). The associated factors are early age of onset (23% with onset less than age one versus 7% with age of onset above two years), duration of the seizure disorder, and type of seizure. Patients with grand mal and psychomotor attacks may have intellectual deterioration, while patients with pure petit mal do not show any intellectual deterioration.[31]

FACTORS "TRIGGERING" SEIZURES.—Although most epileptic seizures seem to happen spontaneously, there are many patients who are apt to have attacks under certain conditions.

Sometimes this is characteristic of the type of seizure disorder, as the induction of absences by hyperventilation, photic stimulation, and anxiety. Many patients with various types of seizures are sensitive to one or more of the following: (1) diurnal cycle—sleep deprivation often induces seizures and some patients only have attacks either asleep, awake, drowsy, or on arousal; (2) emotional stress; (3) menstrual cycle, particularly the several days before each period; (4) infections, even without fever, often exacerbate childhood seizure disorders; (5) alcohol and illicit drugs—seizures may occur as the patient recovers from a "high" and there is often sleep deprivation and failure to take anticonvulsant medication as well; and (6) medications—occasionally an anticonvulsant paradoxically worsens a seizure disorder (e.g., phenytoin in absences), and convulsions can be induced by many commonly used drugs, such as phenothiazines, butyrophenones, antihistamines, local anesthetics, theophylline, and penicillin, chiefly when these are given in large parenteral doses. Rarely are seizures provoked by music or reading.

NEONATAL SEIZURES.—Due to nervous system immaturity, seizure manifestations in neonates are very different. They often are fragmentary and subtle, especially in prematures. Tonic-clonic seizures are rare. Blinks, stares, rhythmic eye movements, clonic jerking, and pedaling movements are usually seen.[32] Apneic spells can be caused by seizures. Sustained tonic seizures are relatively uncommon but can seriously impede ventilation, and have an ominous prognostic significance. The EEG may be helpful in confirming the presence of seizures and estimating prognosis.

The principal causes of neonatal seizures are summarized in Table 2.[33] The major cause is hypoxia and/or ischemia occurring during labor or in the early newborn period, from conditions such as premature placental separation, placenta previa, breech delivery, meconium aspiration, or respiratory distress syndrome. In premature infants, severe cerebral venous congestion, hypotension, and hypoxia are often associated with intracranial hemorrhage and seizures.

Metabolic disturbances (Table 3) are frequently involved in neonatal seizures. Severe systemic neonatal conditions such as anoxia or sepsis are very often complicated by varying combinations of acidosis, hypoglycemia, hypocalcemia, or hypomag-

TABLE 3.—METABOLIC CAUSES OF NEONATAL SEIZURES

Anoxia
Hypoglycemia, hypocalcemia, acidosis, etc. complicating neonatal stresses such as
  anoxia, ischemia, sepsis, or birth trauma
Primary hypoglycemia: small-for-date babies, infants of diabetic mothers
Primary tetany ("benign neonatal tetany") due to hypocalcemia, hypomagnesemia,
  and/or hyperphosphatemia, usually around the second week of life
Hyponatremia: inappropriate ADH syndrome
Hypernatremia
Kernicterus: hemolytic disease, liver dysfunction
Inborn errors of metabolism: phenylketonuria maple syrup urine disease, and other
  amino- and organic acidopathies; vitamin B_6 dependency

nesemia. Infants of diabetic mothers and those with intrauterine growth retardation are frequently hypoglycemic. Although rare, inborn metabolic errors must be considered because some are treatable (e.g., vitamin B_6 dependency and several of the amino acid disorders). Hyperbilirubinemia and intrapartum physical brain injuries are now less frequent due to improvements in obstetric and neonatal management. Some patients with congenital brain anomalies are dysmorphic and have cranial and/or facial abnormalities. When the mother is a drug addict or takes large doses of medication, the infant may demonstrate withdrawal symptoms such as irritability and seizures.

As in other ages, seizures in the neonatal period must be considered symptoms of brain involvement; prognosis for future brain development depends largely on the cause of the seizures. Overall, roughly 1% of all newborns have seizures and of these, approximately one half will subsequently be normal.[34] As examples of prognosis determined by cause, seizures from hypoxia-ischemia, intracranial infection, and cerebral malformation carry a very high risk for subsequent brain impairment, while those due to "benign neonatal tetany" (the primary or uncomplicated type of hypocalcemia, hypomagnesemia, and/or hyperphosphatemia) generally have an excellent prognosis for subsequent normal brain development.

FEBRILE CONVULSIONS.—Fever-induced seizures occur in about 5% of all young children, and are, therefore, about ten times more frequent than afebrile seizures in this age group. Although the pathophysiology is poorly understood, an age-dependent sensitivity of the nervous system (Figure 11) allows

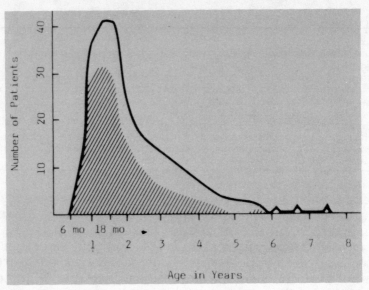

Fig 11.—Age when febrile convulsions occur. *Upper curve,* all attacks, initial and recurrent. *Shaded area,* initial attacks only. (Based on 200 children with initial and recurrent febrile convulsions reported by Frantzen E., et al.: Longitudinal EEG and clinical study of children with febrile convulsions. *Electroencepalogr. Clin. Neurophysiol.* 24:197, 1968.)

triggering of the seizure by fever. Further, the family history is often positive in a parent or siblings and thus indicates a genetic factor.

Over three fourths of patients have *typical febrile seizures* (also called "simple," "benign," or "uncomplicated").[35] The neurologically and developmentally normal child experiences a single, brief (less than ten minutes, and frequently less than two), clonic or tonic-clonic, generalized (nonfocal) seizure with a temperature of 102 F or above, usually within a few hours after onset of the fever. A few children will be briefly unconscious without tonic or clonic activity. The peak age is 18 months (see Fig 11) and the age range six months to five years. Fever is usually from a significant upper respiratory infection, less often gastroenteritis, roseola, or pneumonia,[36] not a primary CNS infection. During high fever, any child may exhibit abnormal lethargy and minor twitching.

The remaining one fourth of fever-triggered seizures are

atypical febrile seizures because (1) the child is not neurodevelopmentally normal or (2) the seizure is "complicated," i.e., over ten minutes long, focal or multiple, or with minimal temperature elevation. The diagnosis of febrile convulsions always excludes other primary CNS disorders and, therefore, tests appropriate to the individual case must be done to rule out CNS infections such as meningitis, encephalitis, and brain abscess; metabolic disturbances such as hypoglycemia and electrolyte imbalance; intoxications like lead poisoning; vascular insults; and unreported head trauma due to child abuse. Also, the many epileptic children whose seizures are exacerbated by infections are not considered to have "typical febrile seizures."

Sequelae of febrile convulsions.—The majority of children with febrile convulsions will subsequently be normal. Those with typical febrile seizures have about a 1% risk for later epilepsy, about twice the risk in the general population.[37-39] The risk for another febrile seizure is age-dependent (see Fig 11).

However, those experiencing an atypical febrile seizure (neurodevelopmentally abnormal child or "complicated" seizure) may have a risk approaching 1% for death or permanent neurologic residua. Rarely, for example, older children or adolescents developing complex partial seizure disorders have a history of prior "febrile status epilepticus" that may have left permanent temporal lobe damage. In general, the child with an atypical febrile seizure is at a greater risk for subsequent epilepsy (up to 15% when both the neurodevelopmentally abnormal and complicated febrile seizure risk factors are present) and here the febrile seizure appears to be the initial manifestation of a preexisting epileptogenic CNS abnormality.

Management.—After a febrile seizure of short duration, the physician's concerns are diagnosis and treatment of the febrile illness and whether to give prophylactic anticonvulsants.

Diagnosis requires careful clinical assessment to find any systemic or intracranial disease capable of causing the seizure. Lumbar puncture should be performed at even slight suspicion of intracranial infection, and glucose, calcium, and electrolyte levels should be checked in most instances. In typical febrile seizure patients, other studies such as computerized tomography (CT) or isotope brain scans are usually not necessary and the value of electroencephalography is controversial because normal and abnormal EEGs do not correlate with subsequent epilepsy. Fever is controlled by tepid baths, antipyretics, and treatment of infection.

Because so many attacks occur soon after the onset of fever, antipyretics are of limited value and anticonvulsants of no value when given at the onset of fever for preventing recurrences during subsequent febrile illnesses. In general, the initial typical febrile seizure does not require prophylactic anticonvulsant treatment in view of the extremely low risk for subsequent CNS injury and the significant side effects of medications for preventing recurrences when given on a daily basis. Indications for prophylactic treatment with phenobarbital 3 mg/kg of body weight/day (2 divided daily doses, blood phenobarbital of at least 15 μg/ml) include: (1) less than one year of age at onset, (2) a second typical febrile seizure, and (3) all cases of atypical febrile seizures (see above), for atypical patients seem to be at a higher risk of febrile status epilepticus and subsequent epilepsy. In the first two instances, treatment, if well tolerated, may be stopped at age 24 to 30 months. Because the side effects of phenobarbital will be relatively common, the indications for this and alternative drugs will often have to be carefully considered. In atypical patients, treatment should be started and neurologic consultation obtained.

DIAGNOSIS OF SEIZURE DISORDERS

Diagnosis of seizures requires a careful history of the events that preceeded the seizure and of the phenomena observed, usually by the parent. Since most seizures have terminated by the time the child is seen by a doctor, the physician is heavily dependent on a description of prodromata (aura), abnormal movements or behavior, incontinence, tongue biting and postictal drowsiness, confusion, or weakness. Sometimes a recurrent, paroxysmal event will prove to be nonepileptic. Careful physical, neurologic, and developmental examinations must be done, particularly to search for other evidence of neurologic dysfunction, for example, signs of meningitis in a child with fever and seizures or signs of cerebral palsy and developmental delay in a child with seizures and a high-risk birth history. A careful examination of skin may reveal café-au-lait spots of neurofibromatosis or hypopigmented spots of tuberous sclerosis.

The principal laboratory test is the EEG, but since it can be normal or nonspecifically abnormal in children with or without seizures, it cannot replace good clinical judgment in seizure diagnosis. An occasional child will have an "epileptiform" EEG without having epilepsy, e.g., siblings of children with absences. The yield of EEG abnormalities can be increased by "activating" techniques, such as hyperventilation, flashing light (photic) stimulation, recording during drowsiness and sleep, and the use of nasopharyngeal or sphenoidal electrodes. In special laboratories video and EEG recording of attacks can be helpful, e.g., in documenting hysterical seizures.

Other diagnostic tests are directed to the cause rather than the physiology of seizures. CT scan (see Figs 1–6) is an advance in the diagnosis of brain disease. Indications for CT scanning in seizure patients are partial (focal) seizures, signs suggestive of focal or progressive CNS disease, and seizure refractory to therapy. CT scanning largely replaces skull radiographs and isotope brain scans. Lumbar puncture must be done if CNS infection, meningitis, or encephalitis is suspected. In other circumstances it adds little to the diagnosis. Other tests that should be done in most patients are serum glucose and calcium, screening tests for inborn metabolic errors, and intoxication with drugs or lead. Angiography may be helpful to assess the vascularity of a lesion that is to be approached surgically or to demonstrate an arteriovenous malformation. Pneumoencephalography is rarely indicated for any reason.

TREATMENT OF SEIZURE DISORDERS

Comprehensive management for seizure disorders should start with a discussion of the diagnosis and plan for treatment with the family, including the patient so far as possible. Proper first aid for seizures (airway maintenance, avoidance of placing objects in the mouth) should be discussed as well as prognosis for seizure control, which is good in many instances.

Long-term oral anticonvulsant medications are the mainstay of seizure therapy. Even if a brain lesion is found and removed, the patient will still require drugs for a prolonged period. It must be emphasized at the outset that it is the child with seizures, not the EEG or drug levels, that should be treated.

The goal of drug therapy is complete seizure control with no significant drug-related side effects. This can be attained in a majority of children, but in a sizable minority one must compromise between incomplete seizure control and drug side effects. Unfortunately, a few children are inadequately controlled even with toxic doses. The choice of drug depends on the seizure type (Table 4). Dosage is a function of body weight (Table 5). The least toxic drug likely to be effective should be started in conventional doses, and blood levels checked whenever seizures fail to respond or drug side effects occur. A single drug rather than combinations should be used whenever possible.[40]

Blood anticonvulsant levels are now becoming widely available and are a cornerstone of good management. Levels should be checked whenever side effects such as sedation or incoordination develop and whenever seizures relapse, fail to respond, or change in type. A therapeutic drug level does not assure good control; an elevated level does not necessarily imply clinical toxicity. Other laboratory tests should be done periodically

TABLE 4.—DRUG INDICATIONS BY TYPE OF SEIZURE

TYPE OF SEIZURE	DRUGS (in order of most likely usefulness)
Convulsive seizure disorders	
Major motor	
Partial	Carbamazepine
Motor	Phenobarbital or primidone*
Sensory	Phenytoin
Complex	
Multifocal	Above + valproate
Nonconvulsive seizure disorders	
Absence	Valproate
	Ethosuximide
	Clonazepam
Myoclonic/atonic	Valproate
	Clonazepam
	Ketogenic diet
Infantile spasms	ACTH, corticosteroids
	Clonazepam
	Valproate
Febrile seizures	Phenobarbital*
Neonatal seizures	Phenobarbital
	Phenytoin
	Valproate

*Particularly when low doses are effective and behavioral side effects are absent or minimal.
NOTE: In individual cases drugs not listed may prove to be more useful.

to monitor possible toxic effects of each drug; the appropriate tests vary with each drug. The frequency of anticonvulsant dosage depends on the half-life of the drug (see Table 5). Most anticonvulsants are best given twice daily, except carbamazepine and sodium valproate, whose shorter half-lives may require three or four daily doses.[41] After early infancy the use of tablets, chewable tablets, and capsules is encouraged for more accurate dosage, provided the pills are crushed for infants beforehand to prevent aspiration. Liquid phenytoin (Dilantin) is particularly prone to dosage errors due to its viscosity and to incomplete shaking of the suspension. When immediate "therapeutic coverage" is desired, an oral loading dose of twice the maintenance dose for two days or a parenteral loading dose should be given.

In many patients psychological stress increases seizures and vice versa. Intervention by a properly trained counselor or psychiatrist often improves seizure control when emotional conflicts improve.[42]

Other modes of therapy include (1) ACTH or corticosteroids for infantile spasms, (2) induced ketosis for refractory myoclonic seizures using a ketogenic or medium-chain triglyceride diet, and (3) surgical excision of epileptogenic foci in carefully selected patients.

Treatment failures may result from problems other than the epileptogenic disorder itself.[43] These problems include (1) medication noncompliance, (2) improper seizure classification and medication choice, (3) misdiagnosis of disorders such as syncope or breath-holding as epilepsy, (4) injudicious drug usage, such as sudden discontinuation (which may trigger status epilepticus), underdosing, failure to obtain drug levels, drug toxicity (which may actually increase seizures), and unnecessary polypharmacy, (5) failure to deal with emotional disturbances, (6) inadequate patient-family instruction, (7) failure to diagnose an epileptogenic systemic disease such as hypoglycemia, phenylketonuria, or pyridoxine dependency, and (8) unrecognized progressive CNS disorder, such as tumor, neuronal degenerative disease, or vascular malformation. All patients with unusual or refractory seizure disorders should be evaluated by a consultant experienced in pediatric seizure diagnosis and management.

Phenobarbital (see Table 5) deservedly remains the most

TABLE 5.—Doses and Pharmacologic

DRUG	ROUTES AVAILABLE FOR ADMINISTRATION	TOTAL DAILY DOSE INFANTS AND TODDLERS (mg/kg/day)	OLDER CHILDREN (mg/day)	THERAPEUTIC BLOOD LEVEL (μg/ml)
Phenobarbital	Oral	3–8		10–40
	IM, IV	10–15		
Primidone (Mysoline)	Oral	15–25	250–1500	(Phenobarbital level of 5–15)
Cabamazepine (Tegretol)	Oral	10–20	200–1600	4–12
Phenytoin (Dilantin)	Oral†	4–10		10–20
	IV†	10–20		
Valproate‡ (Depakene)	Oral	30–60	750–3000	50–100
Ethosuccimide (Zarontin)	Oral	20–40	500–1500	40–100
Clonazepam (Clonopin)	Oral	.03–.2	2–20	.01–.05

NOTE: The "therapeutic" blood level varies greatly among different patients.
*See Physician's Desk Reference or drug literature for more extended lists of toxic and side effects.
†Phenytoin should not be given IM due to poor absorption. Chewable tablets (Dilantin Infatabs) should be used instead of liquid phenytoin due to potentially serious dosage errors with the phenytoin suspensions.
‡Other generic names are sodium valproate, valproic acid, and dipropylacetate.

widely used anticonvulsant in infants and children because of its very broad spectrum of anticonvulsant activity and safety. It is effective in major seizures, prevention of febrile convulsions, and many instances of partial seizures. Occasionally, it is effective by itself in controlling absences and myoclonic seizures. It is absorbed well orally and intramuscularly and, with caution, can be given intravenously. Because of its long half-life, the daily oral dose of phenobarbital may be administered once per day, or in two divided doses. Methobarbital (Meberal) is demethylated to phenobarbital by the liver. It may have fewer behavioral side effects than the parent compound. Side effects include respiratory depression, sedation, hyperactivity, behavioral and sleep disturbances, learning disorders, and al-

DATA OF MAJOR ANTICONVULSANTS

AVERAGE HALF LIFE (hr)	NO. OF DAILY DOSES	COMMON SIDE EFFECTS (AND SERIOUS TOXIC EFFECTS)*
96	2	Sedation, hyperactivity, learning and behavior disorders, respiratory depression (allergic rash)
96	2	Similar to phenobarbital
12	2–4	Diplopia, dizziness, sedation (blood dyscrasia, hepatopathy)
24	2	Gumhyperplasia, hirsutism, ataxia, sedation (blood dyscrasia, hepatopathy, allergic rash, rickets, pseudolymphoma, lupus-like reaction, neuropathy)
10	3–4	GI irritation, sedation, hair loss (hepatopathy, pancreatitis, elevated NH_3)
30	2	GI irritation, sedation (blood dyscrasia)
30	2–3	Very sedative, ataxia, hypotonia

lergic rashes. The appearance of any of these side effects would necessitate lowering the dose or discontinuing the drug.

Primidone (Mysoline), another barbiturate, is unusual in that its metabolites (principally phenobarbital and phenylethyl malonamide) as well as the parent molecule are all effective as anticonvulsants. Primidone is generally used as an adjunct drug, and for psychomotor seizures. Sedation and behavioral changes are important problems. Primidone can only be given orally.

Phenytoin (Dilantin) is the second most widely used pediatric anticonvulsant. It is effective against major motor and most partial seizures but is generally ineffective in preventing febrile convulsions or absence seizures. It is much more variable than phenobarbital in its absorption and subsequent hepatic metabolism, so that much greater variation is encountered in the dose necessary to achieve the same blood level in different children. Some infants require very large doses (10 mg/kg of body weight/day or more) to reach therapeutic levels.

Phenobarbital and phenytoin have an important interaction; phenobarbital induces the hepatic microsomal enzymes that metabolize phenytoin. When using this combination, increased amounts of phenytoin may have to be given to maintain adequate clinical response and blood levels.

Cosmetic side effects occur to some degree in most children who take phenytoin over long periods. They may occur with drug levels in the therapeutic range and include gum hyperplasia (a function of salivary drug level), hirsutism, acne, and coarse facial features. Parents frequently complain of behavioral and learning difficulties, sometimes noted retrospectively after the drug is discontinued. At toxic levels, ataxia, sedation, and even increased seizures (absence) may occur.

Phenytoin may be given orally and intravenously but not intramuscularly because of very poor absorption. Phenytoin, like phenobarbital, may be administered once per day, or in two divided doses.

Carbamazepine (Tegretol) has emerged in the last decade as a highly effective anticonvulsant for a relatively broad spectrum of psychomotor seizures, other partial seizures, and major motor seizures. Many experts consider carbamazepine to be the drug of choice in all these situations, particularly in partial seizures. In comparison with phenytoin, carbamazepine does not have cosmetic side effects and is roughly equivalent in the incidence of grave side effects, such as bone marrow depression and liver damage. There is no parenteral or liquid formulation of carbamazepine. Because of its short half-life, carbamazepine should be given three to four times per day. This may present a problem to adolescents.

Valproic acid (Dipropyl Acetate, Depakane) is a highly effective anticonvulsant that may be the drug of choice in many nonconvulsive seizures, particularly absence.[41] It is also useful in major motor and febrile seizures, as well as myoclonic/atonic spells. Its serious side effects include hepatitis, pancreatitis, and thrombocytopenia. Increased sedation is important, particularly when combined with other anticonvulsants. Valproic acid may increase phenobarbital levels if both drugs are given together. Absence status has been reported due to the combination of valproic acid and clonazepam. Less serious side effects are gastrointestinal upset, hair loss, or sometimes weight gain. Because of its short half-life, valproic acid should be given three to four times per day.

Ethosuximide (Zarontin) and other succinimides are excellent drugs for typical and atypical absence seizures. Although gastric irritation is a problem, it has less toxicity than valproic acid; both drugs are used for the same type of seizures. Many experts use phenobarbital along with ethosuximide to prevent major motor seizures that frequently are associated with absences.

Clonazepam (Clonopin) is a benzodiazepine that has proved useful in a number of refractory seizure states, including infantile spasms and other myoclonic/atonic seizures, refractory absences, and major motor seizures. Sedation is a problem with clonazepam, particularly when it is used along with other anticonvulsants, as it usually is. Diazepam (Valium), another useful drug in the benzodiazepine group, is more sedating than clonazepam.

Steroid therapy (ACTH 40 to 80 units/day or prednisone 2 mg/kg of body weight/day) is specifically used for infantile spasms, with seizure control in about 70% of patients and some improvement in 20%. Despite adequate seizure control and normalization of the EEG pattern (hypsarrhythmia), mental retardation is the most likely outcome in this group of children. Steroids used in these dosages may produce Cushing's syndrome; the appearance of diabetes mellitus or hypertension while on steroids necessitates stopping the drug. Many other anticonvulsants are available but should generally be reserved for refractory seizure cases and used only by physicians thoroughly experienced with them. They tend either to be less effective or more toxic than drugs listed in Table 5. Second line drugs are rarely effective when first line drugs have failed.

Emotional factors and seizures have a positive feedback interaction. Anxiety and stress can bring on seizures or make them more frequent. Frequent seizures lead to anxiety and stress. Psychiatric help for the patient and family, particularly

478   CHARLES B. BRILL AND MICHAEL H. MITCHELL

adolescents, is frequently helpful in dealing with these issues.[42]

Certain seizure situations do not require anticonvulsant medication. These include the first simple febrile seizure, an isolated major motor seizure that may not recur, a brief seizure following a breath-holding spell or syncopal attack, and a questionable seizure, where the history is not clear.

In treating a difficult, resistant seizure disorder, some important contributing factors that may require correction are:[43] (1) Improper classification of seizure type, which leads to incorrect choice of medication; (2) failure to demonstrate a correctable cause of the seizures, such as phenylketonuria or hypoglycemia; (3) failure to recognize progressive neurologic disease, such as Tay-Sachs disease or subacute sclerosing panencephalitis; (4) failure to use anticonvulsant drugs appropriately in terms of dosage level or frequency of administration, interactions of two or more medications,[40] and rapid shifting of drugs; (5) drug toxicity leading to increasing seizure frequency; (6) failure to correct emotional triggering effects; and (7) poor education of patients and their families, which often leads to noncompliance with the treatment regimen. If these factors are corrected, seizure control will often improve.

Tables 4 and 5 will be helpful in choice of medication and give some important pharmacologic facts.

When an operable epileptic focus (tumor, abscess) is found surgical excision should be attempted. This method can be employed occasionally when a physiologically well-defined focus lies in a nonvital brain area and the patient's seizures are refractory to vigorous, prolonged attempts at drug management monitored by adequate drug levels. Excision of such a focus, usually in the nondominant temporal lobe, may lead not only to a marked reduction in the number of seizures, or even complete control, but also allow a lowering of anticonvulsant drugs and dosage. Improved alertness, behavior, and school performance will result.

In children with refractory myoclonic/atonic seizures, it is sometimes helpful to induce a chronic state of ketosis through the ketogenic diet containing large amounts of fats or medium-chain triglycerides. This diet may be dramatically successful and the advantages of lowering or discontinuing drugs may also be realized.

Status Epilepticus

Major motor status epilepticus is a medical emergency in which convulsions continue for more than 15 minutes, or recur so rapidly that the patient does not recover consciousness in between attacks, in contrast to the usual major motor seizure, which lasts one to three minutes, on the average. In status epilepticus, the child becomes hyperthermic, acidotic, and hypoglycemic after approximately 25 minutes of continuous seizure. After this period, cerebral blood flow and oxygen and glucose delivery to the brain can no longer keep up with the demand of increased cerebral metabolic rate. Therefore, increased brain damage or death may ensue.[44]

Status epilepticus occurs most commonly in an epileptic patient who suddenly discontinues medication or develops an acute infection.[45, 46] When it develops without a previous history of seizures, it implies a very serious illness, such as encephalitis, electrolyte disturbance, hypoglycemia, head trauma, or vascular insult. The mortality rate in the group of patients with prior epilepsy is low, 0% to 3%. In the group without a prior history of seizure the mortality rate is 10% to 20% and is related as much to the underlying disease as to the seizures themselves.

Table 6 lists the principles of treatment of status epilepticus. The physician should try to control the seizure with one drug, and if possible, use the drug with which he is most familiar, and in large enough doses that high drug levels are quickly achieved. A common error is to use small doses and repeat them frequently; this may preclude the rapid achievement of adequate levels, and in addition cause respiratory depression.

In any case, the first priority is to establish an airway and oxygenate by proper patient positioning, removal of secretions, administration of oxygen, and, when necessary, endotracheal intubation and artificial ventilation. Next, an intravenous (IV) line should be established for administering medications and glucose and obtaining appropriate blood determinations such as glucose, electrolytes, blood gases, anticonvulsant levels, and toxicologic analysis.

Diazepam is an excellent drug for the emergency treatment of status epilepticus. It should be given intravenously at 1 mg/

TABLE 6.—EMERGENCY TREATMENT OF CONVULSIVE STATUS EPILEPTICUS

Initiate treatment immediately and move to intensive care environment as soon as
   possible
Maintain vital functions, especially *respiration*
   Assure airway by:
      Proper positioning
      Removal of secretions
      O_2 administration
      Intubation if necessary
   Check vital signs
   Remember, a few further seizures are less harmful than brain anoxia
Perform a rapid neurologic and general physical examination, checking in particular:
   Signs of infection
   Trauma
   Dehydration
   Intoxication
   Papilledema
   Focal neurologic dysfunction
   Status of brainstem function
   Spontaneous respiration
   Pupillary responses
   Extraocular movements
Insert an intravenous line
   Draw baseline glucose, electrolytes, blood gases, complete blood cell count
   Administer glucose 25–50 gm immediately
   Administer anticonvulsant drug immediately
      Diazepam (Valium) .3–1 mg/kg, max 20 mg., IV slowly or 1–3 mg/min
         Use only when patient is actively convulsing at the moment of drug
            administration
         Note very short action (about 20 min) and potential respiratory depression
      Phenytoin 20 mg/kg IV *slowly* (50 mg/min)
         Use immediately after diazepam to provide long-lasting treatment, or as initial
            drug
         Note: hypotension and cardiac arrhythmia, especially during too-rapid
            administration
      Phenobarbital 10 mg/kg IV *slowly* (100 mg/min)
         Long-acting alternate or adjunct to phenytoin
         Respiratory depression may occur, especially after diazepam or with too-rapid
            administration
         Give phenobarbital 10 mg/kg IM when IV medications cannot be immediately
            given
      Other possible treatments if diazepam, phenytoin, and phenobarbital are
         ineffective:
         Paraldehyde drip, 1%–10% in dextrose, 5% in water. Dilutional hyponatremia
            may occur
         Induction of coma with pentobarbital, curarization, and intubation with
            ventilatory support; general anesthesia
   Avoid excess fluid administration, which may result in hyponatremia and brain
      edema
Initiate maintenance anticonvulsant medication
   Phenytoin 5–10 mg/kg/day and/or phenobarbital 5–15 mg/kg/day (initially IV in
      divided doses)
   Follow blood anticonvulsant levels closely and adjust doses accordingly

minute until the seizure stops. If diazepam is given more rapidly than this, depression of respirations is likely to occur. This point should reemphasize the need for adequate airway control. IV diazepam will usually terminate the seizure within several minutes. However, the half-life after IV administration is only about 15 minutes, so that a long-acting anticonvulsant, such as phenobarbital, 6 to 10 mg/kg, or IV phenytoin 5 to 10 mg/kg, must be given to prevent seizure recurrence before the effect of diazepam wears off.[47] The total dose of diazepam required to stop an attack of status epilepticus varies greatly. Usually the maximum doses required are 0.3 to 1.0 mg/kg in infants or 5 to 10 mg in older children. IV phenobarbital is another excellent drug for the treatment of status. It should be used in the dose range of 10 to 12 mg/kg, with careful monitoring of the respiratory status. If the seizure stops, phenobarbital may be continued as the maintenance agent.

IV phenytoin is very effective in stopping prolonged seizures. It is not as sedating as diazepam or phenobarbital, and is also an excellent maintenance agent. However, it must be given intravenously, not intramuscularly[48] (it crystallizes in the tissues), and it may cause cardiac arrhythmias. Therefore, EKG monitoring must be done, and the drug cannot be delivered faster than 50 mg/minute in older children; it must be delivered slower in infants. The dose of phenytoin for static epilepticus is up to 25 mg/kg of body weight.

Paraldehyde, administered as an IV drip, is useful in refractory, frequently recurrent seizures. Liquid paraldehyde is diluted with 5% dextrose and water to yield a solution from 1% to 10% and is given as a rapid IV drip until the seizure stops. Water intoxication, hyponatremia, is a danger if large volumes of dilute solution are given.

General anesthesia with curarization is a rarely necessary desperation measure. The seizures may recur when the anesthesia is stopped.

In infants or in dehydrated children, it may be very difficult and time-consuming to achieve an IV injection. Here, intramuscular phenobarbital 8 to 10 mg/kg of body weight often is effective within 15 minutes and allows the nurse or assistant to administer the medication while the physician concentrates on establishing good ventilation and other essential supportive measures.

A continuous focal motor seizure is called partial status epilepticus and may result in depression of consciousness and respiration, particularly in infants and small children. It is treated in the same way as major motor status epilepticus. Petit mal status epilepticus (see "Absence Seizures" above) usually responds well to IV diazepam (5 to 10 mg).

Migraine

Migraine refers to chronic, recurrent, often pulsatile headaches accompanied by visceral symptoms and sometimes neurologic signs. Migraine is very common in childhood, particularly between age five and adolescence. Younger children may also have migraine, but headache is less typical at this age, and the clinician may have difficulty making the diagnosis.[49]

CLINICAL MANIFESTATIONS OF MIGRAINE

The well-known classic form of migraine, which comprises only 10% of cases, displays the characteristic "aura" of visual disturbances such as flashing lights, "colors," or blindness, followed by the intense throbbing unilateral pain of "hemicrania" in the eye, forehead, and temple, with associated photophobia, nausea, vomiting, and abdominal distress. Sometimes the patient will experience the aura without proceeding to headache. Occasionally the aura will be other focal syptoms such as paresthesias or aphasia.

Common migraine is far more frequent but less characteristic, having diffuse rather than unilateral pain and frequently no visual aura. The prodrome of common migraine is more apt to consist of personality change, lightheadedness, or nausea. Typically, attacks of both types of migraine will last several hours, inducing the child to retire to a dark room to "sleep it off."

Light and sound make children with a migraine attack more uncomfortable, therefore, they do not turn on the TV or stereo during an acute attack. The headache usually lasts one to several hours, very rarely days. In a younger child, recurrent carsickness, abdominal pain, nausea, or vomiting may be the harbinger of migraine. Alternating hemiplegia may be a migrainous manifestation.

In complicated migraine, hemiplegia, ophthalmoplegia, or other focal signs accompany the attack. Vertigo, ataxia, dysarthria, and vomiting are attributed to basilar artery migraine. Episodic confusion, macropsia, or micropsia (the Alice in Wonderland syndrome) are behavioral or perceptual manifestations. These deficits or signs usually clear rapidly during the first several such attacks. With repetition the signs may persist for longer periods, hours to days, and may even be permanent, in which case they represent ischemic infarction.

In classic migraine the side of the headache and the auras are likely to vary in different attacks; if these symptoms are persistently unilateral, an arteriovenous malformation or other structural lesions should be ruled out.

PATHOGENESIS

The pathogenesis of a migraine attack is generally considered to be arterial vasoconstriction causing cerebral ischemia and the aura, followed by vasodilation, causing the throbbing, pulsatile headache. The contributions of meningeal and large cerebral vessels are debated. Alterations in cerebral blood flow may be lowered during an acute attack, and a CT scan may demonstrate localized cerebral edema. The aura will depend on the vessel causing ischemia; visual auras, for example, are caused by spasm of the retinal or occipital arteries. The scalp arteries may be tender and appear dilated during the pulsatile phase.

Children with migraine frequently have perfectionistic, hypermature, striving personalities.[50] Attacks may be triggered by (1) no apparent cause, (2) emotional stress (school exams or family problems), (3) nonemotional factors (minor head trauma, fatigue), and (4) dietary factors (chocolate and cheese). A positive family history of migraine is elicited in over half of the patients.

DIAGNOSIS AND TREATMENT

Since there is no specific test, diagnosis must rest on a good description of the attacks, family history, and a negative physical examination, including blood pressure, optic fundi, ears and paranasal sinuses, ascultation for cranial bruits, and neurologic examination. For patients with complicated migraine, where focal signs are prominent, or where the diagnosis is not clear, EEG and CT scan may be helpful.

The most common cause of headache in childhood is anxiety or depression. Therefore, a careful history concentrating on psychosocial forces, particularly in the home, is vital. This may uncover psychological triggering events to the migrainous attacks, or precipitants of depressive headaches, or both in the same patient.

Drug therapy for common and classic migraine is straightforward when salicylates provide adequate relief or when attacks are too short for any drug to be effective. Only severe, frequent attacks should be treated with other agents.

Ergot preparations (Caffergot—ergotamine tartrate 1 mg and caffeine 100 mg per tablet) to cause vasoconstriction and thereby counteract the vasodilation and throbbing headache, are useful in treating an acute, migraine attack. In order to be effective, ergot should be taken at the onset of the attack, and may be repeated once, in 30 minutes. This drug may be taken orally if there is no vomiting. It comes in the form of a rectal suppository for younger children, and in a sublingual preparation for older children. It is contraindicated in complicated migraine, since it may accentuate a focal deficit due to vasospasm.

As opposed to ergot preparations, which are useful in an acute attack, phenytoin or propranolol (Inderal) are useful as prophylactic agents. They should be periodically withdrawn to determine if they are still necessary.

Frequently parents are more concerned about the headaches than is the child due to widespread misbelief that a child cannot have headaches without serious intracranial pathology. In this situation the physician's identification of migraine and/or psychological factors, and reassurance are usually more therapeutic than any medication.

Syncope

Syncope (fainting) is the most common paroxysmal disorder—so common that virtually everyone has fainted or at least felt faint. It results from transient cerebral ischemia or hypoxia. Fainting is often misdiagnosed as a seizure even though a careful history usually indicates the correct diagnosis.

On the other hand, unwitnessed seizures, brief major motor seizures, or akinetic seizures may be erroneously attributed to fainting, especially when the full history is not available.

The usual vasovagal syncope is nearly always precipitated by stress or excitement, such as minor injury or an emotionally startling experience; is found when the patient is upright and is aborted by lowering the head, begins gradually with lightheadedness (the "I'm going to faint" sensation) and pallor; results from temporary loss of vasomotor tone with bradycardia and even asystole; and is typically associated with a normal physical examination, ECG, and EEG. In prolonged faint there can be brief tonic and clonic convulsive movements due to transient cerebral hypoxia, which tends to cause further confusion with epileptic seizures. Important conditions that predispose to syncope are cardiac arrhythmia, anemia, hypoglycemia, Addison's disease, drug side effects causing postural hypotension, anatomic neuropathy, and anomalies of the heart or great vessels.

In cases of straightforward vasovagal syncope, there is virtually no likelihood of cerebral damage, and the neurologic prognosis is excellent. Therefore, therapy consists mainly of reassurance along these lines and advice to abort impending attacks by lowering the head.

Breath-Holding Spells

Breath-holding is relatively common in infants and toddlers and can be very frightening to the inexperienced parent. All infants may hold their breath briefly during crying, but about 5% of all children six to 24 months of age have cyanotic breath-holding spells in which they cry briefly, arrest their breathing in expiration, and do not inhale, and turn blue or pale and lose consciousness for several seconds. If the apnea persists for 30 seconds or longer, there are likely to be several clonic jerks of the extremities. The crying always has a precipitating event, such as frustration or a minor injury.[51] The loss of consciousness and brief convulsive features result from hypoxia, although the mechanisms causing the hypoxia and cyanosis are less well established; among those suggested are glottic closure, diminished cardiac output, increased oxygen utilization, and right-to-left shunting.

In most instances the attacks begin between six and 18 months of age, occur at irregular intervals of days or weeks, and are outgrown by four years of age. About 30% of breath-holders have one to several attacks per day. In spite of this considerable frequency of attacks, the prognosis is excellent; these children are nearly always neurologically normal and do not suffer any secondary CNS damage, including epilepsy.

The diagnosis is based upon the characteristic history. Family history may be positive. If cyanosis accompanies an epileptic seizure, the seizure begins before the cyanosis begins. In breath-holding spells, the reverse is true. In the majority of patients the breath-holding becomes manageable as soon as the benign nature of the condition is explained to the parents, and the child's subsequent neurologic and emotional development proves to be normal. The attacks do not respond to anticonvulsants, which are often prescribed for an erroneous diagnosis of seizure disorder.

In some particularly severe cases, the breath-holding is aggravated by parental overindulgence occasioned by fear of triggering more attacks, or by serious parental psychiatric problems resulting in anxiety or frustration in the child. In these cases psychotherapy may be necessary.

Paroxysmal Vertigo

Benign paroxysmal vertigo of childhood consists of frequent brief attacks of dizziness and inability to stand during which the child becomes frightened and pale and attempts to lie or sit down before he falls.[52] On examination during an attack the child is alert and is likely to exhibit nystagmus, vomiting, pallor, and sweating. The disorder is self-limited and usually disappears within a few months to a year. Functional vestibular abnormalities arise, often demonstrable by electronystagmography with caloric stimulation of the ears.

Unfortunately, some children simply cannot describe what they mean by dizziness. In these instances the associated features may be of greater diagnostic value; for example, fright or pain, including loss of consciousness, in vasovagal syncope, as opposed to sudden inability to stand with preservation of consciousness in typical attacks of benign paroxysmal vertigo.

"Dizziness" is a term so commonly used by children and

adults that some suggestions on how to evaluate this symptom may be helpful. Children often learn the term "dizzy" from their parents and think it has a specific meaning. Usually when patients say they are dizzy, they imply a lightheaded, presyncopal sensation; this should generally be evaluated as a syncope problem. Patients will also use "dizziness" to describe vertigo, that is, the illusion of movement of either the patient or the environment. Diagnostically, it is important to try to establish whether the patient is describing lightheadedness as opposed to "true" vertigo. Although establishing the illusion of movement is very important, the nature of sensation such as spinning, rocking, or falling is of little diagnostic value. Vertigo can be a component of syncope, but when it is persistent and associated with other neurologic signs the patient will usually require more extensive diagnostic investigation because vertiginous attacks can also arise from temporal lobe seizure foci and posterior fossa tumors. Appropriate investigations include otologic and neurologic consultations, audiogram, electronystagmogram, EEG, CT scan, and auditory (brain stem) evoked responses. The syndrome of paroxysmal vertigo usually remits within one to several years. The value of antivertigo agents such as Meclozine and Dimenhydrinate is questionable because of the brevity of the individual attacks, their infrequency and tendency to spontaneous remission.

REFERENCES

1. Jackson H.: On convulsive seizures. *Br. Med. J.* 1:703, 1890.
2. Gastaut H.: Clinical and electroencephalographic classification of epileptic seizures. *Epilepsia* 11:102, 1970.
3. Gastaut H., Gastaut J.L.: Computerized transverse axial tomography in epilepsy. *Epilepsia* 17:325, 1976.
4. Laffey P., Mitchell M., Teplick G., et al.: *Computerized Tomography in Clinical Pediatrics*. Philadelphia: Medical Directions, 1976.
5. Patrick H.T., Levy D.M.: Early convulsions in epileptics and in others. *J.A.M.A.* 82:375/24.
6. Kurland L.T.: The incidences and prevalence of convulsive disorders in a small urban community. *Epilepsia* 1:143, 1959.
7. Cotte-Richard M.R., Courton J.: Semilogical value of adversive epilepsy. *Epilepsia* 3:151, 1962.
8. Penfield W., Jasper H.: *Epilepsy and the Functional Anatomy of the Human Brain.* Boston: Little, Brown & Co., 1954.
9. Lombroso C.T.: Sylvian seizures and midtemporal spike foci in children. *Arch. Neurol.* 17:52, 1967.
10. Daly D.D.: Uncinate fits. *Neurology* 8:250, 1958.
11. Falconer R.M., Serafetinides E.A., Corsellis J.A.N.: Etiology and pathogenesis of temporal lobe epilepsy. *J. Neurol. Neurosurg. Psychiatry* 34:104, 1971.

12. Arid R.B., Yamamoto T.: Behavior disorders of childhood. *Electroencephalogr. Clin. Neurophysiol.* 21:148, 1966.
13. Glaser G.H., Dixon M.S.: Psychomotor seizures in childhood: A clinical study. *Neurology* 6:646, 1956.
14. Gowers W.R.: *Epilepsy and Other Chronic Convulsive Disorders.* New York: Dover Publications, 1964 (1885), American Academy of Neurology Reprint Series, vol 1.
15. Lennox W.G.: The petit mal epilepsies: Their treatment with Tridione. *J.A.M.A.* 129:1065, 1945.
16. Metrakos K., Metrakos J.D.: Genetics of convulsive disorders: II. Genetic and electroencephalographic studies in centrencephalic epilepsy. *Neurology* 11:474, 1961.
17. Sato S., Dreifus F.E., Penry J.K.: Prognostic factors in absence seizures. *Neurology* 26:788, 1976.
18. Meldrum B.S., Horton R.W.: Physiology of status epilepticus in primates. *Arch. Neurol.* 29:1, 1973.
19. Rapport R.L., et al.: Human epileptic brain: Na-K ATPase activity and phenytoin concentrations. *Arch. Neurol.* 32:549, 1975.
20. Meldrum B.S.: Epilepsy and aminobutyric acid—mediated inhibition. *Int. Rev. Neurobiol.* 14:1, 1975.
21. Lott I.T., et al.: Vitamin B_6-dependent seizures, pathology and chemical findings in brain. *Neurology* 28:47, 1978.
22. Glotzner F.L.: Membrane properties of neuralgia in epileptogenic gliosis. *Brain Res.* 55:159, 1973.
23. Fisher R.S., et al.: The role of extracellular potassium in hippocampal epilepsy. *Arch. Neurol.* 33:76, 1976.
24. Falconer M.A., Serafetinides E.A., Corsellis J.A.N.: Etiology and pathogenesis of temporal lobe epilepsy. *Arch. Neurol.* 10:233, 1964.
25. Stewart, L.F., Dreifus F.E.: "Centrencephalic" seizure discharges in focal hemispheral lesions. *Arch. Neurol.* 17:60, 1967.
26. Schmidt R.P., Wilder B.J.: *Epilepsy.* Philadelphia; F.A. Davis, Co., 1968.
27. Penfield W.: Epileptic automatism and the centrencephalic integrating system. *Assoc. Res. Nerv. Ment. Dis.* 30:513, 1952.
28. Wada J.A., Osawa T.: Spontaneous recurrent seizure state induced by daily electric amygdaloid stimulation in Senegalese baboons *(Papio papio). Neurology* 26:273, 1976.
29. Huges S.R.: Bilateral EEG abnormalities in corresponding areas. *Epilepsia* 7:40, 1966.
30. Lennox W.G.: Brain injury, drugs and environment as cause of mental decay in epilepsy. *Am. J. Psychiatry* 99:174, 1942.
31. Currier R.D., Kooi K.A., Saidman L.J.: Prognosis of "pure" petit mal. *Neurology* 13:959, 1963.
32. Volpe J.: Neonatal seizures. *N. Engl. J. Med.* 289:413, 1973.
33. Hopkins I.J.: Seizures in the first week of life: A study of aetiological factors. *Med. J. Aust.* 2:647, 1972.
34. Dennis J.: Neonatal convulsions, late neonatal status and long-term outcome. *Dev. Med. Child. Neurol.* 20:143, 1978.
35. Livingston S.: *Comprehensive Management of Epilepsy in Infancy, Childhood and Adolescence.* Springfield, Ill.: Charles C Thomas, Publisher, 1972.
36. Fischer S.: Convulsions as a complication of shigellosis in children. *Helv. Paediatr. Acta* 17:389, 1962.
37. Nelson K.B., Ellenberg J.H.: Predictors of epilepsy in children who have experienced febrile seizures. *N. Engl. J. Med.* 295:1029, 1976.
38. Freeman J.M.: Febrile seizures: A concensus of their significance, evaluation and treatment. *Pediatrics* 66:1009, 1980.
39. Concensus Development Panel Conference of Febrile Seizures, NIH, May 19–21,

1980: Febrile seizures: Long-term management of children with fever-associated seizures. *Pediatrics* 66:1009, 1980.

40. Shorvon S.D., Reynolds E.H.: Reduction in polypharmacy for epilepsy. *Br. Med. J.* 2:1023, 1979.
41. Jeavons P.M., Clark J.E., Mahesari M.C.: Treatment of generalized epilepsies of childhood and adolescence with sodium valproate. *Develop. Med. Child. Neurol.* 19:1, 1977.
42. Williams D.T., et al.: The impact of psychiatric intervention on patient with uncontrolled seizures. *J. Nerv. Ment. Dis.* 1967:626, 1979.
43. Carter S.: Management of difficult seizure problems. *Brain Dev.,* 3:80, 1978.
44. Blennow G., et al.: Epileptic brain damage: The role of systemic factors that may modify cerebral energy metabolism. *Brain* 101:687, 1978.
45. Alcardi J., Churie J.J.: Convulsive status epilepticus, evaluation and treatment. *Epilepsia* 11:187, 1971.
46. Celesia G.G.: Modern concepts of status epilepticus. *J.A.M.A.* 235:1571, 1976.
47. Dell D.S.: Dangers of treatment of status epilepticus with diazepam. *Br. Med. J.* 1:159, 1969.
48. Wilensky A.J., Coloden J.A.: Inadequate serum levels after intramuscular administration of diphenylhydantoin. *Neurology (Minneap.)* 23:318, 1973.
49. Prensky A.L.: Migraine and migrainous variants in pediatric patients. *Pediatr. Clin. North Am.* 23:461, 1976.
50. Menkes M.M.: Personality characteristics and family roles of children with migraine. *Pediatrics* 53:560, 1974.
51. Lombroso C.T., Lerman P.: Breath-holding spells (cyanotic and pallid infantile syncope). *Pediatrics* 39:563, 1967.
52. Koenigsberger M.R., et al.: Benign paroxysmal vertigo of childhood. *Neurology (Minneap.)* 20:1108, 1970.

Subject Index

A

Abdominal nodes: in lymphadenopathy, 366–367
Absorptive capacity: estimation, in infant, 329–332
Abuse
  child, and drug abuse in adolescence, 17
  drug (*see* Drug abuse)
Adolescence (*see* Drug abuse in adolescence)
Airway obstruction: upper, and hypoxemia, 43
Alactasia, 122–123
Alimentation, enteric, 319–339
  diarrhea and, intractable, 334–335
  economic factors in, 337
  in gastrointestinal problems, 319–339
  heart disease and, congenital, 336–337
  lactose intolerance and, 333–334
  management principles, general, 332–337
  protein "sensitivity" and, 334
  short bowel syndrome and, 335–336
Amino acid sequences: of insulin-like growth factor and proinsulin, 299
Ammonia, aromatic, in self-injurious behavior, 399–402
  analysis of, 406–408
Amylase: ontogeny of, 113–114
Anemia: iron deficiency, in young female athlete, 211–212
Anticonvulsants
  doses, 474–475
  pharmacologic data on, 474–475
  in seizures, 474–475
Antigen(s)
  of factor II, 65–66
  T-lymphocyte surface, and thymic factors, 249–251
Apnea alarms: comparison with TcPo$_2$ monitoring, 41–43

Aromatic ammonia in self-injurious behavior, 399–402
  analysis of, 406–408
Athletes, young, 187–228
  (*See also* Sports)
  fat and, body, 208
  female
    especial concerns of, 209–211
    iron deficiency in, 211–212
    iron deficiency anemia in, 211–212
    iron depletion in, 211–212
  health care needs of, 187–228
  nutritional concerns of, 204–209
Atonic seizures, 459–460
Attitudes (*see* Drug abuse in adolescence, attitudes)
Autoimmune disease
  lymphadenopathy and, generalized, 346
  thymic factors and, 259–263

B

Barium swallow: in gastroesophageal reflux, 168–169
Behavior
  disorder, and generalized seizures, 445
  self-injurious (*see* Self-injurious behavior)
Beikost products: carbohydrates in, 105
Bernstein test: in gastroesophageal reflux, 173
Biopsy
  esophageal, in gastroesophageal reflux, 171
  excisional, in lymphadenopathy, 370–372
Bitter substances in self-injurious behavior, 402
  analysis of, 406–408
Blood
  gas determinations, 35

491